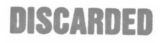

LIGHTS OUT

Lights Out

Sleep, Sugar, and Survival

BY T. S. Wiley
WITH Bent Formby, Ph.D.

POCKET BOOKS
NEW YORK LONDON TORONTO SYDNEY SINGAPORE

The author of this book is not a physician and the ideas, procedures, and suggestions in this book are not intended as a substitute for the medical advice of a trained health professional. All matters regarding your health require medical supervision. Consult your physician before adopting the suggestions in this book, as well as about any condition that may require diagnosis or medical attention. The author and publisher disclaim any liability arising directly or indirectly from the use of the book.

POCKET BOOKS, a division of Simon & Schuster Inc.
1230 Avenue of the Americas, New York, NY 10020

ISBN: 0-671-03867-2

First Pocket Books hardcover printing February 2000

10   9   8   7   6   5   4   3   2   1

POCKET and colophon are registered trademarks of
Simon & Schuster Inc.

Printed in the U.S.A.

For our fathers,
one of whom was taken by the mistakes of
conventional medicine,
and the other, a victim of relentless evolution

ACKNOWLEDGMENTS

The first round of thanks goes to our families for their patience and support. Bent's Florence is in line for sainthood and my Neil is, and has been, forever my very own Medici. I am nothing without him. My children, poor neglected Jake, Max, Zoe, and Ian remain the best kids on the planet. This endeavor took five long years for me and almost three for my partner. In that time, our families put up with more "science talk" morning, noon and night than anybody should ever have to. More often than not, their dinners were late and their misery was palpable, but yet, they still love us and we're grateful.

To my older daughters, Mara and Aja, I am especially indebted for their rare and diverse intellects that served to inspire and expand my own. Mara Raden spent unending hours in insightful debate, provided many evolutionary and neuroendocrine concepts, unconditional encouragement and a lot of the early, tedious editing. Aja Raden, as creative consultant, came up with the title of this book, many of the chapter titles and more than a few of the sound bites/subheads. She also spent countless hours explaining physics, chemistry and math to her old mom.

Wiley Lorente proved blood is thicker than ink by working side by side with me, editing, reorganizing and just plain suffering for all five years and fourteen versions. And to my partner, the incredible Dr. Bent Formby, thank you. Thank you for understanding what I was saying before you gave me the words to say it. Thank you for being the world's greatest teacher and mentor. Thank you for your great ability to grow and change. Without your thousands of hours of research, my theories were just "theories." Bent, you are the other half of my brain.

Many of our other colleagues served as collaborators, too. Dr. Julie Taguchi at Cottage Hospital in Santa Barbara; Dr. Alex Depaoli, now at Amgen; Dr. Eve Van Cauter and Dr. Martha McClintock at the University of Chicago; Ernst Mayr at Harvard; and Anthony Cincotta at Ergo Science all allowed me to pick their brains on more than one occasion. And, of course, the great minds *forced* to collaborate at the NIH, Dr. Thomas Wehr, his post-doc Holly Giessen and Dr. Ellen Leibenluft.

My personal assistant, Chelsey Haskins, labored over edits and endnotes endlessly and our office manager, Krista Silva, compiled Bent's voluminous research. Both of them spent way too many hours at FedEx and on e-mail, and just generally "putting up" with me. The others too numerous to name to whom we owe a great debt of gratitude are all of the voluntary readers and the guinea pigs who have believed in and tried out our theories.

Perhaps the most stalwart soldier of all in our crusade to bring back the night is our agent, Deborah Schneider. She identified and rallied behind the truth years before we had the research to prove it. Without her visionary support and talented representation, we would have never joined forces with the amazing people at Pocket Books. My first conversation with Emily Bestler and Jane Cavolina convinced me that no other publishers would do. Their enthusiasm and rare intelligence that radiated over the phone across three thousand miles that day continues to warm my heart to this one.

"My editor" is a phrase that truly gets me through the night. Jane Cavolina has taken ownership of this project and truly convinced me, once and for all, that we're not "all in this alone." Her self-described "house cleaning" metaphor for the artistry of her editing does her no justice. She made the writing process, version after version, utterly painless and the final product something I am deeply proud of in a profound way.

Thank you, Jane.

And last, but by no means least, we thank Pam Duevel. If you're holding this book it is thanks to Pam Duevel, the absurdly talented, ridiculously creative, hard working leader of the publicity team at Pocket Books assigned to get this information into the hands of the people who need it.

—T. S. Wiley

CONTENTS

We are not here concerned with hopes and fears, only with the truth as far as our reason allows us to discover it. I have given evidence to the best of my ability . . .

—Charles Darwin,
The Descent of Man

LIGHTS OUT

INTRODUCTION

It's all over the news.

In *Life* magazine in January of 1998, 70 million Americans finally admitted that, occasionally, we do fall asleep at the wheel, drop the ball, or take a dive. Books like *Power Sleeping* and news clips on "jet lag" permeate the media. Sleep loss is the new American deficit. This deficit is a yawning chasm we can't hope to close. Apparently, when we lose sleep it's like chasing a moving train on foot. The problem is, with sleep, you really *can't* catch up. Why not?

Your hormones don't spring back like that.

Hormones and *sleep?* That's a new one.

Hormones like estrogen and, occasionally, testosterone are always in the news. DHEA and human growth hormone even surface once in a while, but these hormones are always in news stories about *aging*. The only hormone ever connected with sleep to make the news is good old melatonin, and everybody knows you can buy that over the counter. If you need it you can get it, right?

So why let sleep loss keep you up nights?

Because when you sleep less than you're meant to, melatonin isn't the only hormone affected. There are at least ten different hormones, as well as many more neurotransmitters in the brain, that go sideways when you don't sleep enough. Melatonin is just the tip of the iceberg, so to speak. It is all the other shifts that change *appetite, fertility,* and *mental* and *cardiac* health.

So why isn't everybody talking about hormones and sleep?

Perhaps it's because the news is buried separately in five or six different disciplines in academia. For example, Dr. Eve Van Cauter at the University of Chicago calls the hormonal shift she records in her sleep-studies lab "sleep *debt*." Catchy sound bite. Now losing sleep may get some attention. Somehow relating sleep loss to being owed something or owing someone something, just like money, gives it a new importance. Money always talks: That sleep debt you're acquiring has a direct annual cost to the nation of $15.9 billion, and an indirect cost of more like $100 billion in lost work time and accidents. But we're going to tell you that the cost is really much higher.

It's your *life*.

Sleeping through your alarm, or falling asleep at the keyboard and knocking your coffee over on your desk, is not the major disaster facing the sleepless, it's *death*.

And we don't mean in a car crash.

As a nation, we are sick because we don't sleep. We are fat and diabetic because we don't sleep. We are dying from cancer and heart disease because we don't sleep. An avalanche of peer-reviewed scientific papers supports our conclusion that when we don't sleep in sync with the seasonal variation in light exposure, we fundamentally alter a balance of nature that has been programmed into our physiology since Day One. This cosmic clock is embedded in the physiology of every living thing that exists.

The story we're about to tell you is so obvious yet so fantastic that if it weren't true, you'd never believe it. There's more to the story of sleep loss than anyone ever expected, because until now no one has been able to see the whole picture.

We do. And we're going to show you.

In *Lights Out*, we prove that obesity and the major killers correlated with obesity—heart disease, diabetes, and cancer—are caused by short nights, by working ridiculously long hours, by, literally, burning the candle at both ends, and by the electricity that gives us the ability to do it. *The cause is most certainly not overeating fat or a lack of exercise.*

We have researched the increase in obesity and the diseases known to correlate with that increase for two and a half years. Our conclusions are built on more than a decade of research at the National Institutes of Health (NIH) in Washington, D.C., and on more than one thousand other scientific sources. The new approach to illness may be humbling and unsettling, but that is the cost of truth.

So listen up.

* * *

When extended day length created by artificial light-and-dark cycles became the norm a short seventy years ago with the widespread use of the lightbulb, obesity, diabetes, heart disease, and cancer suddenly became the official causes of death on the coroner's reports, instead of the usual widespread use or injury common before the advent of the lightbulb.

Ever since these diseases began to surface as major killers around mid-century, the efforts on the part of science and medicine to explain the startling rise never examined any other overwhelming environmental change except diet. *And all these years later, as Americans continue to die, the doctors and the researchers all continue to fish in the same pond.*

It's time to see the light.

The biggest change human beings have lived through in the last ten thousand years happened less than seventy years ago. Electricity and the widespread use of the lightbulb qualify along with the discovery of fire, the advent of agriculture, and the discovery of antibiotic treatment as a point of no return in human history.

In 1910, the average adult was still sleeping nine to ten hours a night. Now the average adult is lucky to get a full *seven* hours a night. Most of us don't. Those numbers add up to an *extra five hundred waking hours* a year. In nature, we would sleep 4,370 hours out of a possible 8,760, or half of our lives. Eighty years ago, we were down to 3,395 hours. Now we are lucky to get a measly 2,555. If nature keeps score, and we bet she does, that means we only get to live about half as long. We may have doubled that figure with surgery and antibiotics, but think how long we could live if we slept, too.

In the 1970s, Americans devoted 27 hours a week to "leisure" time. In the 1990s, we're down to 15. And we work at least 48 hours a week, compared to 35 for the average worker in the 1970s. Then we had hobbies, we were players of baseball and builders of model ships, members of the garden club and Boy Scout troop leaders. Now, in the 1990s, although the number of hours we devote to work and leisure are approximately the same, the ratio has shifted considerably. In the thirty years since 1970, we've found new passions to add to the old duties—exercising, going to the doctor, commuting through ever-increasing traffic, watching 150 channels and real movies on cable TV, and the newer time bandits—E-mail and eBay. No wonder there's no time left to sleep or take care of our children.

So why didn't the guardians of our health look at stress and lack of sleep *before* they placed the entire blame on food? Go figure. And even when they did examine the diet of Americans and offered advice, they got it *backward*. They told the public to eat sugar and avoid fat.

By illuminating how your body has evolved with the planet and everything else on it, and by explaining how it uses food to initiate sleep and deal with stress, we will be able to tell you exactly what happens—to your mind, your body, and the planet—when you eat. We're going to show you the light.

The science of circadian rhythmicity explains it all. All the mysteries can be unraveled. We've looked at the scientific evidence in this book through the lens of evolutionary biology and biophysics. The resulting molecular maps show us the way home and retell us what we always knew. Sleeping controls eating, eating and stress control reproduction. Sleeping, eating, and making love control aging.

The hormones melatonin and prolactin are major players in your mind-body-planet connection. They communicate with your immune system and metabolic energy system about light-and-dark cycles. Insulin and prolactin orchestrate the brain chemistry governing serotonin and dopamine in your brain, to control your behavior and mood. Serotonin and dopamine control your behavior toward food and sex. Bottom line: Not enough sleep makes you fat, hungry, impotent, hypertensive, and cancerous, with a bad heart.

The sun's energy is the catalyst for all life. The amount of light that hits you informs your "system controls" about the rotation and orbit of the planet we live on. This global positioning helps our instincts to keep a bead on the food supply. It's this cosmic communication that has been telling us, since time began, when to eat, what to eat, and when to reproduce to maximize food availability. We and all the other organisms on this planet evolved *with the spin*—in and out of the light of the sun.

The fact that you are reading this means the system was successful.

The fact that you *want* to read this means the system is breaking down.

Most Americans are sick and tired of watching their weight and worrying about their hearts. We're about to tell them how to stop.

We could have called this book *Lose Weight While You Sleep,* but it seemed too cheap and easy. We almost called it *Kept in the Dark* after we found out exactly where all the studies proving our premise were conducted—in Washington, D.C. No less than the National Institutes of Health confirm that it is a scientific "given" that light-and-dark cycles:

- turn hormone production on and off

- activate your immune system

- time neurotransmitter release daily, and especially seasonally.

We've just told you that once upon a time we existed in sync with all biophysical cycles and rhythms in nature. Now, not only do we control the food supply, but we have pushed back the night and the weather. In *Lights Out,* we quote you the price for playing God.

Here comes the bill. The unending artificial light we live in registers as the long days of summer on that internal sundial because night never falls and winter never comes. As mammals, we are hardwired to store fat when exposed to long days and then to sleep or at the very least starve . . . for a while.

But now we don't sleep and we don't starve, either; at least, we don't starve for carbohydrates. That's why we're fat and getting fatter. It's endless August.

While fire, with its illumination, extended our day enough to affect intellect and reproduction, limitless electricity may just put us under.

Unless the government does it first.

If the NIH has run most of the studies that provide the evidence that depression, obesity, heart disease, and cancer can be prevented in a great many cases by sleeping more and turning the lights off, why have they kept us in the dark? Why do they continue to insist high-carbohydrate diets and exercise will cure us? Are they *really* trying to kill us?

The truth is always stranger than fiction. Scientists with the MacArthur Mind/Body Foundation at the University of Chicago, at NASA, and at the National Institutes of Health and the National Institutes of Mental Health in Washington, D. C., have been studying biophysics for at least the last decade. This means that the ultimate scientific think tanks in America are researching the same science we have researched for this book. As you read this, they, too, are proving that we are seasonal eaters and breeders with a feast-famine metabolism who develop diabetes, heart disease, cancer, and severe depression on *anything less than 9.5 hours* of sleep a night for at least seven months out of the year.

When we asked Dr. Thomas Wehr, the head of the department studying seasonal and circadian rhythmicity at the NIH in Washington, whether he felt the public had the right to know that on less than 9.5

hours of sleep at night—i.e., in the dark—they will (a) never be able to stop eating sugar, smoking, and drinking alcohol and (b) most certainly develop one of the following conditions: diabetes, heart disease, cancer, infertility, mental illness, and/or premature aging, he said, "Well, yes, they do have a right to know. They should be told; but it won't change anything. Nobody will ever turn off the lights."

Perhaps not.

After all, the light is seductive. The longer we stay up, the more we learn. That's why we Americans are the brightest and the best as well as the sickest people in the world.

But we still think it could happen.

After all, when authority figures told Americans in the late 1960s that they had better find time to exercise or they would die, they exercised. And when they said to cut the fat in our diets or we would die, all of the food factories retooled. When medical science said cholesterol-lowering drugs would be our ultimate salvation as we got sicker and sicker, we tossed the pills back like M&Ms. Of course, many people stood to gain financially from the fitness movement, the low-fat food, and the drugs. *The only person to benefit from sleeping is you.*

Whether or not we want to go to bed earlier and work fewer hours is really what's at stake here. With twenty-four-hour mini-marts, 150 channels of television, and the Net to surf all night, reversing our pace would require a Herculean effort. We know that, but we're just out to make going the way of the dinosaurs a *personal* choice, not a federal one. We think the public deserves the facts, and accurate nutritional advice, from our government.

We pay for it.

Every American knows that Washington thrives on secrecy, but it's a little hard to swallow that while the surgeon general's office is telling the public to eat a low-fat, 58-percent carbohydrate diet to cure obesity, diabetes, heart disease, and cancer, literally *across the street* the NIH is proving that it is the excessive consumption of carbohydrates brought about by sleep deprivation is among the causes those diseases.

Why have we been kept in the dark, when they've had the truth all along?

PART I

SECRETS
AND LIES

WE WANT TO BELIEVE:

The Church of False Gods

At some time in the past, scientists discovered that time flows more slowly the farther from the center of the earth. The effect is minuscule, but it can be measured with extremely sensitive instruments. Once the phenomenon was known, a few people, anxious to stay young, moved to the mountains.

Now all houses are built on Dom, the Matterhorn, Monte Rosa, and other high ground. It is impossible to sell living quarters elsewhere . . . To get the maximum effect, they have constructed their houses on stilts . . . People eager to live the longest have built their houses on the highest stilts . . . They celebrate their youth and walk around naked on their balconies . . .

In time, people have forgotten the reason that higher is better. Nonetheless, they continue to teach their children to shun other children from lower elevations. They have even convinced themselves that the thin air is good for their bodies, and following that logic, have gone on sparse diets, refusing all but the most gossamer food. At length, the populace have become thin like air, bony and old before their time.

—Alan Lightman,
Einstein's Dreams

In Woody Allen's classic film *Sleeper,* Miles Monroe, health-food-store owner and clarinetist, checks into Saint Vincent's Hospital in 1977 for a routine procedure. He has a peptic ulcer. When he awakens two hundred years later, he discovers he's died, and a caring aunt has placed him in cryogenic suspension.

The plot thickens when two renegade scientists illegally defrost him to take advantage of the fact that he is a numerical nonentity and, as such, can help them overthrow the fascist regime controlling America in 2173. We eavesdrop as they discuss his progress:

> "Has he asked for anything special?"
> "For breakfast, he requested something called wheat germ, organic honey, and tiger's milk."
> "Ahh, yes, yes, back then people thought of such things as charmed substances that contained life-preserving properties."
> "You mean there was no deep fat, no steak, or hot fudge?"
> "Oh, no, those were thought to be unhealthy, precisely the opposite of what we now know to be true."
> "Incredible!"

What's most unnerving about this snippet of filmdom? That social security numbers classify every citizen in a Big Brother–like computer bank, that a fascist regime is controlling America, or that *The New England Journal of Medicine* released a study in 1998 concluding that fat may actually *protect* you from heart disease? Could the 1970's nutritional wisdom we've been relying on for decades be completely bogus?

What's next? Sleep more or you'll get cancer?

Consider the last statement prophetic.

Later, Miles/Woody watches Diane Keaton's character light up a cigarette for medicinal purposes and moans:

> "How could we have been so wrong? Everybody knew fat and caffeine were toxic substances!"
> "Miles, everybody knows that the only things that have kept mankind alive are coffee, cigarettes, and red meat!"

Somehow that's not as funny, now that it might be true.

Coffee and cigarettes certainly seem to keep the French alive. They even look better than we do. In this same tragicomic scenario, the wheat grass and tiger's milk are thinly veiled doppelgangers for our salads and Balance bars. In the 1970s, salads and Balance bars definitely would have been classified as "health food" for "health nuts." Everyone was very comfortable with the fact that there were "health nuts" and there were the rest of us. Today, if you're *not* into your health, you're considered nuts.

Today, *everything* is labeled "low-fat," "fat-free," "99% fat free," or

"30% lower in fat," in an attempt to qualify as "health" food. Even fruit juice and dried pasta are sold as "fat-free," because we're all nuts. Your doctor and the media docs on TV all say, even after Dr. Atkins, *Protein Power,* and *Enter the Zone* have proven otherwise, that you can't get enough high-quality carbohydrates to lose weight unless you consume

- 5 to 7 servings of fruits and vegetables a day on top of the

- recommended 5 to 7 servings of grains and breads on top of

- pasta and wine.

They never even figure in the Pepsi, Coke, Snapple, honey in your tea, and the high-fructose corn syrup that shows up as a preservative in almost *all* processed food. Now, let's imagine all of the food they've recommended piled up on the table (because it would never fit on your plate). Doesn't that seem like a lot?

What if all those low-fat promises of a long, cancer-free, diabetes-free life in a beautiful, thin body, run by a strong, clear, non-hypertensive heart, were bogus from the start? What if carbohydrates, not fat, were the cause of obesity, diabetes, and cancer?

THE GOD MODULE

We think it's the exercise that's the key to why you feel so good while you're dying. It's also the reason why some people are able to stay on a low-fat regimen long enough to kill themselves. What could make a person do this?

The desire to be thin and well? No way.

Michael Persinger, Ph.D., professor of neuroscience and psychology at Laurentian University in Canada, has isolated an area of neurons in the brain's temporal lobes that repeatedly fire bursts of electrical activity when one thinks about God or has any feelings of spirituality. We scientists know this from CAT scanning praying monks, nuns, and schizophrenics as they "talk to God." Near the front of these temporal lobes is the amygdala, an almond-shaped organ that imbues events with intense emotion and a sense of meaningfulness.

Because of the way the temporal lobes are structured and hardwired to the amygdala, they are the most electrically sensitive regions in the brain. Dr. Persinger has personal knowledge of this because he created a helmet with coils of wire set just above the ears (picture Woody in *Sleeper*). By passing a carefully controlled electrical current through these coils, the doctor creates a pulsating magnetic field that mimics the firing patterns of the neurons in the temporal lobes. This creates a mystical spiritual experience, complete with a healthy dose of peace. Dr. Persinger's subjects report an "opiate-like effect with a substantial decrease in anxiety, a heightened sense of well-being, similar to reports of enlightenment."

While Dr. Persinger was doing his best mad-scientist impression, Vilayanur Ramachandran, Ph.D., director of the Brain and Perception Laboratory at the University of California at San Diego, was channeling heaven. Dr. Ramachandran announced in 1998 that he had discovered the "God module." This "module" is located in the brain in an area within the temporal lobes that becomes electrically active when a person thinks about God or spirituality or recalls a "mystical" experience. Wow, that sounds familiar.

We also know that stress, grief, and mostly a lack of oxygen also trigger heavy electrical firing in the same neighborhood as the God module. Since lack of oxygen brings on such neural bursts, some scientists believe this mechanism may account for many near-death experiences of euphoria and tranquillity. Also, sleep apnea in people with twitchy temporal lobes may mean that they hear someone calling their name as they fall asleep, or that they have an "out of body experience," such as flying, in their dreams. We're also going to tell you that the hyperventilation resulting from the exercise that goes along with urban yuppie low-fat living kicks the God module into play. That's why a runner's high is such a religious experience.

Your brain thinks you're dying. But you're just out of breath.

We're worried that you might be out of time, too.

The truth is, all of that exercise is doing more than making you high. It's exacerbating the burnout of your cortisol receptors. Running is a fear response. In the real world, it means something is after you; at least that's what your body and brain think. If you run long enough, all your systems believe you're not going to outrun that predator. The brain chemistry that follows extended running has evolved to make your exit from this world more pleasant. This means that oxygen depletion alone will kick in the part of the brain that takes you to heaven or, in this world, gives you a reason to keep running. The mechanism of brain chemistry that causes you to see God as you run out of oxygen evolved from programmed responses—responses to environmental cues that no longer exist, responses that once upon a time might have kept you alive or made dying okay.

Now, they're killing you.

HEALTHY LIVING?

What other modern environmental cues are triggering ancient survival switches? The answer to that question is a chilling scenario worthy of a science fiction novel. Or a book like ours.

Working late in bright lights after dark, or watching David Letterman, or checking late-night E-mail, for even just half an hour, all register as the long days of summer to your inner environmental controls. This means that your brain will force you to seek energy for storage by eating sugar. Sugar (carbohydrates) is the only path to insulin release; insulin's job is to store excess carbohydrates as fat and cholesterol so you have something to live on when summer's over.

The abdominal fat pad common in insulin-resistant, high-cholesterol heart patients and Type II diabetics would, in another time and place, have served to keep internal organs warm and would have been utilized as energy during normal famine (winter). Increased intake of carbohydrates (sugar) is always dumped into increased cholesterol production, too, because the carbs lower the freezing temperature of the cell membrane. In the real world, you'd never have access to that much sugar unless it was summer before winter. You don't live in the real world.

The next time your doctor says your cholesterol is too high and you should cut back on the fat and exercise more, tell him he's mistaken. Tell him you're not sick, you're just going to hibernate and you don't want to freeze. He might laugh.

You, on the other hand, should be crying. You're in big trouble.

All of the systems that have evolved to keep you alive and have brought you to this point are shouting, *"Famine's coming!!!"*

When you exercise day and night to stave off the weight gain your body and mind crave, you kick in your "stress response." The message you're sending to those systems is

"Oh, my God, a famine's coming *and there's a tiger chasing me!!*"

Trust us, this is no solution.

In fact, exercise just might be the last nail in our collective coffins. The stress response enacted when you run for your life on that treadmill causes your cortisol levels to rise. If you do this once in a while, say, every ten days, the natural *episodic* cortisol response will keep your heart and brain healthy. But if you exercise like a maniac more that once a week, the high cortisol levels resulting from all of the chronic exercise actually mimics the stress of mating season, when the long hours of light and the competition (especially for males) kept cortisol at *yearly* highs. Sexual competition is the most stressful situation possible in nature, short of being killed. Mating season would come to naught without a fat base to nourish a pregnancy through the winter. So it's no coincidence that carbohydrate craving to put on fat, and high cortisol and high sex hormone levels all coincide. There must be a bun in the oven for most mammals by August or September in order for the baby to be born in April or May, in the spring, when food is plentiful.

So you're in the gym, it's November, it's anywhere from 6:30 to 9:30 P.M., and at least 3 bazillion watts of fluorescent lights are on and being intensified by reflecting mirrors that are shining right into your eyes and all over the skin of your overexposed body. You lift weights, run or jog on a treadmill or track, and, if you're really suicidal, you're on a StairMaster or you're spinning.

Know that, to your body and mind—which were evolved over millennia to recognize cues in nature—you are in a fight, a death match, just like the head butting wildebeests on the Nature Channel. You are in a fight for an egg, for immortality, or at least for a chance at the next round. This fight seems reasonable to your body because the long light at night (gym glare) means it's late summer and you must mate or go berserk. (Anybody who's witnessed the mating behaviors going on at the Vertical Club can't possibly question our hypothesis.) That's why cortisol is up during the day—to supply glucose to muscles to fight or run away and to keep you calm for decision-making processes—for mating. That's why, when we are constantly bathed in unending light, we all feel so antsy (read: paranoid, aggressive, hysterical, urgent), even those of us not exercising ourselves into oblivion.

In this chronic state, not only are you keeping your blood sugar up, taxing your insulin response system with cortisol's blood-sugar-mobilizing effects, you are actually becoming insulin-resistant as you exercise, too.

This fact means *exercise can make you fat.*

While you're exercising like a maniac and living low-fat, if you even smell a cookie you gain weight—and you're pouring sex hormones, too, causing cancer and suppressing your immune system in the bargain. Chronic high cortisol also skews your time perception, making you feel continually rushed. It's the altered time perception that fosters much of the late-night stalling before bed, while you stay up under the impression that there must be more to do or that you haven't finished your work. Then you stuff yourself with more sugar because you haven't slept, and your insulin is sent even higher. We know this behavior alone makes you fat and sick.

Really, it's not the lack of excercise or the meat or the butter.

It's not fat at all.

Really.

If eating saturated fat caused obesity, we would already be well on our way to reducing obesity nutritionally. Actually, we would all look like supermodels. We're eating less fat and exercising more than ever before, but we don't look anything like supermodels.

In fact, we really look like hell.

We're fatter and sicker than ever before in our nation's history. Not only do we still look incredibly bad, but our plan to eradicate heart disease, cancer, and diabetes is shot to hell, too. The average American has actually *gained eight and a half pounds* since the "low-fat war" on obesity began.

The assumption we've held dear for thirty years has been that losing weight by cutting fat and exercising would lead to massive improvements in the occurrences of cardiovascular diseases, not to mention diabetes and cancer.

But that hasn't happened.

When it didn't happen, the medical establishment said that the scientists said that we hadn't lowered fat *enough.* And that if we lowered the fat content in all processed foods, if we further reduced meat consumption, and if we created fake fats like Olean, the brand name for olestra, the tide would finally turn. Now all these goals and miracles have occurred *and* we exercise day and night, and we are much sicker than ever. There is no "real food" available in the grocery stores and, pathetically, many of us have at least once in the last ten years attempted to become vegans. Every day, talk show hosts, TV documentaries, news anchors, and cooking shows tell you low-fat living is working. You'd never know it's not, unless you took a look at the statistics and the increasing sale of diet drugs. These numbers give a very different picture.

To say the picture is not so rosy would be downright facetious. Recent studies showed a body count of more than 1 million people for heart disease alone. The big rumor among statisticians is that cardiovascular death is now widely underreported. Somehow, although the number of deaths from heart disease has decreased, the actual number of heart attacks has gone up.

That means somebody's playing with the numbers.

It also means people are still having just as many heart attacks and as much cardiovascular disease as ever, but procedures like bypass surgery, angiograms, a clot-busting drug called t-PA, 911, and angioplasty are saving them for the moment and decreasing death rates. That's just cardiovascular *death;* there are still 60 million more people (that's 25 percent of the American population) who will eventually die from heart disease, according to their risk profile.

Some of these "risks" are smoking, age, gender, high blood pressure, high serum cholesterol levels, diabetes, stress, and, of course, almost everyone's own medical nightmare, obesity. (The terror in this society isn't destitution, heart disease, or even violent crime, it's the haunting thought that you might just get up one morning really fat.)

Well, wake up and smell the Slim•Fast.

The average man in this country is not thin. He has 23 percent body fat, and the average woman has 32 percent. Those figures make the average guy 53 percent fatter than the healthy ideal and the average woman at least 50 percent fatter. In 1961, obesity was, so they thought, at an all-time high of 20 percent of the entire population. In 1995, the Centers for Disease Control and Prevention told us that the number of Americans who were seriously overweight had increased to 30 percent during the eighties *alone.* Remember the gym. For twenty years prior to that, these same obesity statistics remained unchanged, holding at one quarter of the population. This is exactly the same twenty-year period that encompassed the bulk of new nutritional research that we now follow. This twenty-year span also saw the end of real food, the forty-hour work week, and the two-week vacation, as well as the advent of cable TV, cell phones, voice mail, and E-mail.

EVER WONDER?

Every year, 80 million Americans "go on a diet." The amount of weight they lose isn't even at issue, because 95 percent of them gain it all back (plus some) within five years. We've been steadily *decreasing* our consumption of fat and cholesterol, and yet increasing our incidence of obesity, disease, and death.

Since the turn of the century, sugar consumption has increased by 150 percent. As sugar became a cheap preservative, it became an additive in almost all processed foods, and, as we know, American consumption of processed foods has increased exponentially over the last fifty years.

In the 1940s, TV was rare. By the mid-1950s, three in ten households were receiving visible radio waves. Even in the heyday of Nickelodeon-derived programming, harried housewives only occasionally poisoned their families with TV dinners. Now the average family has two adults employed full-time and eats out or from the freezer case at least four nights a week. If that's the norm in a two-parent family, imagine how rarely the average single-parent household gets a home-cooked meal.

Mom either picks up the kids at day care and they go out, or she calls the baby-sitter to start boiling the water for the pasta. It's already at least 6:30 P.M. by the time dinner (pasta, juice, or low-fat milk for the kids, plus bread, and dessert) is ready. Mom needs a drink just to keep going and there's still homework, baths, and "quality time" to accomplish. If Mom cooks a real dinner from more than two of the recognized food groups, instead of feeding the next generation Cheerios or pasta, it's even later. And if she does that, Mom needs two drinks.

Now it's at least 9:00 or 9:30 P.M. and she still hasn't had a minute to sit and stare after work. In the summer, this would actually be okay. But the scenario we're describing is during the school year, which means "dark time" in nature, so this single-parent family or working mother with a lazy or, on the other hand, even harder working "absent father" will endure at least five, maybe seven, extra hours of light in a twenty-four-hour period, day in and day out for seven months *out of season* every year, year in and year out, decade after decade—until Mom gets breast cancer, her little girl has acne and is too fat to find her image in *Vogue*, and Junior, who is only 5′5″, has asthma. If our imaginary dad is present, he has clogged arteries, high blood pressure, and high blood sugar.

And how this all happens is a complete mystery to medical science.

The disastrous slide in the health of the American people corresponds to the increase in light-generating night activities and the carbohydrate consumption that follows. Just consider the increase in the average weight of young adults and teens over the last fifteen to twenty years. It has, predictably, increased by more than ten pounds. The percentage of overweight teens rested at 15 percent in the 1970s and rose to 21 percent by 1991. Now it's up to 30 percent.

A recent front-page article in *The New York Times* cited television as *the* cause of the increase of obesity in young people. Its claim rested solely on the "couch potato" premise, pleading a lack of activity (exercise). It is TV, all right—but not the way they think. Most young people today were born into a low-fat/ heavy-exercise world. More than a third of them are self-declared vegetarians and bikers and hikers and Rollerbladers. There are approximately 12.5 million of them in America today. These young adults, when asked *why* they're vegetarians, predominantly say it's for their health; the rest just think it's cool. They have no idea what they're doing to themselves.

THE ENDLESS SUMMER SYNDROME

Besides a steady increase in heart disease and obesity, statistics already show that diabetes and cancer are also on the rise.

Maybe it's not just the food.

In the January 12, 1998, issue of *U.S. News and World Report,* the head of the Harvard School of Public Health's department of nutrition, a very fickle man, Walter Willet, was queried about a low-fat diet's failure to cure any diseases or save any lives. His weak reply, "It was just a hypothesis to begin with," showed no shame.

That hypothesis has cost more lives than the last two world wars and the Vietnam conflict put together. Just check the American Cancer Society's and American Heart Association's statistics for the last three decades. In 1999, it was predicted that 1,257,800 people would die from cancer alone.

If you'd like a future projection, check the American Diabetes Association's mystifying numbers on the growing population of Type II diabetics. Now researchers are on the lookout for genetic markers for obesity, because if there's anything we're sure of, it's that obesity is the beginning of the end. Obesity is *the* precursor for adult-onset diabetes. It's no coincidence that in the year 2000 there will be more than 25 million Type II diabetics. That's about 98 percent of the entire diabetic population. If all 25 million become diabetic, then a great proportion of them will certainly have heart disease and high blood pressure, two conditions that lead to stroke. Those complications are the leading killers of diabetics.

It's been predicted for years now that reducing dietary fat would decrease cancer, but cancer statistics show us an increasing incidence of colon cancer with an associated decrease in death. That means colon cancer is increasing, but people are dying from it less often. This is not a cure. For breast and prostate cancer, both increased incidence and increased death can be seen. These numbers on breast cancer, prostate cancer, and colon cancer are the ones that, most certainly, should have shown a drop, given all the dietary changes Americans have made in the last fifteen years. Instead of acknowledging low-fat's defeat, medical research gave us Mevacor, Provachol, Proscar, and now Tamoxifen and Raloxifene.

Medicine admits that the "improvement" in cancer statistics is derived from early detection, not from treatment or prevention. But early detection only extends the time of awareness—the victim just knows sooner that he or she is going to suffer and die. It doesn't actually change the *date* of death. Early detection never *saves* lives; more often it only prolongs them long enough to skew the numbers. All these numbers prove that we're on the wrong course. We agree that dietary intervention certainly can reverse the course of disease. Cutting carbohydrates would cure obesity and most diabetes, but not heart disease, and certainly not all cancer. The end of this story lies in *extinction*.

Food is part of the equation, all right, but it is not the answer. The answer lies in circadian rhythmicity and evolution.

The answer is to eat and sleep and reproduce in sync with the spin of the planet or go the way of the dinosaurs. The long hours of artificial light that confuse your ancient energy regulation system also destroy the lining of your heart, so excess cholesterol can obstruct blood flow. Your subconscious has, over the course of evolution, been conditioned and fine-tuned to believe and act on the following when the lights stay on too long: "Eat carbohydrates now or die later." Your subconscious, too, has, over the course of evolution, been conditioned and fine-tuned to believe and act on the following when the lights stay on too long: "Mate or die." This light-responsive instinct has been the basis of our feast-or-famine metabolism and ultimate survival for at least 3 million years. All the effects of chronic light exposure and the carbohydrate consumption that follows that exposure would have, in another place and time, prepared us for the worst—for no food and for the shorter, darker, colder days of less sun.

We have always "feasted" to endure the "famine" that always followed—until now. Unfortunately, the truth in our time is that we eat carbohydrates now *and* die sooner. Your body translates long hours of artificial light into summertime. Because it instinctively knows that summer comes before winter, and that winter means no available food, you begin to crave carbohydrates so you can store fat for a time when food is scarce and you should be hibernating. This is the formula:

A. Long hours of artificial light = summer in your head

B. Winter signifies famine to your internal controls

C. Famine on the horizon signifies instinctive carbohydrate craving to store fat for hibernation and scarcity

This storage is accomplished by:

1. Increasing carbohydrate consumption until your body responds to all the insulin by becoming insulin-resistant in muscle tissue;

2. Ensuring that the carbohydrates taken in end up as a fat pad;

3. Prompting the liver to dump the extra sugar into cholesterol production, which will keep cell membranes from freezing at low temperatures.

If you sleep at night for the number of hours it would normally be dark outside, you will only crave sugar in the summer, when the hours of light are long. It is the "perennial adaptation," or the chronic, constant *intent to hibernate,* that causes overconsumption of carbohydrates and obesity and its attendant high blood pressure, high cholesterol, and inevitable heart failure.

Steps 1, 2, and 3 also correspond to the hormonal portrait of Type II diabetes—a disease that, in truth, is the end result of *excruciating* fatigue from light "toxicity." On the way to the end, you'll definitely encounter one of the following—obesity, heart disease, stroke, mental illness, or cancer. The medical community, the FDA, the National Institutes of Health, and your TV will tell you that the cause is a plague from the great beyond that can only be cured by an 80-percent nonfat diet, at least three to six hours of exercise a week, and a cadre of supplements and vitamins.

Who are you going to believe?

The market is saturated with information on low-fat diets: how to eat low-fat, why to eat low-fat, who should eat low-fat. There are only a few dissenting opinions, though the numbers are growing every day. It's slowly leaking into the American consciousness that "for some people, low-fat may not be the best choice," according to Walter Willet. This half-mumbled, hedged recant is too little, too late for those we knew who didn't live through the low-fat movement.

This national health catastrophe has, in real time, been at least seventy-five years in the making. In all those years, countless souls have struggled and failed to follow nutritional advice that never could have led to success. They failed because it was never really about food. We know from history that the diseases of civilization all hit hard after the Industrial Revolution, when electricity made the potential of unlimited cheap artificial light possible. It was the electric lightbulb that turned night into day. The price-performance curve for the lightbulb mirrors the price-performance curve for the laptop computer. A 100-watt bulb costs 33 cents at any Home Depot. In 1883, the same amount of light would have cost the consumer $1,445. The experts have concluded that machines usurped our physical well-being; in reality, it was the refined and sugared processed food that became part of our lives for the first time, at the same time as the lights extended our day and changed our appetites, that did it. Although the instrument of destruction may be food, the cause of death is something much more insidious.

CAUSE OF DEATH

Your appetite is but one symptom of this deathly dysfunction, just as obesity is correlative with heart disease but is not the cause. The real truth is that the urgent need to sleep is also the cause of Type II diabetes. All diseases that are not caused by contagion and injury are born of immune dysfunction by way of metabolism. Your immune system is governed by two substances: prolactin and melatonin, and both of them are controlled by light-and-dark cycles. It's these major biological controls that are deranged. Seasonal variation in daylight, and intensity of daylight, control budding, growth, and dormancy in plants *and in animals;* seasonal changes in ambient lighting control hibernation, migration, and breeding. To expose ourselves to the unremitting glare of artificial lighting for more hours than it is actually daylight is asking for trouble. Until seventy-five years ago, we spent up to fourteen hours a night, depending on the season, *in the dark.*

By the 1920s, most people could afford to keep the lights on for a couple of hours at night after sunset. They could afford a couple of Edison's new light "bulbs" and the electricity to keep them on because the same energy source was building an economy that utilized an enormous workforce. The lights brought jobs to pay for the lights. By the late 1920s, expensive machinery in factories had begun to hum around the clock. Suddenly they were running twenty-four hours a day, when, only a decade before, gaslight was too expensive to use all night. Before electricity, factories ran only ten hours a day. This second Industrial Revolution remapped the economic landscape.

Night-shift work brought more money in countless ways. Not only did it line the pockets of the factory owners, it also provided more jobs and money to an economic underclass of new immigrants. But, more important, night-shift work brought a service economy with it. That service economy spawned transportation, all-night places to eat and all-night grocery stores, night tennis courts and baseball games, gambling joints, and on and on. The electricity powered the telephone, which is the basis of our present science-fiction communications capacity, which has allowed small markets to become global markets. There's even a new piece of terminology in our language for this phenomenon, thanks to the Internet—twenty-four/seven. It was a ridiculously bad piece of luck in an otherwise pretty fair century that, at exactly the same time that sugar started to be used to process and preserve packaged "food," we had the opportunity to stay up all night and eat it.

Granted, there weren't a lot of packaged foods on the market at that point, but the ones that were on the market used highly refined (by machine) corn syrup to prevent moisture loss and extend shelf life. Most packaged foods still do. Even the shrink-wrapped whole-grain low-fat honey-sweetened bran muffins you find next to the cash register in the mini-mart have been preserved with sugar. It's illuminating to note here that the incidence of Type II diabetes dropped sharply during World War I and World War II, when sugar was rationed.

THE INSTRUMENT OF DEATH

To understand why carbohydrates are the instrument of death, we need just a little science. Only recently have science and medicine begun to acknowledge a condition called chronic hyperinsulinemia. That's the term for chronic high insulin made in your own body. This can only occur when you chronically consume carbohydrates. You could *never* chronically consume carbohydrates in nature. Trees and plants fruit only in one season and flower in the other. Living on sugar for more than a month or two in a row would not be possible unless you were preparing to hibernate like a woodchuck for a long winter nap.

The media doesn't talk much about insulin unless it's reporting on Type I diabetes, so most people know insulin as a medicine for Type I diabetics, who for reasons that are viral or autoimmune in origin can no longer make their own insulin. The diseases known as Type I and Type II diabetes are both characterized by uncontrollable blood sugar.

Insulin is at the center of both forms of the disease because it controls blood sugar by binding to cell receptor sites like a key opening a lock. Once the floodgates are open, the blood sugar can enter and energize all of your cells. Insulin resistance is the body's inability to respond to the insulin that you normally produce because receptors have retreated to save your life. Every function of your body, from basic molecule-to-molecule communication to complex operations like appetite control or temperature regulation, is in a tight zone of normalcy called homeostasis. The retreat of your insulin receptors is an attempt to control how much sugar is allowed in. Too much is not normal.

The telling clue to our impending doom is that the incidence of insulin resistance is occurring in younger and younger people. The entire population is aging in "fast forward." The logical response would be to retool all the food factories and advise people to cut out sugar, right? That's the approach we took with fat and the population fell right in line. Believe us, *it wouldn't be as easy with sugar.* It would be more like Prohibition. *We are as addicted to a low-fat, high-sugar diet as alcoholics are to alcohol,* because high insulin levels create the same brain state as alcohol does.

Alcoholics "sleep it off" after a binge, not only because the alcohol itself has a drug-like effect on their opiate receptors but also because the huge carbohydrate load of the grape, grain, potato, cactus, or, in the case of rum, sugar cane in the drink literally puts them to sleep. Remember this as you go for that glass of wine *after* dinner. The spike of insulin after a binge makes the serotonin in the brain turn into melatonin and it's lights out. In our culture, we take in as much carbohydrate in a day as a rummy on a binge. For him and us, the natural recovery is the same.

Sleep it off.

RESURRECTION OF THE TRUTH

Could it really be the loss of sleep destroying the endocrine clock that controls weight gain? Could how much you sleep really control your appetite? Our findings are almost too simple and extraordinary to believe. But here, we remind you of the legendary rule of Occam's razor, which states: "All things being equal, the simplest answer is always the correct one." We know that, for most of you, what we're telling you is like finding out that everything you've grown up believing is a lie. Well, it is. Don't you want to know?

It turns out that everything we've come to know as fact about our health turns out to be no more than wild conjecture. Conjecture that has no science to support it. Conjecture that, to some people, made sense.

Not anymore.

TWO

INTO THE DARK:
An Extinction-Level Event

To sleep, perchance to dream.
> —William Shakespeare,
> *Hamlet,* 3.2.54, 1554

To sleep, perchance to dream,
perchance to mess with reality.
> —Sony Corporation, 1997

You, darkness, enfold the spirit of those who ignored your glory.
Take us now.
> —Mayra Montero, a prayer to be said for
> the dying from *You, Darkness,* 1999

The soft comfort rendered by the sounds of amphibians at night is as deeply buried in the human consciousness as is the silvery music of running water. The pounding of the ocean on the shore, a gurgling Roman fountain, crickets chirping, and frogs croaking all bode well for humanity. And we count on that. Since day one we have felt secure hearing those sounds because they translated into survival: food, water, and company.

Now that's all changing. The frogs are too quiet. The silence is deafening. Amphibians, frogs, and toads are dying under mysterious circumstances. In some cases, not even the bodies are found. According to *New Scientist* magazine, in the Causuco National Park in Honduras, more than one species of jungle frog has vanished without a trace; there are no tadpoles left, either. In Australia, not one, not two, not three, but four species have disappeared from the forests of Queensland. On the Hawaiian island of Kauai, a once plentiful toad is just not there anymore. The locals told investigators that all the toads had "just gone away" one day. These now absent creatures lived in delicate balance between water and land, air and light.

So do we.

It's a chilling prospect to realize that, in the end, our disappearance, like that of the amphibians, will most probably happen from some unspecified and general collapse, not from a careening asteroid or a nuclear holocaust. We know that it's begun already. We, those of us humans alive today, are hurtling toward extinction.

BOOK OF THE DEAD

Is our extinction imminent? The odds against our extinction aren't good. It's happened more than once, and it can happen again. Thirty million species live on the planet with us at present, and many more millions have been and gone. Extinction experts agree that biological diversity is disappearing rapidly, especially when you realize that there have been only a handful of major extinctions in the last 3.5 billion years of life on this planet. Perhaps it's just the natural course of events, the coming Ice Age. More likely, it's of our own invention. Whatever the cause, the historical record verifies the signs, and the signs are everywhere. From declining birth rates to escalating diabetes and cancer, a lot of us are not "fit" to live. Some of us are about to go the way of other less adaptable branches of our family, such as *Homo habilis, Homo erectus,* or *Homo neanderthalensis.* Some of those hominids were outpopulated by other branches of the family. But more of them were just less *adaptable.* When you change the environment, the environment changes you, if your genes will allow it to.

All our current genetic makeup evolved in a time before we had the ability to bring light to the blackness just because we wanted to, unimaginable as that might be. Our first foray into celestial control, firelight, changed those of us who could change. It was the acquisition and use of fire that first lengthened our day and shortened our night. Shorter nights meant less melatonin. Less melatonin meant more estrogen and testosterone, more cortisol, and, of course, more insulin. Those of us who could genetically adapt to live with less sleep, more carbohydrate, and the increased fertility that brought lived on. Those who couldn't adapt died, unfit to survive in the new environment.

The next great death knell was the mass human extinction that we feel must have followed close on the heels of the coming of agriculture. We were born, like every other animal, to hunt in the light—whether it be for fruit and fish in the summer or wild pig and bark in the winter—and to rest in the dark. Cultivating grain near our living sites changed all that. Although a year-round supply of carbohydrate energy did help us out-populate almost everything except the microbes, this new miracle, agri-culture, also gave us our first *self-inflicted* plague. The relatively sudden change in the concentration and timing of our carbohydrate food supply polished off more than a few of us by tipping the balance of our nutrition from 90 percent protein to 80 percent carbohydrate (sugar).

For all previous human time, although carbohydrates were available in the months from spring to late fall, we never *craved* it until *the hours of sunlight changed,* when March turned into April and April into May. By June and July, our nights were only seven or eight hours long, compared to the dead of winter, when the blackness lasted at least thirteen hours each day.

Agriculture meant that we were suddenly living on an ever-increasing amount of carbohydrate (sugar) for even *more* of the year due to our abil-ity to control the growing seasons. After making it through hundreds of millennia and a couple of Ice Ages without sugar out of season, the sud-denness, in terms of evolution, of its arrival caused the same kind of death we're seeing now.

Our most recent unspecified and general collapse began with the dis-covery of electricity. Our first innocent maneuver was to carry away glow-ing coals from lightning strikes. This "fire" had real possibilities. Next we managed to learn how to reanimate coals that had gone cold. We lived like that for maybe a million and a half years, then, less than eighty tiny years ago, we took up residence with the gods.

BRIGHT LIGHTS, BIG CITIES, BIG BUCKS

This round, we've gone ourselves one better: We've learned to re-create the lightning that gave us the magic of hot coals. We hold the god Thor hostage. Harnessing the primal energy of lightning gave us the keys to the kingdom. Now we're going to pay.

From the middle of the 1700s until the late 1800s, Europeans like Michael Faraday, Alessandro Volta, and a few scattered others pursued magnetism until nature, in the form of electrons, lined up and saluted. Now, eight thousand years after farming began, we sorry survivors of agriculture, the last great threat to mankind, face a *new* kind extinction—artificial lighting, brought to us by *Look* magazine's Man of the Millennium, Thomas Alva Edison.

In 1831, Michael Faraday created the electric generator. Edison saw it at the Philadelphia Exhibition and, so the story goes, was inspired—so inspired that he went on to become the Bill Gates of the burgeoning century. The lightbulb, the phonograph, parts of the telephone and its wires, *and* the movie projector all came from the mind of this one man.

In 1877, he took J. P. Morgan's money and promised him a lightbulb. The British team of Sawyer and Mann were very close to producing one, and Edison wanted to beat them. By 1878, he still had no working bulb. One year later, he had lost his family and his money, and still no bulb. At that point, though, he still had his eyesight.

Under the gun, so to speak, he worked around the clock for three straight weeks in only one change of clothes with a team of fifteen men. He smoked twenty cigars a day, drank incessantly, and slept not at all. For approximately five hundred hours, give or take a twenty-minute nap here and there, Edison stared at burning filaments in vacuum tubes trying to find one that could be reliably relit.

Going from platinum to bamboo to baked sewing thread (the burned fibers of which produced carbon), he burned one filament after another until he got one to burn for thirteen hours. Then, half blind, he finally went to sleep on whiskey and a fair amount of morphine. The next morning, he called a press conference and announced a demonstration. Three thousand people came to Menlo Park, New Jersey. Edison had strung wire and one hundred bulbs over the small town. At the demonstration, he promised to light New York City within a year; that alone made him a "personality." Though he didn't make his deadline, two years and miles of wire later, one-quarter of a mile of Pearl Street in downtown New York City had 2,323 working lightbulbs. His quest for the perfect filament cost him his family, at least half of his eyesight, and a great deal more of his health. From that period on, he was never able to sleep, day or night, without morphine. But he won the race.

And his accomplishment permanently remade the world.

In two short years, culminating in one very bright night, everything changed forever. The way we ate, slept, lived, and died would never be the same. Although it's not much consolation, those years changed Edison, too. He partnered with the British in 1900 to found General Electric and lost a bitter AC/DC war with Westinghouse. Although he died lonely and a little crazy, he could count among his close friends men like Henry Ford and Harvey S. Firestone. After all, cars need tires *and* headlights.

WELCOME TO PARADOX

By 1925, all American cities of any size at all were lit; only rural areas lagged behind. It's an important point that rural areas are still the most common sites of exaggerated longevity in Americans. All of the diseases that modern medicine declares war on never seem to touch any of those ninety-year-old farmers who have lived on bacon and eggs and butter for almost a century. The media, following current low-fat medical wisdom, calls that a paradox. We don't.

We see these examples of less disease and longer life span correlating to the delayed arrival of electric lighting. The REA, or Rural Electrification Administration, which was founded in 1935, was brought into being because fewer than 11 farms out of 100 had electricity at that time. In 1950, 30 out of 100 were lit, but it wasn't until the very late 1970s that 99 percent were wired and glowing. The REA is still a viable and active organization, bringing wires and twenty-four-hour lights to U.S. territories and Puerto Rico, so that we can all die together.

Weather, food supply, and sexual competition have all served to "ter-raform" us and all other species to the landscape and the times we live in. It is only in the last half of the last million years or so that we humans have taken it upon ourselves to create the means to our own extinction and that of countless other species. Electricity not only gave us cheap, renewable, unending light; it gave us the means to control all of nature, plants and animals alike. Illuminating the dark meant we could have tractors with headlights and backlit microscopes, as well as control our fellow species with cattle prods and electric fences.

X-PLANATIONS

We can't really fight the future, but we sure as hell can stall. By truly understanding all of the turning points and synergistic mechanisms of life here on earth, it is possible to work the knobs and dials to stave off extinction. Right now, there's no hope of control because Americans are suffocating and ultimately dying under layers of incoherent information.

The TV drones on all day, program after program, about how to "lower your fat intake and increase your exercise," while your doctor repeats the party line. Nabisco puts "the fat" (?) back into SnackWell's. Fen-Phen is pulled off the market, and then put back on the market. Prozac sales soar. The newspapers, of course, confuse the public by prematurely releasing any small hope of salvation . . . Angiostatin, Endostatin, Tamoxifen, Raloxifene, Mevacor, Provachol, Zyban, Allegra, Valtrex ("It's about suppression"), and, of course, Fen-Phen's close cousins, Meridia and Orlistat. For those of us just too tired and too wired to get it up, there's Tylenol PM and ultimately Viagra. Meanwhile, you, your friends, and family get sicker and sicker.

We intend to tell you *what it all means.* In the following chapters, we're going to give you a peek at what lies just beyond the shifting line that defines the limits of our knowledge. The world is stranger than we ever thought. Newtonian physics are just the tip of the iceberg. It's a quantum universe out there, especially when it comes to your health. The incomprehensible aspects of cosmic templates, your behavior, your fate in the form of your genes, and illness are connected at higher and higher levels of interactivity, where it all comes together to make a new kind of sense that has far more meaning than you've ever imagined.

Nothing happens in contradiction to nature, only in contradiction to what we know of nature.

Quantum mechanics is a perfect example. Newtonian physics could never accommodate light. Falling apples, the velocity thereof, even some push-pull in the form of gravity, perhaps, but never the quantum essence of light. Sunlight comes in packets of energy we call photons. These packets of light energy, also called quanta, are simultaneously both a particle and a wave. Imagine a bouncing ball of light that leaves a trail of light as it bounces. That bouncing ball of light—the photon—is a also wave of energy. The light wave left behind can be heat, brightness, or vibrational energy, depending on the rhythm of the bounce. Light, temperature, and gravity control all energy metabolism and reproduction on the molecular level in every venue here on earth. Therefore, they control your health and your very existence.

In the June 5, 1998, issue of *Science,* Jay Dunlap from the department of biochemistry at Dartmouth Medical School admitted freely:

Circadian rhythms and the cellular oscillators that underlie them are ubiquitous—and for good reason. For most organisms, dawn means food, predation, and changes in all the geophysical variables that accompany the sun—warmth, winds, and so on. It's a big deal when the sun comes up, and most living things time their days with an internal clock that is synchronized by external cues. Given this common and ancient evolutionary pressure, circadian clocks must have evolved early, and common elements are likely to be present up and down the evolutionary tree. A series of papers appearing in this week's *Science, Cell,* and *Proceedings of the National Academy of Sciences* reveals an appealingly similar pattern in the assembly of circadian oscillators ranging from fungi to mammals and gives us a close-up view of the way the gears within the clock drive its circadian feedback loop.

What the man said was: We and everything else alive, from plankton and fungus to elephants and ants, are synchronized to the orbit and rotation of the earth in and out of the sun's light to assure us a food supply. All things great and small have internal sundials that measure time with molecular clocks in every cell that switch enormous cadres of regulatory genes on and off. The light, whether a particle or a wave, always sparks biochemical reactions. The whole ball of dirt heats up and cools down, heats up and cools down, over and over again, day in and day out. Plants grow. We animals eat them and each other. We die and become fertilizer. Plants grow, and it starts all over again. World without end. Amen.

All of this wild chemistry is happening on a spinning, gyrating, oscillating earth that, if you could hear the song of the cosmos from outer space, rings like a bell. The sun metabolizes and respires. The earth heaves and sighs, and we and the earthworms make everything fertile over and over again. The ancients were right on. There is an ever-churning circulating flow of energy driven by the light. *Every part of us reads the changing light intensity and spectrum.* When you hold the back of your hand up to the window, cells called cryptochromes in your bloodstream pick up the blue spectrum of the light through your skin. These cryptochromes carry a piece of the sky all through you. That light energy and the carbohydrate (sugar) you eat even keep the symbiotic bacteria that live in the dark deep of your middle thriving. And in return for being a good host, they keep you thriving.

We, and every other living thing on earth are truly beings of *light.*

To make sense of *dis*-eases such as obesity, diabetes, heart disease, and cancer, all you need to understand are our physiological connections to the earth, sun, and sky. Unless a microbe, virus, toxin, or tiger gets you fair and square, all other "disease states" can be explained by identifying the function that the particular "disease" could possibly have had in evolution, and then by locating the modern cultural trigger that has set in motion the ancient physiological response. We, as researchers, have done that with obesity and diabetes in regard to seasonal variation in the food supply and day length. We've done that with mental illness and infertility and sleep loss. Once we looked at eating, sleeping, and reproducing, we discovered cancer and heart disease also have a biophysical explanation. We're willing to bet everything does.

ON DAISY WORLD

Back in the 1970s, a man named Lovelock proposed that all life on earth self-regulates. He called his proposal the Gaia theory. It is, quite simply, the notion that the earth, rocks and all, is as alive as we are. Like our bodies, the earth maintains its own physical equilibrium. At the time, nobody but a few environmentalists really bought it. Lovelock's premise worked to the environmentalists' advantage because it's logical to assume that if we can die, then so can a living earth.

Although it may sound simplistic, the underlying components of the Gaia premise cross many disciplines—meteorology, oceanography, entomology, anthropology, and geology, to name only a few. An easy way to understand the Gaia hypothesis is to look at the Daisy World model. Lovelock realized that all organisms alter their environments just by existing and, in turn, the altered environment changes the organism, which *again* alters the already altered environment, which, of course, further changes the organism, and so on and so on and so on.

Accepting this premise as the fundamental rule of life, let's go to Daisy World, where the only life consists of black and white daisies. In the beginning of our imagined Daisy World, when it is dark and cold, a black daisy has a selective advantage because it can absorb what little sunlight there is. In other words, because it has enough heat to reproduce, it can spread the trait of blackness. The white daisies can't do as well because they can't absorb enough heat to thrive and reproduce.

Now, here's some pure Darwinism: It is the spread of the trait of blackness (the growth of more black daisies) that increases the temperature of the world enough for the white daisies to begin to flourish. Once the white daisies multiply, the world begins to cool again, and again the black daisies flourish.

The important Darwinian principle here is that when white daisies begin to fill the world, the planetary temperature has been brought up to the point where being black no longer confers a selective advantage. In the original Daisy World, the alteration of the environment resulting from the spread of one particular trait ultimately reduces the benefit of that trait. In other words, life self-regulates. Everybody gets a chance.

While this argument would seem to be largely restricted to climate regulation, the principles apply to any environmental variable that can affect growth. And any selective pressure that can affect hormonal release affects growth.

Now you see where we're going.

This self-regulation is a property of the *whole* system of life tightly coupled to its environment. Furthermore, the evolution of organisms and their environment is so closely coupled that they form a single individual process. Plants, people, animals, rocks, and sky are all one thing, one giant physical organism dependent both on the sun's energy and on respite from the sun.

The sun's heat that the black daisies absorb always rises. That causes air movement, which always means wind. The wind stirs up waves in the ocean. The micro-algae in the splashing water can travel to heights of fifteen thousand feet, where the sulfites in them collect the water vapor over the hot spots of black daisies and make clouds. This means that the clouds are alive. As the algae reproduce in the clouds fifteen thousand feet in the air, they produce heat, which makes rain. Those algae fall back to earth in the rain. The rain cools the planet at the same time, so the process can start all over again.

Where do we fit into this heaving, sighing, multi-organ, living system?

Most of us tramp through the world having forgotten we are part of it, but the truth is, we live in Daisy World. When you walk through your garden or through the park, as your legs brush against the plants, the plants send out molecules of communication, pheromones, that warn the other plants that you're coming. When the plants ahead of you receive this molecular message from the plants you've just assaulted, they undergo a biochemical change. The ones ahead become turgid. This rigidity is a self-defense mechanism that protects them from any damage you could cause. For the plants, the sacrifice of some for the good for the many gives them a fighting chance to be the many.

The Darwinian principles of natural selection and favorable traits are an even more powerful combination when you factor this in: The types of life that leave the most descendants come to dominate their environment. Then it truly becomes a case of "be careful what you wish for," because, by spreading the trait that gave you dominance, you assure that that trait becomes the *least* valuable. Always remember the black daisies, and that the changes an organism makes in the environment can be favorable or unfavorable to growth.

That's what's happening to us right now.

When we discovered the uses of fire and brought it inside the caves, the excess light at night suppressed our melatonin. The lack of melatonin, which would normally suppress sex hormones like estrogen and testosterone, increased the fertility of those of us who had been smart enough to tame the fire. Our traits made us, then, naturally selected for, because, with increased fertility, we left more descendants.

However, when those descendants discovered electricity and everybody could keep the lights on all the time, the very same trait that made us the primo survivors—our ability to control the environment has "changed the temperature of the environment" again, so to speak.

By pushing it too far, by turning night into day, we've crossed the line. We've fundamentally altered the requirements for homeostasis again. In the past, the extra hormones—insulin, estrogen, and testosterone—that allowed us to reproduce during the dark time enhanced our reproductive potential by buying us extra "days" that the other animals didn't have. Now all our pouring sex hormones go unsuppressed by normal plane-tary-controlled melatonin because the lights are always on. The sex hor-mones supplied by the firelight that made us year-round breeders now cause the overgrowth of cancer. Now we've tipped the balance again. Just as in Daisy World, the trait that gave us an edge to leave more descen-dants—increased fertility from lack of light-suppressed melatonin—now self-regulates our population with cancer.

Nature hates too much of a good thing.

The same principle holds on examination of the advent of agriculture. Those of us smart enough to grow a year-round supply of plants (carbo-hydrates) and then to save them for famine (winter) were rewarded with more offspring, and, of course, the ability to feed more offspring. In the beginning, too, the increased-carbohydrate diet that increased our insulin also increased the chances that we'd have nuts (body fat) for the winter. However, as the trait for the ability to stay fat year-round spread, the insulin we were meant to live on for only three or four months out of twelve caused new problems, like obesity followed by diabetes. Every time an organism gets the edge, the natural rhythm of life—one step forward, two steps back—keeps it in place. It's all about equilibrium.

Life dances. It never stands still.

ALIEN VOICES

If you bow your head for just a moment in utter quiet you can almost hear a voice emanating from within. That voice is a pattern of neuro-transmitter firings inside your consciousness that has been honed over millennia. That voice is "instinct."

Sleep is an instinct.

When you're tired, your instinct is to sleep.

Why do you fight it?

If you get too successful, nature will just take out your descendants anyway.

Everybody *knows* the truth. We know on such a deep level that in all of our human "art," down to the lowliest cartoon, plants and animals sing and dance and the clouds have smiles. We're not anthropomorphizing them, we're just remembering them. Think of the daisies in *The Wizard of Oz* singing, "Come out of the dark and into the light." It's downright spooky how the "game plan" is intrinsically woven into the fabric of all life. So foreign is the concept, so complete is the amnesia in our species, we offer you a little homily:

If you don't sleep all night, you might get your work done.

If you don't sleep for a week, not only does your work suffer, *you might die.*

ALL LIES LEAD TO THE TRUTH

Isaac Asimov's classic story "Nightfall" is set on a planet that orbits five suns. In this tale, the mystery proffered is why this civilization collapses every ten thousand years. Curiously, the collapse always coincides with a rare astronomical event in which four of the suns are beneath the horizon and the fifth suffers a total eclipse by the planet's only moon. As the story begins, this event is about to happen again.

The solution to the mystery is as inevitable as the sunrise, when the reader realizes that darkness at noon is the ultimate terror to a people who have only ever experienced perpetual light.

The way we fight sleep, it's almost like that for Americans now. When darkness at noon does come during an eclipse, the effect is much the same as the nightfall we never experience anymore. A shadow comes racing out of the west, then as the moon takes its first bite out of the sun, a terrific din is heard as panic-stricken birds fly to their roosts, fooled into thinking that the night has suddenly come. At the same time, the temperature drops precipitously. Without the defense of electric lighting, the experience is both overwhelming and humbling.

In Asimov's tale, this happens only once every ten millennia. So over and over again, the planet's inhabitants are driven mad when night falls for the first time in ten thousand years. They set fire to anything that will burn in a desperate attempt to restore the light, including the records of the last time it happened. The only reason we swim in less irony is that, in our case, record keeping arrived *too late* for us to remember the death that followed the discovery of fire and the arrival of agriculture.

On our planet, ancient cultures in Europe, Africa, Asia, and the Americas were terrified out of their wits by eclipses, which they believed was a monster eating the sun. When this monster plunged all of the earth into cold, utter darkness at noon, our ancestors would gather together to do everything in their power to scare the monster away. This usually involved banging drums, shouting, and screaming as loudly as possible.

Medicine has taken this same approach to curing obesity, diabetes, heart disease, and most certainly cancer. Could their approach to disease and aging ever save your life?

Who knows?

On that far-away planet, in a distant galaxy, the sun returned every time. It's that kind of success that breeds deep faith in bogus miracles.

And science and medicine is full of them.

From *The 8-Week Cholesterol Cure* of the early 1980s to the newest compendium of every current trend, *The Breast Cancer Prevention Diet*, medicine keeps promising one cure after another when they don't even understand the disease. It's only in an overview of the subconscious/ unconscious interaction of all the life with which we coexist that the "contradictions" medical researchers constantly investigate can be explained. The real reason no progress has been or will ever be made in health care on a governmental or institutional level is because they don't get it.

Understanding human physiological dysfunction is akin to repairing a broken vase. You start with the big pieces and, finally, all that's left is the impact point. Those tiny shards will go together in the end, but you never could have started there.

Those tiny shards are the only news the public gets. That's why the newspapers and news magazine shows are rife with "cutting-edge discoveries" that ostensibly will change your world, but, in real time, never provide one single cure.

In the following chapters, we examine the disease state then take into account evolutionary biology and behavior, clinical, anecdotal, or folkloric evidence, cross-cultural practices, and, eventually, statistics. At that point, we make assumptions, to which we apply the science of molecular medicine, genetics, psychoneuroimmunology, and neuro-endocrinology. In essence, we will start with the big picture, then break it down for you until we get to the molecules.

Because God is in the molecules.

MEN IN WHITE

In all fairness to the doctors, it's the system that's twisted. Medical schools assume that something as basic as how the body works is taught before students get there. Most budding doctors entering medical school in the past would have been in a four-year science program at their university. This is universally no longer the case.

These students are convinced by trusted teachers that the body is a static, linear system to be dealt with only in a crisis mode. *Preventive* medicine is thought of as alternative medicine in this country. And young doctors aren't taught the art of healing, they're taught pharmacology. The "drugs and physiology" lectures well attended by these new physicians usually support this crisis approach. Ultimately, doctors in this country are taught that the patient is cured if they have managed to erase the symptoms of the disease. This approach is particularly counterproductive and counterintuitive because all diseases are defined by their symptoms. But this method is all they've got.

That's why Mevacor, Provachol, Tamoxifen, Raloxifene, Meridia, the late great Fen-Phen, and Prozac top the charts of best-sellers. These "remedies" obliterate the symptoms of a larger, more insidious, pervasive malady that has yet to be identified by the people and professionals in charge of your health. The accepted medical wisdom really is just a hodgepodge of inaccuracies pasted together to cover the fact that they don't have a clue about the *real* reason we're all dying. The only hope doctors and patients have is that the researchers will invent a new drug or gene therapy.

SHOW US THE MONEY

The framework in which researchers must function to continue to exist is counterproductive, too. Research in this country is predominantly paid for by drug companies and the government. It's this method that really screws up research and researchers. Even the most dedicated researchers can't really research anything unless it's saleable.

Medicine is big business, like anything else. The truth about research is that research isn't about discovering the truth, it's about making money.

If researchers are earning a living by getting paid to look, they look for whatever the group who's paying them wants them to find. By focusing on the drug company's market potentials or trendy money from government sources, they end up doing experiments in tiny pieces that can never fit together. They constantly find answers without asking any questions. Doctors and the public, however, assume that the researchers are doing what we are doing here—reverse engineering. They're not.

All the incoherent information the public receives via the media in the form of news releases and television comes from fishing. Researchers just keep fishing from the same very limited pond, trying to get funding for the flavor du jour of guaranteed-to-be-paid-for projects, so that they can guarantee themselves a salary. Then they try to fit what they come up with into the rest of the data that everyone else has already collected. Think of it as the crossword puzzle approach: Researchers deduce the answer to a clue, then fill in the blanks, one clue at a time, until all the blanks are full. They've finished the puzzle, but even with each answer to each clue, individually, the entire endeavor still *says* nothing. They then present to the public a lot of answers that don't in any coherent way relate to each other. That's why panic and free-floating angst in the population keeps mounting. *Nothing ever makes sense.*

Since researchers are working without a hypothesis, they have no road map back home. With this approach, there's no hope of actual recovery for us; just a steady diet of pills until we die. The big-money drugs can't possibly cure any of our diseases, because the diseases, on an evolutionary scale, are an "environmental pressure" response. They are not actual plagues of any kind.

The new "miracle" drugs are the worst of all. The premise of drug intervention is this: If A is healthy and B is sick and C is drug therapy, C will somehow return you to A. On no planet can C ever be A. C is always even farther from A than even B was.

The reason conventional medicine uses the ABC formula of drug therapy is because the first drugs invented were antibiotics. Since antibiotics work to subdue another species, ABC actually worked and we survived. But it's insane to attempt to defeat *all* disease states this way, because most disease states are *not* derived from pathogens like bacteria.

Doctors' assumptions might be valid if they were dealing with viruses or germs and anti-viral agents or antibiotics. However, when diseases such as obesity, diabetes, heart disease, or, ultimately, cancer arise from metabolic dysfunction rooted in biology and physics, drugs are not only useless, they are actually counterproductive. The drugs cause new problems, but rarely solve any. That salient fact never seems to come up at the FDA. Many of us are a testament to that, especially those of us who have already gone missing. Like the frogs.

SLEEP OF FAITH

We're dying today because we've lost the faith. Man always looked to the heavens to decide his fate. Doctors and medicine men always looked to the heavens to decide *your* fate. Everyone knew how it worked. The very word "influenza" referred to the "influence" the sun, the moon, the planets, and the stars had on our health. We always knew that there were certain rules for staying alive in harmony with all other living things—how much you could eat, how long you could stay awake, and how much stress you could endure. In our hubris, we've flaunted the rules.

We used to *know* better.

There is an enormous difference between *knowledge, information,* and *understanding.* In our time, we've gained enormous *understanding* of the natural world through a wealth of *information,* but we've lost the *knowledge* of how we fit into that world. Because of this fall from grace, we're losing our lives prematurely. The devotion we give to the world of medicine and drugs is misplaced. Recovery can come from inside ourselves. We, the people, have the power to cure these "incurable" diseases with the flick of a switch.

Early Greek doctors like Galen and Hippocrates, more than two millennia ago, "modernized" medicine by insisting that the causes of disease are *not* attributable to displeased and vengeful gods like the sun or the moon.

Well, we're here to insist that they *are . . .* and that it just might be time to get religion.

WE
ARE
NOT
ALONE

EARTHLING AUTOPSY:

Environment Controls the Genetics of Obesity

The ideal reasoner would, when he has once been shown a single fact, in all its bearings, deduce from it not only all the chain of events that led up to it, but also all the results which would follow from it.
—Sir Arthur Conan Doyle, *The Five Orange Pips of Sherlock Holmes*

We were supposed to roam for food and sex, get some, and then head for the hills, where there were caves when it got cold and dark at night. Not very complicated. Exactly the same scenario was lived out by the ancestors of your dogs and cats, and it's what mountain gorillas still do today.

Think about it.

You don't see a lot of squirrels farming or snakes and birds barbecuing.

Mother Nature still tucks in the rest of the animal kingdom when night falls, but man has become an orphan. On a planet inhabited by trillions of life forms, we humans *alone* can control the light.

And, believe us, it's expensive. Owning the night did not come cheap.

The use of fire for protection, warmth, and cooking has left a mark on our reproductive and immune systems that requires human sacrifice to this day. By altering the rhythms of light and dark exposure, we who control the light never get cold, and fend off the night and any predators, human or animal, that might be lurking in the shadows. We have also, literally, altered the spin of our planet as far as our minds and bodies would record it. We've virtually stopped our planet's orbit around the sun, as well as stopped its spinning.

We've abolished winter.

Now only we, in the galaxy and the universe, stand still.

Winter, or any period of chill, is a big deal in evolution. Adversity (in this case, the cold) is a prime motivator. Think about how you, personally, deal with being cold; you strive to stay warm. If your car breaks down in the snow, you find a place to wait for help, you make a plan to fix it, and the memory of the incident sticks with you, changing your behavior forever. The winners in any evolutionary lottery are the problem solvers. If all of those changes occurred in you because of the one-time inconvenience of your transportation/shelter breaking down, imagine what millennia of ice and snow did for our species intellectually.

All of our evolved physiology and intellect is, literally, geared to light and dark, hot and cold. Just as the mineral content in our bones, identical to stardust, testifies to our extraterrestrial origins, the photoperiodic cells in our blood tie us to the sun and the moon. We are always, every minute of every day of our earthbound existence, a complete part of it all. Even the purported "global warming" we beat ourselves up about is out of our control. When our planet heats up, as it does every ten to fifteen thousand years, everything germinates and proliferates until it reaches a virtual fever pitch, then, predictably, the fever "breaks" and chills set in to cool off and kill off the overgrowth of life. Think of this grand swing of the pendulum as a cosmic reset button to begin the dance all over again.

In the last century, after surviving many, many ice ages, we began to live on a planet with multiple "suns," like the folks in Isaac Asimov's story. Instead of the eclipse's darkness at noon that drove them mad, however, we've created morning at midnight. And trust us, it's driving us mad. All life forms must go dormant to survive the dark and cold or they lose the ability to plan and adapt. Hibernation studies prove that learning and retention are enhanced in animals who are allowed to find respite from life.

During long cold periods, our ancestors dozed off and on for weeks at a time in dark caves, slowing down metabolic functions to save energy when food was scarce. This system mirrored, during one revolution around the sun, the same game plan that we use every rotation in and out of our sun's light. Fractally speaking, day and night are the "short version" of summer and winter. Over the millennia, we evolved hibernational and gestational periods that always ended in the spring, when food was fresh and plentiful. Our first encounter with "energy control," or fire, changed all that forever. The light from the fire was enough to create summer in our ovaries all year round. The minute all of those flowing sex hormones for mating kept us awake all winter by suppressing melatonin, we left earth's family, never to return.

QUANTUM LEAP

We are interconnected physiologically with every other life on earth. Life is a quantum entanglement. Quantum entanglements are what physicists call a problem of "perfect order." Perfect order is the theory that all matter is alive and connected through a continuous flow of energy. *Everything is one.* All of us together are then further connected to the sun, moon, and stars by biophysics. That means that our biology is a product of photons, magnetism, and gravity.

There are light-sensitive monitors built into the cells of our eyes, skin, blood, and bones. We've always, way back to the primordial ooze, registered the spinning of the earth as it circles the sun. Mammoths, man-eaters, mice, and microbes, all from the same humble beginnings, evolved physiologic controls based on light and dark. The plants and we are one. The molecule heme, that structures the faction of our blood called hemoglobin, is the same molecule that structures the blood of plants—chlorophyll.

We really *are* all one.

The energy the sun puts out supports the biochemistry that is the foundation of the biological systems that are all of the life here on earth. Hence, biophysics. The energy of sunlight—as photons, the heat (temperature) photons produce, and electromagnetic gravity we are subject to—controls every bit of energy metabolism and reproduction, *on the molecular level,* here on earth. The light, no matter what form it takes—a particle or a wave—sparks massive cascading biochemical reactions globally in all life, except at night, when all things rest from the light.

The big problem with canceling the night and winter is one of duality: yin and yang, up and down, here and there, left and right. Day needs night to exist. The first half of any equation rests in the existence of the other half. In the universe, symmetry is all there is. Summer/winter, spring/fall, light/dark, black/white, hot/cold, man/woman, dead and alive all have each other to thank for their existence. Cutting-edge quantum physicists believe the universe is constructed out of energy in patterns that conform to an "order of symmetry." Makes sense to us. The leading quantum theory is even called supersymmetry. If supersymmetry is a *cosmic* quantum law, you can bet it's a *biological* law, too.

All life as we know it rests on principles of biology that rest on the principles of biochemistry. In any biochemical reaction, the way molecules bond to other molecules or the way cells display polarity inside and outside all chemical reactions abide by rules of electrical attraction. The bonding and polarized reactions that are the hallmark of biochemistry are defined by the principles of the physics that they employ.

All that we are pointing out in our theories of energy metabolism is that in this hierarchy the sun is the generator of all basic energy and life. The sun is the principal controller of all life simply because of the structure of matter. There are two main branches of physics—Newtonian and quantum. Newtonian physics is concerned with mechanics—the falling apple *always* hits Newton on the head, and if you close your fist and punch something there's an equation to measure the force of the thrust.

Quantum physics is more likely to explain Qi and telepathy. The theoretical difference between the mechanical predictions of Newtonian physics and the predictions in quantum mechanics is that the same experimental conditions can lead to a variety of very different final outcomes in a quantum world, but never in a Newtonian one.

The unpredictability of life beyond the mechanical Newtonian realm is explained by string theory. It's a romantic notion, but not a wholly unfounded one, that the music of life is truly a function of a universe constructed of strings, all vibrating.

In string theory, all life emanates from the same fundamental structure—an extended string. An infinite number of outcomes to any situation are possible because of the different ways in which the fundamental string can vibrate, just as different harmonics are present in the sound coming out of a guitar string. Since there are an infinite number of possible vibrations, it stands to reason there are an infinite number of outcomes to the same set of initial conditions.

Understanding supersymmetry and string theory gives new meaning to the notion that life is a crapshoot.

The only hope of having any leg to stand on (all puns intended) rests in something called chaos theory. Chaos theory holds that the events or

occurrences that seem most random or senseless are really quite pre-
dictable if you can stand far enough back to observe them; that over the
very long haul everything has a genuine, albeit difficult to discern, pattern
of behavior. Employing this premise, we can understand the conundrums
of disease in medicine. We just need to learn the melody to appreciate the
music.

STANDING ON A BOARD ON A LOG

Since we are, part and parcel, down to our bones, just a small piece of this
universe, which exists within a framework of laws like chaos and symmetry, our physiology and spirits must abide by them, too. This duality or
symmetry exists for us as balance.

Harmonically, we are part of a larger song. The tune we sing is written
by the natural rhythms in our environment.

The only way to stay in the game or remain stable is to be able to roll
with the punches. All of the systems now in place to perform the constant
compensatory actions necessary to survive were developed by adaptive
"intelligence" in response to environmental pressures over millennia. No
trait or behavior is capricious. Living or staying alive is just like standing
on a board on a log. But in this case, if you lose your balance, it's a long
fall.

There are no survivors at the bottom.

Our viability as a life form means that our responsiveness to the seasons in terms of food supply and reproduction are really all there is in
regard to ending up on top, in the Darwinian sense. That's why our genes
have "on and off" switches, controlled by hormones, that respond to environmental cues. We are finely tuned to survive by responding *event to
event,* because the only sure thing in nature is changing circumstances.
Without this system, we couldn't vary our behavior in sync with the
immediacy of the occurrence. Life's a dance.

We listen to the music and sway.

The vibrations from the environment are picked up by the hormonal
interface that we call the endocrine system. This endocrine system is acting as the software that runs an organic computer we call the body/brain.
The amount of light (brightness, temperature, and electricity) and gravity
(magnetism) you are exposed to is the program that runs the software.
Through the auspices of this hormonal software program, which throws

switches on genes that control the machine nanosecond by nanosecond, you balance on the board on the log.

This whole "human sub-machine" is an integrated part of the larger machine of the environment, or biosphere. Every living thing is an interactive machine or biocomputer programmed for adaptive intelligence. That means the definition of life is the ability to learn and change in response to experience. This experience-based decision system allows each life form to change in response to every other life form, because hormones control your behavior and your genes.

The actions you take in a day are not really derived of free will. They are, rather, a product of *thoughtware*. The elements in the environment control the hormonal processes in your body that program your brain to control your behavior. So a brain without a body is mindless, but a body without an environment is brainless. *The fluctuating fat base on that body is really an immune response that protects and makes you viable in all seasons.* Your behavior with regard to food cravings and appetite is simply an immune response, too.

Everything we coexist with is balanced in tension with us. Imagine two people at a gym throwing a heavy ball back and forth. When two people play "catch" with a heavy ball, they are sort of pushed apart because of the weight. The constant exchange of weight keeps the game going. It's the same with life. Back and forth, back and forth. To stay in the game, we have a circumscribed existence with a narrow set of options. Consider these options a "playing field." The hours of light you are exposed to control actual genetic "on and off" switches, enzyme activity, and, most important, the growth of four pounds of *symbiotic bacteria* that live in your gut. These guys are the keys to life and death and dress size.

WE ARE NOT ALONE

Your "personal bacteria" are constantly at war with other bacteria and viruses over **you.** How this Armageddon creates and maintains your immune system—the same immune system that controls your metabolism and fertility—is the key to the whole shooting match between light and health. But this battle only rages at night, when you sleep. Every morning, the outcome of the war predicts not only your immunity, fertility, and weight but your mental health, too.

Our lives, you see, are not our own.

We are symbionts, controlled by a different life form with priorities of its own. When we're in the light, we pick up the light through our skin and carry its energy, in cells called cryptochromes, down to the symbiotic bacteria that live in our middles.

They love light and they love sugar.

We think they love reproductive hormones, too. The common observation that young people and the elderly have weaker immune systems is a misinterpretation. The truth is that *reproductive* adults have stronger immune systems than the elderly and little children because the bacteria in our guts love sex steroids for breakfast and because when we reproduce we make more condos for the bacteria to live in. That principle is the reason women often have diarrhea during a menstrual period, when their hormone levels are flat and the bugs are leaving a sinking ship.

ONE IS THE LONELIEST NUMBER

Carsten Korth, in his article "Co-evolutionary Theory of Sleep," published in the *Journal of Medical Hypothesis* in 1995, agrees with us that the development of sleep as we know it was an evolutionary strategy to keep us even with the microbes.

The mat of bacteria in your gut exudes endotoxins that control your physiology. The endotoxins exuded are cell-wall constituents that are sort of like pheromones or germ sweat. As the bacteria thrive over the course of a day, the endotoxins build. At a certain level, your immune system kicks in to take them down, so you continue to thrive. It's what's known as a host response. We *only* go to sleep when a substance called *endotoxin LPS* is exuded over the course of the day by these friendly bacteria in our guts. We go to sleep when LPS reaches a critical enough concentration in our bloodstreams to trigger an immune response. Sleeping is that immune response. White cells called macrophages and leukocytes multiply and kill some of the bacteria in your system. It's well known that sleep is induced by an immune "expression," or a cytokine, called interleukin-2, which happens in response to the LPS put off by our gut bacteria.

These "neighbors" have become active participants in our entire immune existence as it relates to the spinning planet and all of its other inhabitants. There's more of them than us. They're everywhere. Our gut alone contains 1 kilogram of bacteria. There's more in your mouth and on your skin. All evolving species had to evolve around, or, more to the point, *with*, bacteria. They owned the joint way before any of us got here.

We had no choice but negotiation.

Our coevolution is just a case of domestication on both parts. Over the millennia of symbiosis between them and us, our human immune systems have evolved in response to their orchestration. They gave us an immune system as a self-controlling mechanism and as defense for their turf. For us, sleeping is actually just "thinning the herd." Bacteria ranching is just like a successful cattle ranch operation, in which homeostasis is achieved by eating or selling off just enough of the herd to keep it manageable. Our domestication of bacteria works the same way. The herd and the rancher both benefit. The evolutionary tactic of sleep is just a sneaky adaptation that allows us to get the edge on them, *once every planetary rotation*. The inequity in any tug of war only arises when one side stops pulling; therefore, *no sleep, no edge*.

The immune expressions, or cytokines, that ensue from high levels of endotoxins can act as neurotransmitters and literally take you down, too. By rendering you unconscious, they close your eyes. Closed eyes means melatonin happens and later, at midpoint in the night, prolactin. Both these hormones mediate immune function through other cytokines called interleukins. Interleukins have numbers like IL-1, or 2 or 3, instead of real names, probably because there are a bazillion of them. High levels of IL-2 are always found in sleep states, even those that result from illness. Once you fall asleep, the surging melatonin encourages white-blood-cell activity specifically designed to respond to pathogens like the bacteria living in your middle.

Needless to say, whether it results from closed eyes or the sun being on the other side of the globe, dark is dark; and the darker the better for melatonin production. Sick sleep is more intense and related to the phenomenon of fever through IL-1 and IL-6. You must sleep when you're sick or you won't survive an onslaught by the "other." Sleep is when the melatonin and prolactin kick in to make white cells, T cells, and NK (natural killer) cells. A gut "out of whack"—meaning having too little or the wrong kind of bacteria punching a broken time clock—means a seriously impaired immune system.

So not sleeping on purpose, when it gets dark, means destroying an ancient ecosystem.

Remember, coevolution means we're supposed to be dancing, not stepping on toes.

These bacteria keep you alive—granted, it's for their own purposes—but it's still life. All they ask is a little sugar and a little light and maybe a few sex hormones to control your internal environment, which controls your external environment.

INQUIRING MINDS WANT TO KNOW

All of your hormones—melatonin, prolactin, cortisol, insulin, and sex hormones, too—are the interface between your central nervous system (thoughts and reactions) and the environment. The queries cycling in the "big picture" between you, the bacteria, and the environment boil down to: *Is it light? Is it dark? Is it cold? Is it hot? Where's food? What's after me?* and *Who's mating material?*

All of the information relating to these queries is acquired through sight, hearing, taste, touch, and smell. The same way baking cookies or bread evokes a reaction from your salivary glands, light hitting your eyes and skin activates other glands and tells the bacteria in your middle what time it is. The melatonin clocking the hours in 24, trips the prolactin timer to tell your brain what to have an appetite for. Insulin levels are synergistic with sex hormones like estrogen and testosterone for mating. All of these bytes of information are squeezed through the prism of your hypothalamus (timekeeper), pituitary (sex controlling), and adrenal glands (stress meter). This HPA axis serves as a built-in timer, not unlike the one that automatically turns on your coffemaker every morning, except that the HPA axis is turning on and off biological functions. This "HPA axis" acts in concert with the environment to synthesize and disseminate the translated "rays" of information that have been gathered from environmental cues. Without this constant synthesis between the environmental cues and your physical reaction to them, there is no way to surf with the fluctuations in the environment and stay alive.

Big secret: Life is based on a paradox. The stability of function needed to stay alive is only possible through constant change in response to the environment.

The hormones from these glands, your HPA hormones, are, in turn, called into play. These hormones run the gamut from sex steroids like estrogen and testosterone to cortisol, human growth hormone, and leptin from your fat base. These hormones throw the switches to turn vital functions on and off instantaneously. Hormones do this by locking on to "promoter regions" on strings of DNA called genes, and throwing the switches that trigger genetic action.

Whether or not the gene produces its protein product is a function of whether or not it's turned on by a hormone, growth factor, the sun, or an electrical impulse. The proteins produced by these genes, when they're on, fit into receptors on all of your cells, which then send the messages to the nucleus of said cell to throw other switches, and so on, and so on. These communiqués are ephemeral. Split-second decisions are made by your hormonal network in response to environmental pressures. If any of these switches gets stuck on or off, nature percieves you to be too sick to be part of the project.

It's when your switches are stuck—open or closed—that disease happens. High, sustained levels of any hormone are instinctively maladaptive to maintaining your balance on the board on that log. Any sustained hormonal note in the chemical symphony destroys the harmony. So high estrogen without a progesterone chaser to turn it off can cause cancer, and chronic, day-in–day-out, high levels of insulin lead to heart disease, diabetes, and cancer. Because once you've lost the rhythm, you're out of step and you lose your balance. Then comes the fall—from Grace.

STRANGE VIBRATIONS

As above, so below. The same strings throwing off the electrons, quarks, and neutrinos in ten different dimensions that make up the atoms that make up the molecules that make up the hormones that receive vibrations from the waves of light and gravity play the music of the cosmos to our bodies through our hormone receptors.

We're like tuning forks. We literally vibrate on impact with the environment.

The vibrations we know as *actual* music cause actual vibrations that reach neurons in the brain via the eardrum, provoking emotion. In *The Medusa and the Snail,* Lewis Thomas said: "Music is the effort we make to explain to ourselves how our brains work. We listen to Bach transfixed because this is listening to a human mind." In 1976, Leonard Bernstein attempted to apply Noam Chomsky's work in language to his effort to find a structure for the human response to music. Chomsky found that babies as young as four months old always prefer music with constant pitch intervals; so does nature.

In his book *How the Mind Works,* Steven Pinker uses the musical terminology of "prolongation reduction" to define the way that melodies are dissected. He defines the process as: "Musical flow captured across phrases, with the buildup and release of tension within longer and longer passages over the course of the piece, culminating in a feeling of repose at the end . . . tension builds up as the melody departs from the more stable notes to less stable notes and is discharged when the melody returns to the stable ones."

In the words of the late Frank Sinatra, "That's life."

You can also quote us: "That's chaos."

In the same way that music satisfies by conveying tension and resolution across unstable and stable intervals, your feast-or-famine metabolism has the same need for interval and rhythmicity or you get sick. Your immune system and bacteria, in a twenty-four-hour period, have the same need for tension and resolution. So does your mind. On your CD player or on the molecular level, there is and must be a rhythm—whether it's your heartbeat in 4/4 time, your circadian rhythm, or your menstrual cycle—that rolls high and low to measure your turn on the planet. Otherwise, you can't roll with the punches. And finding a way to roll with the punches is the key.

Your consciousness and will are comprised of complex environment-hormone-behavior interactions, all of which are driven by chronometers. We're telling you that these same interactions exist between you and the environment, and that all the feedback loops do is monitor and register the melody. The song may sound like Wagner or it may be Pachelbel, but it must be music, it must pitch and roll, or it is maladaptive. Maladaptive, according to our previous definitions, pretty much always ends in death, even if it comes by your own hand. When schizophrenics hear voices, the voices invariably say, "Kill yourself." As a precursor to death, maladaptive more often than not means *nonreproductive;* and it's nonreproductive that sounds an alarm in nature. When you're nonreproductive, you don't count in the grand scheme of things here on earth. That's why cancer, Type II diabetes, and heart disease always follow obesity, which always means accelerated aging in planetary years. In the *real* world, life lasted as long as reproductive potential. Twenty-five to thirty years was long enough to replicate DNA and culture. Now we live too long and eat too much for our antiquated set points.

THE MAN WITH TWO BRAINS

It is your central nervous system in the form of your brain and gut that responds to your endocrine system. Your hormones report changes in your HPA axis to your immune system, which uses cytokines or neuropeptides to direct all traffic with regard to homeostasis. The immune system is much more than bone marrow or spleen, peyer's patches or thymus cells. Even the lymph system is only a part of what we call the immune system. Those sites are actually just factories for the production of white cells, lymphocytes, or the now infamous T cells. About eighty percent of the full force of your defensive immune system resides in your intestines or gut. This makes sense, since most toxins will enter through your mouth.

Even though we're led to believe that the immune system is *our* defense system, nothing could be further from the truth. The immune system is planetary, not individual. Our hormonal interface with the world in the form of the HPA axis means that the immune system is really "the man behind the curtain" working the knobs and dials that make the brain seem so competent. The elements of the immune system—gut, skin, fat, lymph, brain, and glands—all recognize, communicate, memorize, react, and even plan to survive earth changes that have been timed into our programming by millennia of experience. These capabilities mean that the immune system is as sentient, on its own, as you think you are.

It also makes sense that eighty percent of the immune system is located in the gut because the gut was your original brain. As we slithered across a rock, pre-"head brain," the neurotransmitters we know, like dopamine, serotonin, and norepinephrine, and hormones like adrenaline and insulin ran The Project from your midsection.

The real clue to the overwhelming power and control the immune system has comes in the realization that it is completely mobile, so like the free thinking individual you perceive yourself to be. The immune system *within* is, at least, your equal. Your immune system controls your behavior by controlling neurotransmitter activity. All immune cells have receptors to read both neurotransmitters and hormones controlling energy regulation and sex hormones. By the same token, the immune expressions called cytokines are active in your gut and your brain and your fat base and gonads.

It's the immune system, locked in step with environmental pressure and the bio-ecosphere, that can spell Judgment Day, either by a lack of defense or an all-out attack on your body. If you lose your balance with other life forms or the cosmos, the immune system reacts to compensate. Sometimes it's really just the compensatory mechanisms that are the real causes of what we perceive to be disease. When you experience a sore throat in the throes of a viral infection, the pain you feel is not borne of the virus at all. It is, instead, the pain of dying cells sacrificed (killed) by your own immune system. The same goes for the body aches, fever, and headache. *It's not the pathogen at all* making you sick. It's the planetary immune system in you making you sick in an attempt to rid you of the virus-infected tissue at the point of origin, which is your throat or nose, all to restore order to all living things. If the virus makes it all the way to your stomach, your immune system will sacrifice the lining there, too, to shed the virus. Then you'll have a stomachache and diarrhea to add to your misery.

JUST CHILL

Temperature regulation during sleep is another antibacterial strategy we've evolved. While a very warm organism has more of an adaptive advantage through flexibility in acquiring new habitats, the constant heat provides optimal conditions for the growth of most bacteria. The best bet is to cool down. That's why our temperature drops at night.

Since you can't find food in the dark—in fact, it's more likely you'd become food—melatonin acts as a rheostat that lowers body temperature during NREM (Non-Rapid Eye Movement) sleep in order to slow metabolic processes and stave off hunger. The bonus is that the bacteria also respond to the less than balmy temperature: The cold that slows our metabolism also slows theirs.

At the beginning of sleep, you dream a little, while you cool down as melatonin rises; you dream again during the predawn hours before you wake up, as melatonin falls and you warm up. Mammals in cold climates sleep for months at a time, or hibernate, to slow metabolic processes during food scarcity and darker days. Cooling us down in the dark, melatonin does antioxidant work, times ovarian and testicular function, and revs up the immune system for the next waking period, when we must keep harmful microbes out from behind the front lines.

Sleep is the biggest immunological defense scheme we've come up with yet, because not only does it defend us against other organisms in our environment, it defends us against starvation by the insulin-melatonin system. Insulin is produced only when your body senses sugar or stress. Since stress is heralded by cortisol, and cortisol is elevated as long as you're bathed in light, circadian rhythmicity, or day-night cycles, along with carbohydrates, control your insulin production. Light-and-dark cycles control insulin so you can store fat for hibernation, or dormancy. Long days meant the end of summer and food supply. The short sleep cycles of long days translate hormonally into an increased need for carbohydrates to store fat and cascade other hormones to put you to sleep. Carbohydrate craving is a precursor to sleep that we all still respond to every night that we're up late. Hibernation "drives" drive us to eat ice cream or have a glass of wine after a long day. Remember, a midnight snack is never a hard-boiled egg.

That last thing you think about, the last thing you want to eat before surrendering the light, is always any kind of sugar you can get your hands on.

Insulin secretion is controlled by the food you eat, but the food you *want* is controlled by your immune system responding to perceived seasonal variation in the light. When your body and brain need sleep to maintain immunity and reproductive capacity, melatonin and prolactin must surge. We even have melatonin receptors on our ovaries and testes that "read" light-and-dark cycles.

Melatonin is a potent antioxidant that, along with prolactin, controls immunity while you sleep. Without sleep, you become defenseless and autoimmune. Your immune system, too, like every other mechanism of life, is comprised of a sacred duality. Th1 and Th2 cells stand on that board on the log as the two halves of your immune function. One side controls defense and the other side controls offense, because what we term "your immune system" *doesn't really belong to you,* per se. The real entity that serves as your immune system is a sentient, spooky, intelligent force, reminiscent of the proverbial Grim Reaper, that keeps *score*. This spiritual policeman/gatekeeper really exists to even the score for all living things. It's actually the *biosphere's* immune system, not yours.

You only get to be a part of the whole scheme if you play ball.

That means: Get up with sun, sleep with the moon, eat only your share, and be fruitful and multiply. That's it. That's what you were built for, no more, no less. Evolution has fine-tuned you for, really, nothing more.

SEX FILES

The prime survival trait is reproduction. Life goes on. So, after hearts beating and lungs breathing, all energy is directed to reproduction. Life, without all we do to kill time, is only sleeping, eating, and sex. These activities must be maintained at all costs or nature perceives you to be a liability. Sleeping, then eating, is the prerequisite for reproduction, *in that order.*

Human primates were always seasonal breeders until fire came in to stay. Seasonal breeding, needless to say, is run by a clock that is wholly dependent on light-and-dark cycles. Reproductive function depends on metabolic clocks and mechanisms. You can't reproduce without enough fat to survive. That's the reason why lean female athletes often stop ovulating and having menstrual periods. No fat, no future . . . for you or your offspring. So why waste the eggs? That's how nature reads it. Fertility and sleeping are as closely linked as eating and sleeping because in the end it's all one thing.

In the real world, perfect function—whether it be reproductive, a good night's sleep, or weighing the right amount—exists in a *tight boundary that is dynamic with all other living things.* There's really no margin for error. The "give and take" among the life forms on our ball of rock creates our bio-ecosystem, our world. The life force of the bio-ecosystem is all the energy of the sun circulated in what's known to science as the food web. Simple food chains interlace through their interaction with each other to web all substances and species into smaller "feedback loops," wherein each species affects another. Big fish eat little fish, who eat littler fish, who eat plants that suck nourishment from the rocks, and so on and so on. This is a positive feedback loop. Many feedback loops are "negative," or fail-safe feedback loops.

All feedback loops work like the automatic transmission in your car. If you increase the pressure on the accelerator, as the car goes faster, the transmission will jump up a gear to compensate. If you glide downhill, slowing as you go, the transmission naturally drops down a gear to slow you down. The transmission works perfectly well unless you keep up the pressure on the gas pedal while you hold your foot down on the brake.

Keep that picture in your head.

Not only are you going nowhere, but you're destroying your car. Feedback loops are delicate mechanisms that read a signal from one system in the body and send it back to another. Negative feedback loops read a signal and control the reaction in that system, like the transmission in a car going downhill. Usually, the signal sent back in a negative feedback loop will be *stop*, or at least *slow down*. These loops feed back within you and all other species and then feed back to the larger ecosystem. All the whiny Greenpeace people are right. The cosmos, the planet, the little animals, and the people are all connected biologically in one big feedback loop, just like on Daisy World.

If you were out in your local park in a loincloth, these systems would have a chance to do their job accurately. Sitting at a desk or in meetings under fluorescent lights wearing Calvin Klein way past sundown totally screws with your feedback loops. According to a recent study in the journal *Nature,* even too much or too little sex changes the size of your neurons. If that's true, then we can certainly conclude that the amount of sleep you get affects appetite and fertility, which affect metabolism. All of these actions together are part and parcel of the immune system.

SELF-CONTROL

Remember that adaptive intelligence continues to evolve by reacting to input from the environment provided by information-driven feedback loops. These feedback loops are really just streams of information that report back from various "outposts" to their points of origin to control the process.

Let's take a trip to an imaginary place, the natural world, where you don't live anymore. You're just knuckle-ambling along with your buddy when you see a big breadfruit. The fact that you saw a big breadfruit means the trees are fruiting, not flowering, and that it's late spring or summer. The smell gets your juices going and you remember eating one before and, since it was a good experience, you make the decision to eat another. The sugar hits the portal vein between your liver and stomach and your pancreas kicks in with a big shot of insulin. Just as the sugar from the fruit is crossing the blood-brain barrier, sending you to Happy Land, that big shot of insulin simultaneously sends the excess sugar to short-term storage.

Short-term storage in your liver and muscles can't take in too much more because you ate that other kind of fruit with the larvae in it and that shrub with the thorns and berries on it about an hour ago. So, instead, insulin converts some of this breadfruit to cholesterol and the rest is sent to your inner thigh for fat storage because if you're eating breadfruit and berries and whatever that other fruit was your immune system knows winter must be around the corner and, as every immune system also knows, that means no more breadfruit.

So the insulin and stored sugar, in the form of fat, hits your leg (long-term storage). You're a big eater and you've already got about twenty pounds of fat, so leptin from your fat cells sends a signal to your brain. This leptin nails a button in your brain called neuropeptide Y that controls the appetite for carbohydrates. That appetite now goes off.

You stop eating because you have enough energy in short- and long-term storage to make it through tomorrow. That's a negative feedback loop. A negative feedback loop is a self-controlling program that works day by day.

There are also self-perpetuating feedback loops. They tend to work year by year and season to season. For example, if it's late summer and the days are long and you already have more than twenty pounds of fat plus a full supply in short-term storage, it's a different story. It's a winter's tale. Instead of a negative feedback, a positive one will ensue. A different adaptive hormonal and behavioral scenario kicks in, because different environmental buttons have been pushed. September's days are shortening, so instead of just counting on the "light signal," nature's evolved a bonus system for a literally rainy day. The positive feedback loop on your newly gained twenty pounds means you can continue to gain, self-propelled by your own expanding fat base, until all the carbohydrates are *really* gone.

This will circumvent the light response and buy you a month or two more to get *really* fat. Only then will the food definitely be all gone for good until next spring, when the planet wakes up again. So the end of summer is the *only* time in actual nature you would ever have full stores *and twenty extra pounds,* which the long light and short nights have provided.

Prolactin pushed into the daytime by short nights suppressed leptin and left your appetite for carbohydrates (neuropeptide Y) turned on. This gave you the twenty pounds to get the ball rolling. Then the leptin from your own fat base took over to create leptin *resistance.*

This leptin shutdown mechanism serves the purpose of saving you from longing for something (sugar) that's long gone until next summer. Your leptin receptors on the NPY button go dead from overload. With no receptors to read the leptin, it's as if you have none, and your appetite for carbohydrates stays permanently switched on until all of the carbohydrates run out. This mechanism exists because in nature you would never get that fat unless you needed to, *because all the food will be gone.*

The problem in the world we live in is that the food (sugar) will never be gone.

In our *un*natural world of endless summer and sugar, this leptin "overdrive switch" gets flipped. In our world all you have to do is get twenty pounds overweight for the leptin streaming from your expanding fat base to cause the leptin receptors in your brain to retreat, creating leptin resistance and causing the fat to get fatter, *because fat people are always hungry people.* Why? Because their negative feedback loop is broken: their leptin receptors burned out, and there is no longer a curb on their appetite for sugar.

HIDDEN AGENDA

Insulin and the counterregulatory hormones cortisol, human growth hormone, and epinephrine deal with the ultimate *use* of food you take in. They also control sleep, along with melatonin and prolactin. Food for human primates exists in a sum total of three possibilities: protein, fat, and carbohydrate.

The pathways of protein, fat, and carbohydrates through the body are all distinct. And three distinctly different neurotransmitters control your appetite for the three different substances. The control of carbohydrate intake by the neurotransmitter NPY (neuropeptide Y) is not at all like the controls on your appetite for protein or fat. Carbohydrate consumption is part of a planetary energy metabolism that holds true for *every* organism with insulin. Carbohydrates are energy that can be stored, and they can only be stored by insulin. That's why *you can't eat fat and get fat;* but *you do eat sugar and get fat.*

No other substance that you can eat provokes an insulin response. These different paths for dietary fat and sugar are always and have always been dictated by the interaction of hormones responding to the environment and your stress levels.

Insulin is on one side of the board on the log and epinephrine, cortisol, human growth hormone, and glucagon are on the other. The balance between the two sides of the board is accomplished when a hormone molecule heads for a receptor—often its own, but not always. Remember, survival rests on the cross-talk. Hormones *and* their receptors are single molecules of different weights.

"Ligand" is another term for any molecule that binds to a receptor—not just hormones, but brain and gut neuropeptides and immune system cytokines, too. Remember the lock and key metaphor. Receptor molecules are large and ligand molecules are small. *Ligare* is Latin, meaning "that which binds." *(Ligare* is also the source for the word "religion." It's not a coincidence.) Receptors float up from within the cells like water-lily pads with really long roots. As the pads answer a call to "surface" for an interface, the roots reach to connect with the cell's nucleus. A mechanism called chemotaxis guides the prospective partner molecule to the rendezvous with the receptor on the lily pad. Chemotaxis works like a tractor beam on *Star Trek.* When the hormone, neurotransmitter, or immune expression (cytokine) molecule drops into the lily, the "petals" respond.

The receptor changes shape in the presence of a ligand. The receptor molecule actually *embraces* the ligand's chemical key. When this happens, the receptor begins to wiggle and shudder, and the shimmy or message is passed on as both the receptor and ligand literally, not figuratively, vibrate and hum. In *Molecules of Emotion,* Candace Pert says that "a more dynamic description of this process might be two voices—ligand and receptor—striking the same note."

There's the music again.

Hormones, neurotransmitters, and cytokines are ligands whose message is translated by the effect of a molecule tickling a receptor until the disturbance creates a conformational change. Once the receptor is mounted and the crescendo is past, the ligand molecule's message travels along the root of the "lily" deep below the surface to throw switches on the strand of DNA in the nucleus.

When you leave the lights on, you eat sugar; your hormones respond appropriately to the carbohydrate you've consumed, eventually affecting the DNA in every cell in your body. That's how a species can adapt to the environment and to what's available to eat. If the availability of one of the three choices changes, ultimately the animal will change. So if you try to live on only one food group to the exclusion of the other two, bad things will happen. In essence, those of us not yet able to handle the change in the light cycles and/or the food supply will die.

Exposure to artificial light was minimal for most of our existence, a glowing ember here, a candle there. We slept more and had no access to the caloric power of refined sugar and flour. Now our twenty-four-hour well-lit day-for-night existence means to our controls that it's endless summer, and that signal demands continuous feasting.

So we feast.

Because the sugar never ends.

ON ICE:

Evolution, Biophysics, and the Dark

I am part of the sun as my Eve is part of me. That I am part of the
Earth my feet know perfectly and my blood is part of the sea.
                                        —D. H. Lawrence

Sugar is captured sunlight. The life-giving energy of the sun is locked away in the plant life of the planet. When we eat sugar, the molecules of carbohydrates become ATP (adenosine triphosphate) energy in the power centers of our cells. Any of the sun's energy that is not immediately used is reassembled in storage form as body fat against the day when the plants are dormant.

Survival is having enough sugar to store some for when there is none available.

Survival was never about eating fat, it was always about *making* fat.

Survival, thy name is sugar.

That's the only truth there is, here and now in America, and as far back as anyone can imagine. It was the same all the way back in dim prehuman history. At least as far back as the origination of a worm with no brain and no heart called *C. elegans,* survival was always about sugar.

Sugar's scientific name is carbohydrate. Carbohydrates are the only food we can store, contrary to what you've been told. Many of the carbohydrates we eat today "came with" the planet—apples, peas, pinto beans, carrots, sugarcane, and beets, in their original form. We humans, always eager to improve upon nature, have invented quite a few more—Snickers, bread, sucrose, Snapple, wine, pasta, rice cakes, and the ever-popular SnackWell's. It doesn't really matter if it's a complex carbohydrate or a refined simple one, it's all just sugar, and to any organism with the magic molecule insulin, that means survival.

The worms would tell you that if they had brains.

It's up for debate what exactly constituted a carbohydrate for *C. elegans*, but we do know he used them to survive because he had almost exactly the same gene to produce insulin that we do. Which means the great-great-great-great-grandfather of our common origins hundreds of millions of years ago, ran on the same fuel as we do because it's what the planet had to offer. Insulin is the reason our own blood sugar can be used as fuel by our cells. Without insulin, our tissues starve, and cellular, mitochondrial mechanisms grind to a halt. If life is *lux*, being without insulin is dark.

TIMING IS EVERYTHING

To most Americans, insulin is a medicine. Certainly, all diabetics know that we can't live without it. People who saw the movie *Reversal of Fortune* know that too much insulin poisoned Sunny von Bülow. But for the majority of Americans, insulin is a nonissue, or so they think.

Insulin is a fairly small molecule made in the beta cells of your pancreas. Insulin has the dual job of giving your cells access to the sugar in your blood and throwing the switches to store the rest of it in a "lighter form" as body fat. Insulin is the storage hormone. Besides giving the muscles, brain, and liver access to blood sugar, insulin's big job is to handle the overload. We have this insulin-receptor mechanism for dealing with excess sugar intake because we were *always* supposed to overeat sugar any time we could. Overeating sugar is, survival-wise, *instinct*. In nature, which for us barely exists anymore, animals always overeat carbohydrates whenever they find them, just in case they don't find them the next day.

All the sugar you eat is very heavy, because carbo-"hydrates" are hydrated. Carbohydrates are fuel and water together. Without the water attached, the carbon molecules weigh a lot less. Those two-carbon molecules left over after the water dissipates through crying, sweating, or urinating are body fat. You can pack on a lot more carbohydrate energy as lightweight fat. How much fat you actually need to store as a mammal depends on how long you plan to go without food and how long it takes you to reproduce. That brings us back to survival.

Prolactin is the survival hormone. Most of us would assume prolactin only makes human milk. It does, but its most important role is to keep us surviving throughout our lives by controlling our appetites. As newborns, our first taste of survival is sweet. We must make fat from sugar from day one. The milk of all mammals has an astronomical sugar content. Breast milk is a carbohydrate-rich body fluid laced with some protein to create the molecules necessary for immune function and a huge array of molecular fatty acid chains to make hormones that will interface with the infant's new environment. It's Mom's prolactin that not only creates our "first-one's-free" addiction to the taste of sweet, but also creates our link with the *planet's* immune system by fostering that addiction. Equally important, Mom's prolactin goes through the roof while she makes this juice because sky-high prolactin means an autoimmune state of being. Autoimmunity just means that Mom's immune system is in overdrive, pouring immune functions into the breast milk to program the baby's immune system with all the collective memory that Mom's, and her Mom's, and her Mom's immune systems have been passing on about their environments since before time had a name.

While insulin makes us capable of rolling with the punches when wrestling with nature by storing sun/sugar energy for later, it's the prolactin that truly controls our appetites for the rest of our lives—by suppressing leptin, which, of course, is the switch for NPY, which is in charge of our appetite for the foods that can be stored. Even with the ability to store carbohydrates, survival—before grocery stores and freezers—was completely dependent on timing, especially during scarcity brought about by weather changes. Our feast-or-famine metabolism gave us the edge.

Our celestially driven internal light-responsive genes actually "clock" how long melatonin is produced, to give prolactin the "weather report" to time our appetites in sync with the spin cycle. The resulting length of prolactin production from melatonin's report will determine whether or not prolactin is produced the next day.

In winter, the "melatonin clock" keeps the "prolactin timer" going longer at night, which in turn means that you secrete no prolactin in the daytime. Because if prolactin happens in the daytime, not only will it suppress leptin's action and leave your sweet tooth exposed (at a time when there is no sweet available), but it means in nature's glossary that you're (men and women) "lactating," so thanks to aging and broken clocks, we are all very autoimmune, at this point. (This is this side effect of being out of rhythm that creates huge profits for the makers of antihistamines like Claritin, Zantac, and asthma and arthritis drugs, like Advil.)

Leptin production from our fat base is the "dipstick" that tells NPY what our fat levels are and whether or not to make us crave sugar. The premise is that if you have enough fat, the leptin it produces will turn off your appetite for sugar. Remember the Breadfruit Guys. When prolactin happening in the daytime suppresses the leptin from your fat base, it reads to NPY as "no fat" and your appetite for sugar stays turned on all day and some of the night. If you don't sleep, and the light (or its absence) that would time your melatonin clock through all of those cycles never goes off, you just continue to eat sugar and make fat until you explode because your clock is running so fast.

Your mainspring is broken.

That's about where *we* are, folks.

This feast-or-famine metabolism embodied in the insulin/carbohydrate system facilitated our survival by storing those carbohydrates as fat. This programmed connection to the environment made the adaptation to a starkly different climate possible, as we headed north out of Africa. As we moved into colder and colder climates, with ever-widening variations in seasonal abundance, our body's ability to clock light-and-dark cycles took on even more importance.

Having a solar connection controlling the timing that directed our appetite for carbohydrates and our arousal for reproduction was not only what kept us alive day in and day out, but what actually kept us *living*. Survival as a species depended on eating enough to reproduce and on timing that reproduction to coincide with spring, when there would be food to keep mother and baby alive.

The sudden appearance of a sun that never sets is killing the slower evolvers among us in the no more than eighty years it's existed, which is not even—by today's standards—an entire length of a human lifetime. The irony is that we managed to use fire for at least 45,000 lifetimes added together.

Archaeological site-work has unearthed 300,000-year-old wooden spear points that appear to be hardened by fire. It was a long time before we domesticated it, though. Sometime during the next 230,000 years, we began to "live" inside, not just to seek shelter for sleep or from the weather, but we have no evidence that fire was used for cooking until 70,000 years ago. It's in about the same period that the cave art of the Paleolithic era shows evidence of charcoal drawing.

Until now, after the cold, dark, sleepy winter of short days and long nights, the sun came back, plants grew, and babies were born. The days mirrored the years: With one revolution of the planet, out of light and into the dark, when the sun dropped, everything lay dormant until it rose again, just as summer always turned into winter and then back again. It was a perfect system, until we mastered the art of portable fire. Once we could carry away and eventually re-create the aftermath of lightning strikes, it all began to change. With portable energy, we could extend the day for our own use inside—at night. No other living thing could do that. We, the children of Prometheus, had set ourselves apart from all living things.

It was this light after nightfall on a regular basis that shortened melatonin cycles enough to let testosterone and estrogen surface, big time, all year round. This seemingly simple change removed the normal seasonal cues for the timing of breeding. Our estimate is that we stopped "hibernating," or dozing for days or weeks at a time, during food scarcity in cold climates then, too, because fossilized remains of shellfish and small game are found in Ice Age caves.

So now we were inside, away from the ice, fairly warm, and, no doubt, incredibly bored. This period produced the first cave art, perhaps storytelling, and religion. We were probably praying for something to do besides blow ochre handprints on the wall. Instead of sleeping or dozing to reduce metabolism and physical needs and increase immune functions, we were hanging around with nothing to do but eat and get laid. Just like today. As with all positive feedback loops, less torpor meant more time awake and more time awake meant increased use of fire, and so on and so on. This self-propelled increase in the use of fire meant, of course, even more light to screw up melatonin's report of rotation and orbit. You can see how evolution just gets out of hand.

For all time, before now, not just human or even hominid/primate time, we evolved successful survival strategies to deal with the forces of nature. We went from experiencing seasonal rhythmicity tied to food supply for breeding—just like every other animal on earth—to a new place, alone, without the rest of our family.

Out of Eden, there was no turning back.

The light would change us more than we might have dared to imagine. The light itself was far more seductive than any serpent with a carbohydrate. The light bought us more learning time than all the other species could ever have and ultimately gave us the ability to outbreed them, too. Of course, there would be trade-offs. People began to die in new ways. Things like the smoke in the enclosed spaces and increased sex hormones took a lot of us out right away.

SPECIES II

But those of us who remained after the miracle of mobile fire slept less, imagined more, and started to talk during the dark, cold time because it wasn't as dark or as cold inside anymore, thanks to the fire. We didn't know that the fire, through its light, could kill without leaving a mark, without so much as a blister. We had no idea then, nor do most of us now, that being bathed in artificial light during those hours of the night when it had always been pitch black was changing us *inside*.

Molecules like melatonin, a hormone that we know is secreted during dark time, report on the planet's angle and orbit. When the hours of light stopped varying *acutely* with the seasons, thanks to the light of fire, our "sentinel molecules" became stuck in a springtime report. It was just enough, at first, to make us a little brighter, too. Dreams that used to come in the night sometimes came in the day, thanks to the shifting of prolactin production toward morning. We began to *imagine*. The urge to communicate and symbolize those daydreams gave us language.

It was reproduction after the acquisition of fire that set us apart from all other living things by artificially increasing our numbers. Babies no longer waited for springtime to be born. We were fertile all year round because it was eternal summer in our ovaries and in our minds. Although a lot of the babies starved at first, there were such a great many more that it was, somehow, easier to bear.

Memory, too, thanks to more dopamine from the light, began to criss-cross our expanding brains with "reward pathways" to give us an intellectual edge. That phenomenon, along with all of the meat we ate in the winter, made brain expansion a physical reality, too. Imagine the homeostatic mess that all of the up-all-night, up-all-winter, multiplying-out-of-control, big-brained, small-minded, eternally hungry, sex-crazed, *sensitive* artists must have created for the rest of the earth's creatures still living in sync with each other and the cosmos.

ICE, ICE, BABY

For the last few hundred thousand years or so, our Family of Man hunted for protein in the form of fish, animals, nuts, and insects and gathered fruits, edible roots, bark, and weeds in season during the dormant period we call winter. For much of that time, climatic conditions were slowly chilling the planet and a lot of its inhabitants into a many-millennia-long deep freeze that rendered vast amounts of vegetation permanently out of season. If we hadn't already had fire, we wouldn't have made it, either. The most recent of these 100,000-year-long cyclical glacial periods ended about 10,000 years ago. This last Ice Age buried most of continental Europe and North America, reaching south past New York City and Chicago, in a layer of solid ice that was in some places almost three miles deep. We humans didn't experience any of the previous ages of ice because we hadn't moved north until the last one. The large boulders in New York's Central Park come from a vast plain at the top of the North American continent called the Labrador Oon Gala. The native term for the boulders—in the Inuit language of the people who live where they originated—is *nuno tacs,* or "lonely stones." Whenever a glacier retreats, these boulders remain.

The ice will come again. It will crush cities and suck up the seas. But we will survive, as our ancestors survived. The ice will always come again until the end of the earth's time in the universe because its arrival is timed by our trip around the sun and the angle at which we travel. Our position relative to the sun, or the *inclination* on our axis, varies every 41,000 years or so, and our "wobble" (think of a top spinning) causes a major perturbation every 20,000 years or so. When both of these variations overlap, they create a major event—an orbital shift from *circular to elliptical,* which happens every 100,000 years like clockwork to plunge Earth and us into another Ice Age. The combined effect of the three orbital cycles alters the angle and distance at which the sun's light strikes the earth at northern latitudes. *Northern* is the key to the process happening. The less sun up north at the poles, the more ice, the more reflective ice surface, the more the sunlight is reflected away from the earth, meaning less sun, and more ice, and so on and so on, . . .

These Ice Age centuries changed our metabolism *permanently.* During very short, not terribly warm summers, we scored enough carbohydrates to barely get by. Those who were exquisitely light sensitive and had great storage potential lived, and we are their children. Now these traits are a death sentence.

Had Paleolithic man not eaten a predominantly protein-and-fat diet for the better portion of each year, it would mean that he would have had to go without food for thousands of years at a time. Sorry, vegans, but that's not very likely.

Those thousands of years of heavy protein and fat intake directly increased brain weight, which fostered the evolutionary neural expansion we've cited. For all human time, man lived and thrived on a diet comprised of *eighty to ninety percent protein* and its attendant fat content at least seven or eight months out of the year, and the rest of the time on vegetation foraged only *in season*. The total absence of grindstones and mortars and pestles makes a definite statement on Ice Age nutrition. They never had enough to bother to invent grinding.

Their skeletal remains also testify to their diet. In 1988, anthropologists at Emory University took a look at diet and lifestyle then and now in *The Paleolithic Prescription:* "By studying the skeletal remains from the Late Paleolithic period and analyzing the attributes of recent hunter gatherer groups, it's possible to develop a detailed anatomical and to some extent a biochemical profile. With as little as one limb bone and a formula which relates overall height to limb-bone length, the stature of early man has been deduced. Thirty thousand years ago, Eastern Mediterranean males stood an estimated average 5'10", but the Leakey-Walker fossils indicate more like an average of 6'2"."

These people attained heights comparable to or greater than those reached by today's "well-nourished" populations.

They go on to say, "These skeletal remains also reflect strength and muscularity; the size of joints and sites where muscles are inserted into bones indicate these people's muscle mass and the amount of force they were able to exert. The average Cro-Magnon was easily as strong as today's superior male and female athletes. They worked many fewer hours than the coming Agriculturists, but were significantly more robust."

Even 50,000 years ago, the hominid *Homo sapiens sapiens* was biologically indistinguishable from us. If he were wearing a hat and sunglasses, you couldn't pick him out in a lineup. Culturally and socially, the same traits that kept them alive keep us alive today. We made stone tools, passed down a cultural framework, learned skills, and practiced solutions, all within the accepted notions of family and kinship structure. These qualities of life are still recognized today as important to functional mental well-being. Anthropologists and forensic experts who re-create actual faces from fossilized jaws and skull parts say Cro-Magnon faces were completely modern.

Although people living between 40,000 and 10,000 years ago had not altered the natural world around them to continue their existence for one million generations, one day some woman, tired of making and remaking camp, said, "Honey, what if we just try *growing* this stuff right outside the door?" That day, the world changed forever.

It was only 10,000 really short years ago, give or take a millennium, that we became capable of controlling the interactive earth-given food supply that assured our survival. Until this last century, from that distant point ten millennia ago—i.e., during our entire prehistoric existence—we could eat only the carbohydrates that we could steal and tame from the planet's cornucopia. What that means is we've eaten the same kinds of "natural" carbohydrates for the last 9,900 years, and the same amounts.

Not anymore.

No other species has ever had unlimited access to carbohydrate energy without regard for effort, season, competition, and natural disaster. Farming forever altered the balance of nature.

If we were in trouble before, from that moment on, we were in serious *danger.*

The coming of agriculture 10,000 years ago as a viable alternative to hunting and gathering effectively ended the Paleolithic period and pretty much eliminated the hunter-gatherer lifestyle worldwide. The Neolithic Revolution meant the end of our coexistence with everything else on the earth's terms. From then on, all interactions would be on *our* terms. "Revolution" implies an intentional overthrow of one institution for another. In reality, the sudden abundance possible when the food supply became controlled by the consumer also provided enough calories to further support the changing patterns of reproduction.

SETTLING DOWN

After we learned to grow "this stuff right outside the door," we stopped moving as much. Instead of following the herds to eat what we needed, we started to store the increasingly tame grains and fruits and meat. These provisions were too heavy to travel with, but we could feed all the new little mouths, so for the sake of the children we began to settle down. In the old days, one hunter could support himself and one pregnant woman and maybe two children and even an aged parent. Pregnant women and the elderly, along with a child or two, added to provisions by gathering insects and nuts to supplement protein.

The hunter-gatherer, man-woman pairing was an economically "equal" division of labor. When we settled down to farm, however, the dynamic became weighted toward male economic control. This is where sexual inequity was born.

One farmer could not only nutritionally support more children; sometimes he could support more women and their children. A land "owner," in fact, could support all that *and* the men to defend the land and the women that these men owned. Somewhere along the way, the big farmer-landowner evolved into a sultan owning 16,000 virgins, *because he could feed them.* Agriculture translated not only to farmers outnumbering hunter-gatherers; it also became the means for any man to be unimaginably reproductively successful.

The Bible tells us so.

We began to work together in bigger groups, too. This domestication extended beyond our little human band. We had finally tamed the animals by taming the plants. What we could get to grow near our settlements attracted animals to our door—two species for the price of one.

For the first time since we learned to lie to one another, we were eating on a regular basis by duping other species with offerings of food. All the extra light and learning was evolving a new kind of memory and instinct in us, one the other animals couldn't share. This pact with the devil we call farming fostered an enormous population explosion. We human monkeys weren't just annoying anymore, we were a force to be reckoned with. There were enough of us to "terraform" the earth to our needs and enslave most other living things. This in no way resembled our humble beginnings as hunter-gatherers.

B.C.-O.D.

Because the glaciers were slowly receding and the globe was warmer and wetter and because our ancestors' timing was impeccable, civilization turned a corner that day. In the beginning, when we stayed awake longer, we fooled reproductive machinery into working "double shifts," leaving us reproductive all year long. Melatonin suppression and increased exposure to estrogen and testosterone had already changed our ability to reproduce. Now insulin would be tested. How much sugar could we take?

Farming had flipped the nutritional balance to ninety percent carbohydrate and ten percent protein and fat—almost a low-fat diet. Centuries of death and disease followed. Humans, over the course of the last 7,500 years, have lost an average of six inches in height. We were very tiny people overall until recently.

That's why in museums you see those tiny little suits of armor and those Cinderella-sized Victorian shoes, and on the street outside the museum, you see very tall Japanese Americans who've abandoned their predominantly rice-based diet since living in America. Only in the past century has our diet caused a return to a recovered dormant phenotypic potential. In English: With more protein in our diets, we have almost gone back to our original size.

The disease consequence of an agricultural diet was only mitigated by the backbreaking physical effort it took to maintain it. Farming is labor-intensive—labor-intensive enough to burn off most of a ninety-percent-carbohydrate diet if you do all the work personally, you and maybe your ox. The fact is, the expenditure of calories necessitated by farmers pulling their own plows and working ten-hour days explains how we survived as well as we did while we were eating all the bread that we ate.

Farming also brought a new mindset to our view of nutrition: economy beyond need. The biggest reason the greater percentage of our diet was made up of carbohydrates was that killing the animals for just meat seemed shortsighted. Sharing the grain with them meant less for us in winter stores, but if we kept them alive, they could give us milk to make cheese and even continue to make more of their own kind. We had a sort of pyramid scam going. Not only were we conning two other species, we were conning Mother Nature.

Farming, like fire, not only isolated us from all other living things, it also made us very sick again, too. Just as when the babies began to come all year round, the death rate increased, but this time it was barely noticed because of the great increase of the population in general. The value of life was getting cheaper because of the ubiquitousness of man.

Another Daisy World déjà vu.

MACHINE AGING

Our next giant step out of Eden (this is number three) was to create simple machines to enhance our physical strength and abilities. This pushed our pyramid scam of conquering lightning, then plants, then animals, a step higher. It all started with a mortar and pestle. If we ground the grain into smaller and smaller pieces, it went further. A loaf of bread made from two handfuls of grain could feed more than two people, and the increase of man meant many, many more people wanted more and more bread.

This increased continuous consumption of carbohydrate for a people who had evolved to eat them only a few months of the year killed just as many then as it does now. The real plague began for them, and still continues for us 10,000 years later, when they *refined* carbohydrates. Ground grain and, later, the dried, powdered sweet juice of beets and sugarcane registered to our insulin/blood-sugar system like birds on the bottom of the ocean. We had no reference point for it; it made no sense. There was no place where so much energy coming in all at once could fit into our systems. More and more people were wearing their winter coats of fat through spring and summer, too.

BRIGHT IDEAS

All the extra mouths to feed, although they slowed us down, also demanded creative solutions from their parents. A man very fond of electricity once said, "Necessity is the mother of invention." For humans, necessity tipped the balance. To this day, we are unparalleled by any other species on earth when it comes to food production and the supply we can store. We human primates separated ourselves from the others on the planet not by walking upright, but by staying awake longer to learn and by heating our environment when it was too cold to live. We widened the abyss between "them and us" with farming or, more truthfully, with their capture and confinement.

There's no way to go home again.

THE TRUTH IS IN HERE

FIVE

DENY EVERYTHING:

*Sleep Controls Appetite, Therefore Obesity,
Adult-Onset Diabetes, and Hypertension*

*"I have only a bare working knowledge of the human brain but it's
enough to make me proud to be an American. Your brain has a trillion
neurons and every neuron has ten thousand little dendrites. The system of intercommunication is awe-inspiring. It's like a galaxy that you
can hold in your hand, only more complex, more mysterious."*

"Why does this make you proud to be an American?"

*"The infant's brain develops in response to stimuli. We still lead the
world in stimuli . . ."*

—Don DeLillo,
White Noise

America is the home of the brightest and the best and the sickest people
in the world. We hold the lead in productivity, eating disorders, SAT
scores, diabetes, cutting-edge technology, heart disease, and cancer. What
do all of those accomplishments have in common?

It's certainly not a high-fat diet.

In our culture, people boast how little fat they eat and how little sleep
they can get by on. These two accomplishments are an outward declara-
tion of our ambition and stamina. Our national motto is, "You snooze,
you lose." The word "overtime" is now archaic. In order to apply such a
measure to time, we would have to acknowledge a stopping point in the
workday. It's the notion of "quitting time" that's the real artifact.

Look at how many sound bites we've invented to describe the stress of
success, from the benign "type A personality" and "go-getter" to more dis-
paraging terms like "burnout case" and "success freak." Europeans don't
call each other names like that. In this country, we work at least ten hours
a day, try to exercise a few hours a week, and suffer. Dean Ornish says love

will keep us together and Dr. Andrew Weil even suggests a toke or two for medicinal purposes. In this culture, when we're young, we take drugs to relax; when we're old, we take drugs to survive.

Has it always been that way? Only for baby boomers.

By the 1940s, postwar America was describing our unique lifestyle as "keeping up with the Joneses," "climbing the corporate ladder," and our success to the self-congratulatory "good old-fashioned hard work," as though we were the only people on the globe trying to accomplish anything. To acquire the worldwide lead, Americans have, metaphorically speaking, pulled an eighty-year-long "all-nighter."

We live in cities that never sleep in a country that rocks twenty-four hours a day.

It turns out that acquiring the lead in obesity, diabetes, heart disease, and cancer was just a *bonus*. Of course, golf had to go and those Sunday picnics with the family. We Americans only have time for one serious hobby in the 1990s—worrying about dying. Now that maintaining our failing health has usurped whatever time we had left after work for our spouses or children, something as negligible as sleeping is truly unthinkable.

STEPPING OUT OF EDEN

Americans have all but given up sleeping. At most, we get a solid five to six hours a night. We all believe we're doing fine on that. We use alarm clocks, coffee, NoDoz, and, in the 1980s, when we wanted to be Masters of the Universe, coke. And we do mean the *real thing*, not the beverage. We might be tired, but we're not showing it. Or are we?

According to studies on work-related incompetence, it seems we're starting to crack. The National Commission on Sleep Disorders Research (NCSDR) has estimated that the annual direct cost to employers is, as we've mentioned, $15.9 billion, and they're only talking about money. Seventy million Americans report trouble sleeping, but what does that mean?

In 1982, the *Journal of the American Medical Association* published the results of "Project Sleep" from the Association of Sleep Disorders Center. The cases represented the study of 5,000 patients over two years. The most common disorder was "disorder of *hyper*somnia," or excessive sleepiness. Forty-two percent of people in 1982 were too tired to stay awake. Twenty-six percent couldn't get to sleep or stay asleep.

The study concluded that hypersomnia is a result of sleep apnea. Sleep apnea is when you forget to breathe. Forgetting to breathe means you have a very tired brain. Only those of us who can lose sleep and not get fat and sick or forget to breathe will continue to evolve past the evolutionary speed bump induced by artificial light. The descendants of those who can will be able to live in twenty-four-hour bright light and eat the plastic wrappers.

Those people won't be most of us.

Lucky for the rest of us, though, the light remained limited for millennia. Although we could burn anything that would burn, the quality of the light that was produced varied. And the supply of combustible material also controlled the hours and the quality of light past darkfall. The best light came from the wax of bees and the animal fat called tallow. Neither of these substances came cheap.

Even thousands of years after we had made cities and countries, the world at night was black as pitch. Individual dwellings had dim light past sundown, but the world outside the door was still a void full of scary noises. Travel was dangerous. People never ventured out after dark if they could help it. If they did, they paid someone to escort them with a torch. This old "protection racket" became what we know as the police. *Our* police work at night in virtually re-created daylight; but they still carry wooden sticks.

How long have we owned the night?

We evolved in one kind of illumination for 70,600 years. Then, only four hundred years ago, the duration of light in only one place substantially changed. Paris became the first city on the planet to hang tallow candles across the streets at night. Our word "curfew" is really two French words, *couvre feu*, meaning "cover fire"—lights out, go back home. Until the French idea caught on, the average citizen in all big cities hired a chaperone with a torch to accompany him after dark. Except in Paris, domestic lighting in the 1600s was the same as it had been for thousands of years.

Paris retained her title as the City of Light for almost two hundred years, until gaslights were installed in some other cities in the mid-1800s. It was expensive and messy. While the quality of gaslight was certainly brighter than single candles and easier to use, it was nothing like the artificial light we know today. Still, the gaslights of the Victorian era were bright enough to illuminate the scientific minds like Faraday's and Volta's that have brought us to the brink of extinction.

SLEEPING, DREAMING, AND DYING

What happens when we don't get enough sleep? Not just fatigue, but obesity, Type II diabetes, depression, heart disease, infertility, and cancer are on the horizon, if you don't fall asleep at the wheel first. Mental and computational insufficiency are garden-variety symptoms of fatigue. But everybody knows the signs are really physical. When you get really tired, you actually ache all over, your eyes burn, and some people actually get a stomachache. These flu-like symptoms would support the bacterial endotoxin-LPS buildup theory. As the endotoxins from the bacteria living in your middle build up from no sleep, you actually get sick from it. But that's just what we cognitively feel as symptomatic cues. Feeling lousy when you lose sleep is a symptom of much bigger, life-threatening things that are unraveling inside of you.

You're losing the beat.

All living things must be part of the *project*. On the big screen, molecules called chemophores are present in all animals, plants, and bacteria. Think of them as transducers of energy. When hit by light, chemophore cells capture the energy and pass it along. The photons of light enact chemical and electrical changes to the nuclei of all cells. This is a bolt from the blue. This electrification by radiant energy takes place everywhere inside you. Each of your cells is a clock that times exactly one revolution around the sun. All the molecular machinery that you need to keep the beat of the cosmos resides in each individual cell. Every cell in your body is a clock.

You have a gene expressed in every cell of you called dCLOCK. And another one called dBMAL1. The proteins that these two genes code for build up in the cell and join together. The proteins from dCLOCK and dBMAL1, as they join, bind to and throw the switches on two more "clock genes" called per and tim. Per and tim, once bound and activated, begin to produce proteins of their own that in a very general way accumulate inside the cell, just floating in the cytoplasm, around the nucleus, where they join as the hours of the day wear on. That's the "tick."

It's the "tock" that rocks. The tock happens when the proteins of per and tim reach a critical mass floating in the cytoplasm and reenter the nucleus, where they block the function of good old dCLOCK and dBMAL1. And the clock stops—to reset. This negative feedback loop, by stopping dCLOCK and dBMAL1, self-limits per and tim's protein production. In a mechanical clock, the swing of the pendulum to one side and then the other involves an ever-so-brief halt before it returns to the other side. In the cell, this evanescent hiccup only lasts as long as it takes for the proteins of per and tim to dissipate in the nucleus. Then it starts all over again. Like a Chinese water clock that drips from one bowl to the other, as soon as one gets full, it trips and pours into the next.

Of course, in your cells, it takes exactly *one day*, or one turn around the sun, for a complete feedback loop.

This cellular metronome was evident when scientists found photoreceptive cells on the legs of flies called drosophila. To test the same location in humans, researchers at Cornell University put a fiber-optic cable behind the knee of a study subject. They illuminated a patch of skin no bigger than the size of a quarter. The subject was otherwise in complete darkness, yet this small amount of light affected the subject's temperature and melatonin secretion. Imagine what sunbathing, all-night TV, air travel in and out of brightly lit airports at all hours, and staring at computer screens do to confuse your life-support systems.

Since you are no more than clocks upon clocks upon clocks, if the duration of light changes it's only a matter of time before ancient switches on millions of genes controlling your physical and mental states are turned on. All of you, every cell in your body, ticktocks. So just turning off the lights at 11:30 P.M. and closing your eyes to the street lights shining in your windows, the green glow of the VCR, or, ironically, your alarm clock isn't fooling even one of your cells.

THE HIBERNATION HYPOTHESIS

This unending artificial light constantly glaring around you all hours of the day and half of the night, which registers as the long days of summer prior to winter on your internal sundial, is the reason it's so hard to stay thin or sane. *As a mammal, you are hardwired to eat sugar, make babies, store fat, and then sleep it off, and then do it again and again.*

The diseases that we know to correlate with obesity—high blood pressure, heart disease, diabetes, cancer, and depression—are all really the result of a *vestigial hibernation instinct* brought on by too much artificial light. Mammal studies concur that once you start the hibernation preparation cycle, *hyperlipidemia (high cholesterol), high blood pressure, and insulin resistance (leading to obesity) are normal states that resolve them-*

selves with the extended sleep that follows in nature. In other words, all God's creatures get fat and have high cholesterol and high blood pressure and then go to sleep, or at least starve for sugar for a while. That's why only our pets have heart disease, get too fat to walk, and have cancer.

They live with *us.*

In the hormonal state brought on by long hours of light, the urge to consume carbohydrates or drink alcohol to put on a fat base for upcoming winter becomes metabolically and psychologically impossible to resist. In order to control our appetite for carbohydrates to lose weight, bring insulin levels down, and stay sane and fertile, we must sleep more. That's why Americans are eating themselves to death and killing each other.

They're tired. Dead tired.

THIRD-EYE BLIND

In this chapter, we begin to dissect the physiological and mental effects of sleep loss on the American public and all of the people around the world now approaching our technological level. We can tell you why cancer, heart disease, and depression, which go hand in hand with diabetes, all *do* correlate with obesity. We contend that obesity, as we know it in our time, is the prelude to hibernation. Obesity, as prehibernatory physiology, inevitably evolves into Type II diabetes because the end result of prolonged insulin resistance is no insulin action. With no insulin action, there is no way to disperse incoming blood sugar resulting from carbohydrate consumption.

In such a state, you are exactly as diabetic *as if you had no pancreas.*

This mechanism of end-stage insulin resistance is nature's way of stopping weight gain and keeping you from freezing in the winter that never comes. In Type I diabetics, whose pancreases produce little or no insulin because of damaged insulin-producing beta cells, gaining weight is an impossibility. Insulin action on insulin receptors is the only way to put carbohydrate energy into fat cells.

A businessman from Michigan who had received a diagnosis of Type I diabetes in 1907 called it "a hole inside him." He lived in a painless state in which no matter how much he ate, he lost weight, just as though the food was "dropping through" an opening in his stomach. The report of this man says, "He became a shadow of himself, in stature, strength, and coloring, and he died in 1917." Not a surprise.

The cutting-edge treatment for Type I diabetes in 1907 was a low-calorie diet. The premise behind this approach was that the fewer calories the diabetic ate, the more would be utilized by the body. It didn't work. Patients already emaciated from the disease were put on regimens of 500 to 1,000 calories a day, so either way Type I diabetics starved to death. The treatment truly added insult to injury.

Diabetes, Types I and II combined, was the twenty-eighth leading cause of death in 1900, the twelfth in 1920, and the seventh in 1940. In 1999, it was the third most common cause of death in the United States. It could be argued that a rising increase in longevity countrywide due to surgery and antibiotic use translated into a population that was suddenly living long enough to develop the disease, or that the good life and attendant eating habits in Europe and North America had suddenly become sweeter.

What we see is that America's and Europe's appetite for sugar increased at exactly the same time and in exactly the same pattern as the spread of electricity and artificial lights. By 1925, all of America's major cities were wired and Type II diabetes was on its way to quadrupling.

The statistics in the previous paragraph cite a breathtakingly rapid expansion for Type II diabetes, from the twenty-eighth leading cause of death in 1900 to the twelfth in 1925. From 1920 to 1940, the increase was just as startling. The only happenstance to put the brakes on this "epidemic" was World War II's sugar rationing here and in Europe. Even so, Type II diabetes in the last century has grown from a relatively obscure disease to one of the three biggest killers in the Western world. When you examine the numbers that divide Type I and Type II diabetes into two different diseases, the contrast is even more glaring—Type I insulin-dependent diabetics only account for about ten percent of all diabetics. That means the other ninety percent fall into the category we like to call victims of the light. But this is now. Let's look at then.

SURVIVAL OF THE FATTEST

How does end-stage insulin resistance stop weight gain *and* keep you from freezing? Well, we know that when it was too cold and too dark to sustain the plants and animals that we feed on, the unpredictability of the food supply left evolution only one solution—obesity.

Obesity was the key to survival, the key adaptation for all mammals. In order to put on enough fat for the winter, you had to become insulin resistant. The insulin receptors that allow glucose or blood sugar into your muscle cells after your liver is full have to close up shop so all of the sugar you eat can be sent to fat cells for storage or turn into cholesterol. Insulin's immediate purpose is this dispersal.

Insulin's evolutionary purpose is *insulation.*

The point of being really fat is to keep you from starving and freezing. Insulin stores excess energy as internal fat around your vital organs first, before you ever see it ripple under your skin. The purpose is to insulate your heart, lungs, and digestive system from the cold, just as the fetus in a pregnant woman is protected with a layer of fat energy.

In the hibernation scenario, the higher-than-normal cholesterol production from higher-than-normal carbohydrate consumption would protect the exterior membrane walls of all of your cells from freezing, too. But, being truly diabetic is the real evolutionary strategy. The eventual out-of-control blood sugar of Type II diabetes is the end result of this hibernation preparation. If you were diabetic, you wouldn't freeze to death because of the natural antifreeze effect of glucose. A higher-than-normal concentration of blood sugar would keep the interior of your cells from freezing because of the effect carbohydrates have on water molecules.

All antifreeze, even what you use in your car, tastes sweet.

THE FROGS ARE TOO QUIET

Off the coast of Antarctica, fish play at the feet of the glaciers pouring into the sea. If you could take the temperature of their blood, you'd find it to be below freezing, yet unfrozen. On the other end of the globe, at the water's edge of an icy pond in Canada, wood frogs sit absolutely still, with not even a sign of smoky breath in the frozen air.

They are frozen stiff.

If you picked one up of these frogsicles in a gloved hand and hurled it against a tree, would it shatter? Thankfully, no one's tried it, but it would at least make a resounding *thud.* Believe it or not, as soon as the ice on the pond melts, so will the frogs. The blood in their veins will warm up as soon as their hearts start beating again and, within a day, their blood will run hot enough to mate.

The Antarctic fish and the frogs, along with cold-resistant insects and people, all share the protection of blood-borne antifreeze in the form of glucose. In the fish, it has another name—glycoprotein—but it functions the same in all of us. As blood starts to freeze, the formation of ice crystals actually *dehydrates* the red blood cells by sucking all of the water out of them.

Once frozen, the ice crystals are as sharp as microscopic shards of glass. These sharp crystals are formed when V-shaped molecules of water lock together at hydrogen bonding sites to form a snowflake-like latticework. The sharp points on the daggers of ice slice through the cell membrane walls, and the animal dies. This end would follow hypothermia and exposure, not hibernation. Hibernation is very different from hypothermia. In hypothermia, an unprepared animal *not in a diabetic state* just freezes.

In the hibernation scenario, the glucose from end-stage insulin resistance protects cells by lowering the freezing temperature of blood—just as it does the water in a car by coating the water molecules with sugar to keep them from sticking together to form jagged crystals. All of the extra cholesterol production from the consumed carbohydrates completes the mechanism by plugging leaks that would occur when the fat molecules that control the gates for ions and water going in and out of the cell membranes begin to congeal like cold meat drippings. The cells are then leak-proof and filled with antifreeze.

So the wood frogs only look hard as a brick; in reality, only the water *between* their cells has frozen. The frogs, like any other living thing with a sugar based antifreeze blood system, freeze in slo-mo. The colder their extremities get, the more sugar their livers pour into their bloodstreams to circulate as antifreeze.

When the frogs begin to thaw, the organs that were the last to freeze are the most syrupy with sugar and therefore the first to thaw. The heart actually begins to beat in order to pump warmed blood to thaw the extremities. That way, no part of the frog is ever deprived of oxygen. They literally thaw from the inside out.

Researcher Dr. Kenneth Storey at Carleton University in Ottawa says, "The frogs start out with the same amount of glucose we have, and then go right to being diabetic," just like people who never get out of hibernation mode—Type II diabetics. The constant consumption of carbohydrates can mean only one thing to ancient environmental controls—get ready to starve or freeze. That's why Type IIs become insulin resistant, to make fat; but when they have made enough, the next step is for their livers to pour more sugar into their bloodstreams than their pancreas and insulin system can handle. All of that glucose keeps the cells syrupy inside, just the way it does in the wood frogs, even though sixty-five percent of the frog has turned to ice.

TUNGUSKA

The results of the experimental freezing of human organs for later use also supports our premise. In one study, after six hours of being frozen solid, human liver cells were still able to produce bile in a culture dish. This means they were resoundingly resuscitated. Just as frogs and mammals use glucose as antifreeze, Arctic brine shrimp use a sugar called trehalose. Trehalose was used in an experiment at the University of California at San Diego by Dr. Gillian Beattie and Dr. Alberto Hayek, who in 1998 preserved human pancreatic beta cells in a trehalose solution. Every few months, Beattie revives a few cells to see if they're still viable. They are. They still produce insulin in a test tube and when implanted into a mouse and a rhesus monkey. If beta cells can still produce insulin after freezing, then blood sugar can still be dispersed back into other organs and limbs after the big chill for the big thaw. Remember, these are *human* beta cells.

Not so science fiction, now, is it?

The record for longest-frozen revived cells goes to the Russians. A bacterium discovered in Siberia near Tunguska in late 1980 was resurrected by Dr. David Gillichinsky, a microbiologist at the Russian Academy of Sciences in Moscow. He extracted frozen soil bacteria from 150 feet below the surface in permafrost that has been no warmer than 14 degrees Fahrenheit for at least 3 million years. Within hours of their arrival at the surface, they were happily dividing—because life goes on.

In 1992, the cryogenics company BioTime in Berkeley, California, chilled a baboon named Daniel down to a body temperature of 34 degrees Fahrenheit for 55 minutes. Although Daniel was physically unscathed, no one has, as yet, thoroughly examined his mental faculties. That's gotta leave a mark.

Our point is simply that Type II diabetes only occurs because the prehibernation phase of carbohydrate storage and the ensuing insulin resistance never results in actual hibernation. Instead, we stay in the state of fat accumulation, insulin resistance, and subclinical hypertension in the heat indoors, year-round. Most people maintaining this state for decades will eventually become Type II diabetics, and their doctors will blame it on aging.

WHILE YOU WEREN'T SLEEPING

Carbohydrates and insulin comprise the tools we need to survive scarcity *only if* we know when the time is coming. There must be a clocking mechanism in place to prompt us when scarcity is around the corner. The hormones melatonin and prolactin are the drivers of our body's time perception—our clocking mechanism. The public has no real idea what effect that over-the-counter melatonin they're buying for jet lag really has. It just compounds the problem. It actually decreases natural production by shrinking the gland in your head that makes melatonin—the pineal gland.

In order to view the clocking process as it was meant to be, let's jump on the merry-go-round (feedback loop). The handhold to grab for this ride is the time of day. If you were to jump on at 6:00 P.M., depending on the time of year and your latitude (location), the light of the sun would be starting to fall, or diminish. Just prior to sundown is dinnertime in all cultures. The *quality,* or spectrum of the light is shifting, too, as the sun makes a break for it. In this daydream, we've had an okay day hunting and are now joining the group for a bite.

Let's assume you get a bite.

Insulin would rise to deal with the incoming carbohydrates you had dried last summer to eat later and cortisol would start to fall because you've been fed. That's why we all go for sugar when we're stressed. Remember, we're imaging the mythical *natural* world here, not ours. In our world, cortisol never falls until we're completely, unconsciously asleep—and even then, because of light leaks, not completely.

As the sun sneaks off, you and your significant other might try to prolong the day and warmth by huddling around a small fire entertaining each other. By reliving the day's events, you further commit them to memory and exercise your imagination by embellishing them. Sex could be an option, depending again on the season, the climate, and how charming you are.

You'd have to expend too much energy to collect enough wood to waste very much of it on late-day procrastination around a campfire. So your evening reverie won't last very long. As the pink light of sunset comes over the landscape, you start to get really sleepy, because while the reflected "green" bright light of day shuts off melatonin production (at the preoptic site connection to the pineal gland in your brain), the "rose" light of the setting sun *blocks* the green spectrum, causing a release of melatonin to ease you into the night's altered state. Having evolved *with,* not "in response to," the changes in light-and-dark cycles and weather and food supply, it makes perfect sense that the reflected green-and-blue light of day and the rose-yellow-orange of sunset elicit hormonal and neurotransmitter responses we can identify as common behavior.

Of course, Western medicine doesn't accept our premise of neuropeptide cross-talk being the basis of the mind-body connection, so to them the illumination of the interaction between us and cosmological events is like reading them their horoscope. At the opposite extreme, Eastern medicine rejects the linear perspective for a more dynamic and accurate synthesis, but it is unintelligible to Western researchers, who insist on dividing and categorizing parts of physiology in the living as though they were dealing with a cadaver built from mechanical parts like a car.

But back at the Paleolithic campsite, you'd look for a warm spot to settle down because rising melatonin is already cooling you off. Huddling together for warmth also reinforces pheromone communication. In those days, you would literally have been able to *smell* an enemy or a lover. Early sleep is usually REM sleep, so premonitions or hallucinatory "visions" continue the evening's earlier entertainment as your brain sorts and tags the mind's perceptions. Drifting into even deeper NREM sleep as your melatonin surges shifts your brain activity to immune maintenance.

All reproductive activity is slowed at night. That means a better chance for pregnancy would be offered by *daytime mating.* At night, sex steroid hormones take a backseat to increased prolactin production from the pituitary. Both prolactin and melatonin are powerful players in reproduction, too, due to the simple fact that melatonin controls the production of estrogen and testosterone and prolactin makes milk. Melatonin and progesterone are both master-switch hormonal controllers. If either one is out of sync, it reads to nature as "pushing the red button." A chronic lack of melatonin or progesterone, such as that which occurs with aging, tells nature you are not viable anymore.

When you're not a player, nature takes you out.

Because of melatonin, any increase or decrease in dark time triggers physiologic and behavioral changes via sex hormones in many species, like changes in molting, breeding, and migration. Seasonal distribution of conception and birth rates in humans supports the theory that the function of melatonin is to regulate the time of readiness for reproduction, even today. Readiness for reproduction, in turn, determines the amount and timing of progesterone release in women and dihydrotestosterone (DHT) secretion in men.

So going to sleep with the sunset means a whole-body melatonin bath, and a sharp increase in prolactin. Prolactin is not only active in human milk production, it is essential in all mammals for lactation. In birds, nursing takes the form of "brooding behavior," the stillness needed to incubate the eggs. The most major effect of prolactin in all species is to enhance production of T cells and NK (natural killer) cells. These are the first lines of cancer defense. Since there is no cancer in nature among other species except our pets, you, belonging to the pantheon of global life, won't have cancer, either, if you sleep fourteen hours a night in dormant periods. But could you really stay asleep that long?

Sort of. First of all, caves are dark, our bedrooms aren't. We try to sleep with the lights on all of the time—if we even go to bed at all. Not only do we live in endless summer, we live at endless lunch. There's always food, usually carbohydrates, and, lightwise, it's always straight-up noon. Not only have we lost half a year every year to lights and indoor heating and cooling, we've lost the night to blinking digital timers, police sirens, streetlights, headlights, illuminated billboards, restaurants, motels, night baseball, and TV, the Internet, and movies, which used to be our stories around the dying campfire. The real problem is that the campfire never dies because the TV is always on.

THE TRUTH REALLY IS OUT THERE

Studies in 1993 and 1994 reported that human volunteers at the NIH were monitored for hormonal release and brain activity by Dr. Thomas Wehr. The volunteers slept eight hours (a short night) and fourteen hours (a long night). The first result was the obvious: Longer periods of melatonin secretion upped white cell macrophage and lymphocyte production.

This is a good thing.

The second most obvious difference hormonally between short and long nights was the amount and length of prolactin secretion. This change in melatonin and prolactin secretion reflected the long night's fragmented sleep pattern. The long-night subjects spent as many as five of the fourteen hours lying *almost* awake. Wehr's group slept in two nightly bouts, each preceded by up to two and a half hours of wakefulness, with a high secretion of prolactin throughout. That means they got a total of about nine hours of actual sleep as we know it. And, in our time, nine hours of sleep is all we know. The sleepless five hours were very much like the awake-alert quiet state infants display repeatedly in a twenty-four-hour period. The brain-wave readings were akin to those observed during transcendental meditation. Interrupting the subjects' reveries—by talking to them—*caused prolactin levels to drop.*

Wehr's study goes on to suggest that "prolactin in humans probably facilitates a switch to 'quiescent wakefulness,' just as it prompts brooding behavior in birds." The NIH doctor does agree that the fourteen-hour dark period in winter, or at least seven months out of the year, is exactly what our ancestors would have experienced before the invention of artificial light sources. This awake-alert period in adults is now an *extinct sleep state.*

It is statistically proven that ninety or so percent of all babies are born between midnight and 4:00 A.M., the exact time their mothers would, in nature, be in a meditative state with high endorphin (painkiller) levels, just like yogis who are able to walk over beds of nails and hot coals without any effect. In this state, an unmedicated birth would be far more tolerable. It was in this period of time, which we no longer have access to, that we solved problems, reproduced, and transcended the stress, and, most likely, talked to the gods.

In follow-up standardized tests designed to evaluate mood and fatigue, subjects exposed to fourteen-hour nights rated themselves as happier, more energetic, and more wide awake during the following day. But those tests were designed to uncover only debilitating sleepiness. Sleepiness is only a cognitive symptom. When you're tired, you really are experiencing massive metabolic derangement between you and the bacteria controlling your immune system and reproduction, which is translating to mental aberrations.

Short nights that mimic summer mean:

- Reduced melatonin secretion, which reduces white cell immune function;

- A severe reduction in the most potent antioxidant you have—melatonin;

- Less prolactin at night and way too much in the daytime (prolactin secretion at night means more and stronger NK and T cells. Prolactin secretion during the day means autoimmunity and carbohydrate craving).

But the biggest problem with short nights year-round, beyond appetite derangement, is that insulin will stay higher during the dark, when it should be flat, and cortisol falls so late it won't come up normally in the morning. This is a *reversal* of normal hormonal rhythms. You *should* wake up with elevated cortisol to deal with stress during the day. You *should* wake up hungry with low insulin and cortisol rising. Instead, your cortisol is low and your insulin is still up.

In this state, breakfast is easy to skip; with high insulin, you're not hungry.

The reversal you've created by staying up late—making your insulin and cortisol stay high at night, when they should be low—continues into the daylight hours. The first symptom of melatonin overflow is needing an alarm to wake you up. When you have a melatonin "hangover," you're still too sleepy to wake up even though morning light should suppress melatonin spontaneously. The real problem is that without a rise in cortisol, you have no dopamine.

Your cortisol is not high enough to deal with stress during the day and even whacks time perception. Without cortisol to enhance dopamine, the day seems to go *too* fast.

Tell us you've never experienced this.

With your prolactin abnormally high in the morning, and no dopamine, you're kind of stupid, too, with no memory or ability to plan. The same scenario reruns in the afternoon. Prolactin abnormally suppresses leptin again; so around 3:00 P.M., you really crave carbohydrates and get impatient and even dumber.

Does any of this matter?

What's the difference *when* you have hormones surge, as long as they surge?

Unfortunately, timing is everything.

You can't make melatonin in the daytime or with the lights on. So how are you still sleeping with the light of the sun shining? Well, hunger should be your alarm clock. One of the evolutionary functions of melatonin is that it enhances the appetite-suppressing effect of leptin so you *stay* asleep instead of roaming around hungry all night. It's a feedback loop: Melatonin enhances leptin and leptin keeps your brain in the "fed" stage, so you stay asleep and make more melatonin.

Unfortunately for us, less sleep at night—and therefore less melatonin and less leptin—makes you eat more, day and night. Just losing sleep at the beginning of your night is enough to make you hungrier for sugar and you get fat. That's what we said: Sleep loss makes you fat. But really, that's not the half of it. Once you start to eat carbohydrates day in and day out, you start to retain water.

This is a bad thing.

WATERWORLD

Almost everybody in the Western world, male and female, has at one time or another gone on a high-protein, low-carbohydrate diet and seen a weight loss of anywhere from ten to fifteen pounds in two weeks' time.

The biochemical principle that these eating regimens have stumbled upon is the very first phase of the prehibernation process—water retention. The minute you cut your carbohydrate intake down to less than 45 grams a day, you signal your entire endocrine system that famine and winter are coming and you unwind the clock. That, too, is exactly what a high-protein, low-carbohydrate diet does. The calorie counters and low-fat advocates have dismissed high-protein diets for years as nonscientific and dangerous. The naysayers usually point out the potential for kidney damage to the unwary public. The potential for kidney damage would be remote even if the diet went on for more than seven months with absolutely no carbohydrate intake, but that's not possible; even cashew nuts have carbohydrates. In this world, staying completely carbohydrate-free for seven months is not only very unlikely, it's not possible.

In fact, contrary to popular medical wisdom, not only won't you damage your kidneys, but without the incoming carbohydrates, you will drop ten or so pounds of retained fluid, dropping your blood pressure and burning your fat base, a process that throws off ketones and reduces your serotonin too, so you're not as paranoid and depressed. The blood pressure drop is a respite for your kidney function. But even if you stop eating carbohydrates, your cortisol, insulin, and your prolactin won't drop to winter levels *unless you sleep at least 9.5 hours a night,* starting as close to dusk as possible.

This means that the long hours of artificial light alone, without massive carbohydrate consumption, can raise your blood pressure *somewhat,* because cortisol, which is always up when the lights are on, is part of your sympathetic nervous system control of blood pressure. So you're really not out of the woods unless you increase your sleep.

When this ancient clocking system kicks in, you crave the foods that will spike your insulin to create "resistance" to insulin in your muscles, so that you send all the energy to store as fat for the long famine you would endure in the real world. When this goes on day after day, week after week, decade after decade, *even if you never get fat,* your cortisol is up and you're retaining the ten or so pounds of water weight that you would need to hibernate.

That ten pounds of fluid will change salt and glucose absorption in your gut and kidney function for hibernation, but in reality causes what we identify as the subclinical hypertension most Americans experience today.

These states of being—carbohydrate consumption, insulin resistance, cholesterol production, water retention, subclinical hypertension—are all prehibernation preparations that add up to heart disease because kidney function controls blood pressure through the hormones called angiotensin I and II, which read back to your heart to gauge calcium ion flow—or how hard your heart pumps. This cascade is another ancient mechanism that's tripped on your way to "virtual freezing." The calcium changes that gauge how hard your heart pumps also are in play to protect your brain from oxygen deprivation when you freeze by pouring calcium out of your cells to prevent hypoxia, or oxygen deprivation.

APOCALYPSE PRETTY DARN SOON

All of us lie awake when we should be sleeping pondering that same question: *How close are we, really, to "death's door"?* Assuming our statistics in the first chapter are accurate, pretty close. The solution medicine has latched on to is really just an antidote to their low-fat regime. It is, quite simply, to exercise hysterically. All that medicine ever suggests you do is live on sugar and run like hell to burn it off. Of course, burning off all of the carbohydrates you've taken as a result of sleep loss by hysterical exercising does *seem* to reverse the process physiologically. As your weight goes down, so does insulin production, because you produce insulin in a relationship of grams to body weight.

When insulin goes down, your insulin receptors go back up; then blood sugar also falls because your muscles soak it up as you exercise through the now-functioning insulin receptors. This is the way exercise lowers blood sugar. When your insulin is lower, you can't make as much cholesterol and that number goes down, too. Then the doctor declares you cured. *But you're not cured.*

Now you just have a new disease—because it never occurred to them that you don't have to work off what you don't take in the first place. In reality, running, jumping, or StairMastering is, to your body—which still responds with ancient subroutines—a "fear response" that throws your cortisol into the stratosphere while you see God. High cortisol is a blood-sugar mobilizer, so it throws your blood sugar up again; when your blood sugar goes up, insulin follows. That means the continuous rebounding of excessive exercise *alone* can made you insulin resistant over time. Here's how it looks:

- Running, jumping, climbing = being chased

- Chase = stress response

- Stress = Cortisol release = blood-sugar mobilization

- Blood sugar up = insulin up = insulin resistance = fat storage and hypertension

Face it, you would never go from your chair to the door *really fast* unless something was chasing you. This cortisol fear trigger is the big key to mental illness and heart disease. When the lights are on too long in twenty-four hours, it's summer. During summer we mated and ate until we burst. The light, fighting, and eating sugar meant our cortisol never dropped for three to five months out of the year. You, on the other hand, live, in your head, in constant fear and panic on the verge of death.

In the next two chapters, we'll show you how it is the *mental panic* of constantly running away from nothing that really destroys your heart and mind. Just think about what you're doing, in a day, in your life, and how it must be perceived by your body. Obviously, stopping for a low-fat Power Frappuccino at Starbucks on your way to the gym after work, say, at seven or eight at night, and then exercising like hell in bright lights for an hour or so is probably not really accomplishing what you hoped for, is it?

In fact, we're willing to bet that by the time you get home (it's got to be 9:30 or 10:00 P.M. by now) you've probably been awake for sixteen hours already. You are beyond tired and the lights are *still* on. It is at this point that your psyche will kick in to try to save you from yourself and put you to sleep by telling you to look for a "snack." Your mind will now send you to the refrigerator for sugar or, worse, looking for a drink.

When you do find yourself standing at the refrigerator, like a zombie, in that blast of cold air not even sure how you got there, *know* that the reason you're there *is staring right back at you.*

The same artificial light illuminating your way to that last piece of cake started the whole process—from the need to exercise to the "need" for a sweet midnight snack.

You're not hungry, you're just too tired, but inside, your body knows that the cake will send your insulin up to turn serotonin into melatonin and—finally—put you to sleep.

A good ten years of the behavior we just described and you may not recover.

IT *IS* ALL IN YOUR HEAD:

No Sleep and Too Much Sugar Make You Go Crazy

"Jesus, didn't they think it might do damage? Didn't the public raise Cain about it?"

"I don't think you fully understand the public, my friend; in this country, when something is out of order, then the quickest way to get it fixed is the best way . . . It's absolutely painless."
—Ken Kesey,
One Flew Over the Cuckoo's Nest

As you already understand, if you stay up too late, your hormones shift and cause your appetite to change. The sugars you crave send your insulin up to create the insulin resistance you need to get fat. On your way to tubby, you convert all the carbohydrates you've eaten into cholesterol as VLDLs, and you retain water, which alters your blood pressure. At this point, any doctor would tell you there's heart disease on the horizon.

We agree.

But we're going to tell you the first symptom of heart disease isn't high blood pressure and high cholesterol, it's *depression.*

FARSCAPE

When you live in prehibernation mode, but never get to go dormant, you go crazy. You go crazy because you have stayed up so long. You see, in nature, staying up that long would mean you've eaten half of the planet, which is way more than your share. And you are most likely no longer fertile from swimming in all that insulin. Therefore, you have no business living. So nature takes you out by altering your reality so you won't want to live anymore. You actually go crazy so *you* will take you out.

It's the "less work for the hostess" principle manifested in Mother Nature.

The way nature effects this mechanism in your body is by ultimately creating a bipolar state of mind. Nature doubles the odds of your suicide with a bipolar state, inasmuch as your mania means a complete loss of impulse control—so if you don't do yourself in while in the throes of despair during the depressive state, you'll probably make some dangerous, life-threatening move while you're high as a kite. Either way, nature wins.

And don't forget the cortisol principle: When the sun never sets or you never turn the lights off, your cortisol never drops. High cortisol only occurs in nature when you need it to run away or deal with pain. High cortisol is meant to be episodic, not chronic. In nature, chronic high cortisol would mean you're a reproductive loser (the best reason to take you out) and social outcast.

However, in depression, it works more surreptitiously. Having chronic high cortisol and chronic high insulin together puts your mind in the constant "panic" state of summer mating. The lights are on, the food (carbohydrates) must be plentiful because your insulin's up, and, naturally, because of the light and all of the exercise your cortisol is up for competition. You've triggered ancient programs and subroutines that would only ever switch on in true states of peril—like "run for your life," or "your DNA won't show up in the next generation." When your seasonal insulin/cortisol "clock" is off, *real mental illness,* not just gross mood swings, but true manic depression and schizophrenia can occur.

PSYCHO KILLER, *QU'EST-CE QUE C'EST?*

The National Institutes of Mental Health agree with us that the primary cause of depression, manic depression, and schizophrenia is simply being out of light and dark rhythmicity. The NIMH completed a recent (1996) fifty-page study reviewing the effects of the most widely prescribed antidepressants. The purpose of this massive undertaking was to understand exactly how these drugs—selective serotonin reuptake inhibitors (SSRIs), monamine oxidase inhibitors (MAO inhibitors), and tricyclic antidepressants—affect depression. It seems that their efficacy, *all of it,* rests solely in their ability to reinstate normal sleep rhythms in distraught, tired, out-of-sync brains. When you sleep, you feel better and more sane. Well, duh. Your mother told you that.

This document is very important because in it the researchers admit that all mental illnesses, from garden-variety depression to schizophrenia, stem from the common "symptom" of sleep dysfunction (read: loss). All the drugs known to positively affect depression and its many forms show results simply because they put your sleep cycles *back in rhythm.*

It seems they conclude, as we do, that when you can't sleep, you go crazy.

And, conversely, when you're crazy, you can't sleep.

Think of it as The Secret of NIMH.

See, your mind is *not* your brain, it is the echo that follows one beat behind the biochemical and biophysical actions in the body and brain. Your mind is a receiver that amplifies and gives a context to everything going on in your body and in the environment. It is like a television set of sorts, which receives signals from a remote source (body and planet and other living things). When we watch television, we all know that there are no little people in there. It's hard to realize, but the same is true of your head.

There are major players and trendy buzzwords—serotonin, dopamine, GABA, and melatonin—to identify the loops in the machinery, but the bottom line is still the same: *Sleep controls food supply and reproduction, which control your mental state.* In this chapter, we're aiming for the same impact that the Reagan-era antidrug campaign had, only here, we're illuminating your messed-up mind and showing you that "this is your brain on high insulin and no melatonin."

Nancy told you to "just say no." Our advice is:

Just say good night.

Mental illness is the western hemisphere's second most disabling illness after heart disease. That's no coincidence. The important words in the last sentence are "western hemisphere," "mental illness," and "heart disease." We know how both mental illness and heart disease are caused in tandem by overexposure to light on our half of the planet.

ALIEN VOICES II

The most debilitating form of mental illness is schizophrenia. This disease affects 2.7 million Americans. Schizophrenia is, most often, an extreme form of manic depression, which is also known as bipolar disorder. Schizophrenia is, simply put, an excessive, unregulated amount of dopamine in the brain leading to episodes of mania that come complete with hallucinations, including sounds and smells. We've found research to support the supposition that schizophrenics' over-the-top dopamine production means they are, in the truest sense of the word, unbalanced.

When you overeat carbohydrates, not only does your body become insulin resistant, but your brain can, too. In the brain, serotonin and dopamine stand on opposite sides of the board on the log. If one's up, the other's down. It's the duality again. Too much serotonin and you're paralyzed, too much dopamine and you're stuck to the ceiling. Serotonin and insulin are on the same side of the equation (or board on a log) in metabolism. They are also on the same side of the brain. Insulin, therefore—because hormones can be neurotransmitters, too—can suppress dopamine levels, just as serotonin does. But neither serotonin nor insulin can suppress dopamine if there are no receptors to register their presence.

If the only controls on dopamine in our brains are taken out of play, and there's no keeper at the zoo, the possible scenarios you can concoct are legion. Schizophrenia is the ultimate state of insulin resistance in the brain. It is, in effect, cerebral diabetes (Type II), the result of endless summer in your head. You see, sleep loss really *can* drive you nuts.

In support of our theory, schizophrenia has recently been linked to the time of birth.

Works for us.

Until now, it was believed that family history (genetics) was the best predictor of whether or not a person would develop schizophrenia; but now the experts are willing to concede that environmental influences like place and season of birth may be more significant factors than they ever thought possible. A study, in the February 25, 1999, *New England Journal of Medicine* found that people who are born in the dead of winter, particularly February or March, and especially in urban areas, have a significantly higher risk of schizophrenia than people with a familial history of the disease. The study was done in Denmark and covered 1.75 million subjects, all of whom were born between 1935 and 1978 and are the children of Danish women. This time period concurs with the advent of electric lighting in Europe and an increase of carbohydrates year-round. We think that's why people born in Copenhagen, Denmark's capital, were 2.4 times as likely to develop schizophrenia as those born in rural areas, where it gets dark at night and a smaller selection of imported fruits and vegetables is available. The alteration of the evolutionary process must originate in the fetal arena. Some factor of genetics is severely affected by long hours of light during pregnancy.

We think that those of us with the greatest genetic predisposition to a very low threshold of light toxicity (extremely light intolerant) would also probably be leftover seasonal breeders from the time before fire. Therefore, giving birth during the season when hibernation would normally occur probably holds some evolutionary penalty.

Obviously, gestational illumination, followed by being born "out of season" and then being reared in an urban environment (twenty-four-hour light, year-round, and never-ceasing carbohydrate consumption), is enough to push some of us over the edge of the seesaw to brain-derived insulin resistance, or cerebral diabetes. While the rest of us just get depressed, overwhelmingly, bone-crushingly depressed, some of us actually slip the tether.

When the light that controls appetite, which controls insulin, stays permanently switched on, the production of neurotransmitters like serotonin and dopamine, which are controlled by insulin (the food supply), become wildly unstable.

On the way to garden-variety exhaustion, *so do you.*

ZOMBIES

Seventy million Americans admit they are tired. Seventeen million of those seventy million are on Prozac and a few million more are on Paxil or Serzone. This means they're depressed, too, or that a little more than a fourth of those tired people are already over the edge. We think the real numbers are even higher because just about everybody in America takes something to sleep once in a while, which says that there are a hell of a lot more who are clinically depressed. For those who do seek help beyond the over-the-counter remedies, doctors prescribe antidepressants to raise their serotonin levels and they come back feeling better.

That's where the confusion starts.

Depressed, tired people *do not* have low serotonin levels.

Depressed people have low dopamine.

Dopamine, throughout evolution, stayed high in the light, just like cortisol. It's dopamine that lays in reward pathways for memory and controls time perception with cortisol. While the lights are on and we can see, dopamine stays up and we continue to learn and remember. This mechanism is why the light is so seductive, why it's so hard to turn it off and go to bed. The blinking lights from video games, the TV, and your computer are all addictive simply because of the dopamine release they cause. The blinking lights can have the same addictive potential as drinking, gambling, or drugs.

The evolutionary edge the light from fire gave us was to extend the day. An extended day increased learning and brain size, increased reproduction, and, when we brought it inside the cave, its warmth gave us the upper hand with the weather, too.

The trade-off for our seat at the table of the gods is the havoc wreaked with our brain chemistry and our heart physiology. Remember: Light is the eternal *zeitgeber,* or timer, that controls dopamine and cortisol release. Cortisol is the stress hormone and dopamine is the daytime neurotransmitter. Dopamine and serotonin, just like cortisol and insulin, rest on that board on the log. Dopamine and serotonin are balanced and rebalanced in the brain according to environmental cues. So when you screw with dopamine, you screw with serotonin, too. It's part of the plan.

When the sun jacks up your dopamine, you become impulsive and hungry. It's daytime and, depending on the duration of the light, it could be summer. Dopamine controls protein craving just as neuropeptide Y controls carbohydrate intake. With your dopamine up, your serotonin falls, so you want meat. Dopamine gives you the competitive edge to get it and trade it for sex. To have a libido, dopamine must be high. That's why serotonin enhancers cause impotence.

People with genuinely low serotonin levels are happy people because low serotonin levels mean high dopamine levels on that board on a log. Everybody likes to be high on dopamine. It's an experience somewhere between taking speed and being in love.

It's serotonin, in any great amount, that's a *downer.*

And if you don't make melatonin out of your serotonin by sleeping . . . well, you know.

MIND CONTROL

Serotonin is much misunderstood in the media. Most people in this country and probably a fair number of doctors believe that low serotonin levels in the brain are the cause of depression and anxiety, when just the opposite is true. Higher-than-normal levels of serotonin mean danger because the food supply is up and it must be mating season, so the readiness for competition rules all your systems.

Serotonin is the neurotransmitter in charge of impulse control—because to have serotonin you must have high insulin, which means there's carbohydrates and it's summer, which means *be careful,* don't screw up mating or fighting or it might be the end of you. The way serotonin controls your impulsiveness is very sneaky. Serotonin does it by reducing your ability to make connections. Memory retrieval is blunted because high serotonin filters out sensory input. Dopamine, on the other hand, puts everything in sharp focus. Primitive drives and emotions that govern sleep, mood, appetite, arousal, pain, aggression, and even suicidal behavior are all under the control of serotonin and dopamine. Neurotransmitters are molecules akin to hormones in their action, in that they have a target (receptor)—and once they hit that target, your behavior is changed.

Although serotonin is very much a seasonal controller of appetite and sleep, the trouble starts physiologically, at least for your heart, when it comes into play as a panic response, which would only happen when the light is long. Serotonin levels *always* match insulin levels, and there are receptors for it all over the body and brain. You feel serotonin's effects on cells in the gastrointestinal tract when you're worried or actually afraid. Not only is there the butterfly effect (think stage fright), but actual gut motility slows to a crawl because our cave guy couldn't stop to defecate if he were running for his life from a tiger. And it's serotonin that causes your veins and arteries to clamp down, just in case you don't win the race with the tiger or the fight for the egg. There's another timer in play in panic mode, too. If the panic goes on long enough, the surface of your blood platelets will get sticky due to serotonin resistance, which ensues from the panicked outpouring of serotonin. Then the platelets clot faster so you don't bleed to death. Symptoms of higher than normal daytime levels of serotonin, which are classic in panicked animals and depressed people alike, are:

- *Withdrawal,* which can be defined as avoiding danger or escaping from it

- *Immobility,* which means freezing or seeming paralyzed

- *Defensiveness,* implying both aggression and submission

All of these behaviors are evident across all species and in human depression as well. The term "scared stiff" says it all. High serotonin causes a rigidity of behavior that can be repetitive, as in people with obsessive-compulsive disorder (OCD), or paralytic, as in the severely depressed. All the symptoms of high serotonin—a tight stomach, a pounding heart, high blood pressure, clammy hands and feet, and the big tip-off, dry mouth—are textbook symptoms in our world of a classic panic attack.

In real danger, serotonin would make our cave guy run faster, breathe deeper, and bleed less. When a rat is caught in the open by a predator, the serotonin rises in his brain and he freezes, apparently *paralyzed* by fear; in reality, this behavior has been time-tested over eons to save his life. By freezing in suspended animation, the rat believes he is evading all the predators whose vision depends on motion for detection. Most depressives describe their state as "withdrawn and paralyzed." These feelings are absolutely accurate—thanks to high serotonin.

When it is functioning at "normal" levels, serotonin keeps the instinct for drives like eating, sex, and aggression subdued enough for survival. The only reason pop culture has defined serotonin as the "happy" neurotransmitter is the Rodney King mantra. The world we live in requires excessive impulse control to " just get along."

There is no room for impulsive, instinctive behavior in a crowded world dependent on interpersonal relationships like ours. However, in the real world where most of us came from but now never go to, low levels of serotonin are adaptive, because the real world is a threatening place. Until now, we have evolved very nicely on low levels of serotonin during daylight hours. With low impulse control, you can get out of the way faster or respond more quickly to a threat. None of us would be here to debate the merits of high or low serotonin if we hadn't come from low-serotonin stock. In this world, half of us are miserable because we have no impulse control and this life requires it, and the other half of us are, literally, paralyzed and paranoid from carbohydrates and light.

So is the answer for those of us who are paralyzed to find a drug to lower our serotonin?

You don't have to.

Nature will do it for you, whether you like it or not. All you have to do is stay in any chronic state of hormone overload long enough to lose our rhythm and nature asks us to sit down. This process is called homeostasis. We've encountered it before.

Since every system in nature, including evolution itself, is an iterative algorithm or infinite feedback loop, there exists the necessity of *negative* feedback. There has to be a stop mechanism to keep balancing on that board on a log. In the case of stress and serotonin or cortisol, if we get too much of a good thing the receptor becomes resistant to the action of said hormone or neurotransmitter. So unending stress can make you numb to cortisol or serotonin. And the only *true stress* in the natural world comes from too much mating, eating or being eaten, and, of course, not sleeping when everything else does. Losing sleep would be an impossibility in the natural world, unless you were nursing a baby or watching out for that nocturnal predator who made off with your buddy Eddie's arm last night, because with everything as black as pitch, there's nothing else to do.

We live on an entirely different plane of existence. Too bad our bodies and minds haven't caught up yet.

BLITZED NEW WORLD

Serotonin is very important in the modern world. You need impulse control on the subway or in an office or stuck in traffic. Those of us with very low serotonin pull guns on each other and plan massacres. That's also why we all self-medicate with sugar in times of stress. When you're stuck in a traffic jam and pull off at the exit out of frustration, the substance to ease your pain is more likely than not a Big Gulp or a candy bar. Few of us buy string cheese or beef jerky to cope. The insulin produced as a result of the carbohydrate you've eaten makes serotonin, and you get instant impulse control. This is an ancient balancing mechanism.

- When the light was long, we ate sugar (carbohydrates).

- The high sugar meant high insulin.

- It takes insulin to convert the protein that you ate (because your dopamine was up) into serotonin.

- The serotonin balanced the dopamine and diminished during sleep.

- The next day, like every day then, was a new day. And we'd start all over again.

Now, existing only in endless summer, we're caught in only one phase of this particular feedback loop—serotonin making. In nature, this balancing act between serotonin and dopamine would only happen when the hours of light were long, and the hours of light were never long—unless it was mating season or there was impending danger.

There is hardly anyone left in America who is in a nice, normal, low-serotonin/high-dopamine state during daylight hours. Today, those of us not paralyzed from serotonin up to our eyeballs or in complete bipolar rebound are completely *fried*, receptor-wise.

Nature says if serotonin is high, dopamine must be low.

The only time this rule is broken is when receptor burnout occurs. Then the negative feedback loop, or off switch, is broken. When we are under chronic, inescapable stress, serotonin output eventually drops altogether from the feedback loop of serotonin resistance and allows dopamine to search for an escape. The chronic high serotonin of our chronic high-carbohydrate diets creates serotonin resistance wholesale in this country. You remember from our description of insulin resistance that receptors resistant to the action of the hormone read none of the hormone. So you have virtually none.

When scientists first tested serotonin-lowering drugs, which had the potential to treat depression, on rats, they seemed to act as aphrodisiacs. In a serotonin-absent state, the rats displayed terrifying sexual frenzy. Unfortunately, bottomed-out serotonin didn't signal just high times sexually, the low-serotonin state of nonexistent impulse control also unleashed lust's longtime companion—aggression.

Love and hate are really sex and defense in socially acceptable forms. Both activities require a loss of impulse control (no serotonin) and a huge hit of dopamine. Remember that high dopamine brings everything into sharp focus. Complete serotonin resistance means that aggression, or release of inhibition resulting from the complete lack of serotonin, will be layered with the "sensory overload" of rising dopamine. The resulting *in*sensitivity is compounded by perceiving every sensory stimulus *over*-sensitively, creating in the human mind a constant twitchy, aggressive, paranoid state.

This formula—no sleep and an all-sugar-all-the-time diet—could alone account for our particular brand of American violence. Living on a ninety-percent-carbohydrate diet not only signifies the stress of mating season to your whole being and creates the serotonin resistance that begets aggression, it means cortisol burnout for your brain, too, so there's no way to cope with the stress. At that point, we end up with road rage, vandalism, heightened racism, and the next generation killing each other. If everyone in the country witnesses this endless violence three times a day on TV and is exposed to simulated violence (movies) late at night, when we should all be sleeping, the situation is further compounded. Look at the children who witnessed the peer-group massacre in Littleton, Colorado, in 1999. They'll never be the same.

Children exposed to ongoing generation-to-generation violence have the same burned-out stress-response system seen in war veterans with post-traumatic shock syndrome. The normal evolutionary switches that prime the body and mind for danger stay switched on and *experience becomes biology.* Will the Littleton, Colorado, witnesses lead violent lives and thereby "infect" their children?

Remember that whether or not a gene (in this case, the gene for serotonin production) will be expressed is wholly dependent on environmental cues—or what kind of early life experiences an individual faces in his household.

Whether he lives with hostile or violent people or whether his early experiences are calm and reasonable can make all the difference in the world. This pronouncement crosses species barriers, as seen in a vivid snapshot of animal behavior captured in *Inside the Brain* by Dr. Ronald Kotulak. This vignette provides clear evidence of the environmental-genetic link to violent aggression. In the Grand Canyon tiger salamander, we see nature's version of our own Dr. Jekyll and Mr. Hyde.

The salamanders live in ponds along an isolated rim of the Grand Canyon. When food and water are plentiful, the salamander is in its Dr. Jekyll form—a gregarious, peace-loving insect eater. But when the water begins to dry up, food becomes scarce and living conditions become unbearably competitive and cramped, some of the salamanders go through an amazing Mr. Hyde transformation.

Environmental pressures rapidly alter the function of some of their genes, creating changes in their physical shape and making them aggressive. Muscles enlarge to make their heads and mouths bigger and they grow a new set of huge teeth, adaptations that allow them to attack and eat their fellow salamanders.

They become cannibals, but only for a short time. Once they've gobbled up enough salamanders to reduce crowding, they turn back into Dr. Jekyll. Their heads shrink to normal size and they dine on insects again.

Now, that's environment controlling gene expression.

THAT'S WHY THEY CALL IT DOPE

Never-ending higher-than-normal serotonin (produced from all the carbohydrates we consume because the lights are on) makes you feel so sad because you live day in and day out as though you are under threat. If that threat lasts too long, homeostasis rebounds you back to a state of very, very low or no serotonin to leave you ultimately exploding in violence or completely schizophrenic.

In garden-variety depression, your symptoms are responses that are ancient manifestations of fear and panic resulting from high serotonin. A chronic high serotonin state reads as endless stress or a threat you'll never work your way out of, no matter what. The lives we lead and the food we eat create, through a high-serotonin state, a permanently hopeless state of mind.

That's why an increasing number of us seek medical help for depression.

Antidepressants work on serotonin levels through selective serotonin reuptake inhibitors (SSRIs). The term "reuptake" refers to the return of serotonin to the neuron after its message has been sent. The way these drugs work is to increase the already higher-than-normal serotonin to an even more excessive over-the-top state by blocking the receptors that reuptake (suck up) serotonin and take it out of the space between neurons for reuse. A selective serotonin inhibitor works to inhibit serotonin's return to only certain receptors. The actual amount of serotonin you produce is not increased; what you have hangs around longer, giving you more bang for the buck. With a more constant level of serotonin around, your receptors aim for homeostasis and they get it. In this "maxed-out" state, you experience serotonin receptor resistance, which quiets those receptors.

Serotonin resistance, in this case, means that the physical and mental panic and paranoia brought out of genetic collective memory by a chronic high serotonin state ends, or is at least dulled. Because you no longer register the high serotonin at the receptor level, the danger is, in virtual reality, over.

The same feeling of well-being sets in as if serotonin were, in reality, at a normal low level.

The way to turn "as if" into reality is to turn the lights out.

Sleep normalizes serotonin levels because the melatonin produced during sleep can only be made by using up the available serotonin. That's why people who are depressed tend to self-medicate by either sleeping all the time or not sleeping at all. Both options work just like antidepressants. Not sleeping at all in a twenty-four-hour period causes the serotonin to build up to antidepressant burnout levels because it never gets to turn into melatonin. When it gets high enough, it "washes over the top" and the overload causes your receptors to go down and—*voilà!*—it's just like it's low, or just like you're on Prozac.

"Escape sleeping," or sleeping all day and some of the night, works even better, because the serotonin you're soaked in will cascade into melatonin, putting you in a low- or normal-serotonin state, at least for a while. But most of us don't have the latitude to sleep all day, unless we've been fired or divorced, so we need a little "something" just to survive. As Aldous Huxley lamented in *Brave New World:*

> Civilization has absolutely no need of nobility or heroism. There aren't any wars nowadays. The greatest care is taken to keep you from loving any one thing too much. There's no such thing as a divided allegiance; you're so conditioned that you can't help doing what you ought to do. And what you ought to do is on the whole so pleasant, that there aren't any temptations to resist. And if ever, by some unlucky chance, anything unpleasant should somehow happen, why, there's always Soma to give you a holiday from the facts.
>
> And there's always Soma to calm your anger, to reconcile you to your enemies, make you patient and long suffering. In the past you could only accomplish these things by making a great effort and after years of hard moral training. Now you swallow two or three half gram tablets, and there you are.

Soma is Prozac to you.

Prozac is the most famous SSRI, or selective serotonin reuptake inhibitor. People are so changed by Prozac that they've actually written lyrical devotionals about the stuff. The variation of the selectivity of return is why Prozac seems, for so many people, to alter the nature of the self; or why, as Dr. Peter Kramer said in his best-selling book *Listening to Prozac*, "it lends the introvert the social skills of a salesman." Okay.

By hitting only certain receptors, Prozac is essentially a custom-made antidepressant, the effects of which are not at all the same in everyone. Bulimia, for instance, is now being treated with Prozac, because by raising serotonin levels in certain receptors, the serotonin action actually drops the sky-high dopamine levels in the gut, which in turn prevents vomiting.

Seventeen million Americans have taken Prozac since it hit the streets ten years ago, a lot of them for almost a decade. Eli Lilly and Company, the proud and rich manufacturers of Prozac, just announced a new advertising campaign designed to increase Prozac's customer base. Apparently, doubled sales between 1990 and 1999 and twenty million new prescriptions in 1998 weren't good enough. Their profits were $1.73 billion in the U.S. alone that year. Seventy percent of Prozac prescriptions are written by primary-care physicians. Primary-care physicians are family doctors. While it's reasonable to assume that someone in the throes of mental illness might contact a legitimate psychiatrist, your HMO doesn't agree. That would cost too much. So now, thanks to managed care, if you feel less than perky enough to go to the gym because of all the glaring lights and Nutri-Grain power bars in your life, all you have to do is pay the freight for that yearly physical and ask for a little pick-me-up while you're there. Any general practitioner of medicine will do.

Seven hundred thirty-five thousand prescriptions for Prozac for children were filled in 1996. (Eli Lilly still can't market it as a children's remedy, however; because the FDA says they're still exploring it.) The most sinister fact is that Eli Lilly has designed a version flavored with *peppermint* for potential customers who are children. That means any doctor will be able to prescribe peppermint Prozac for a child without even a psychiatric evaluation.

FIRST ONE'S FREE

People who haven't heard of Prozac (there are about four in the world) often survive by other over-the-counter methods—which include nicotine, caffeine, and everybody's favorite, alcohol. Or they procure their panacea from more unsavory sources. Sir Arthur Conan Doyle, in *The Sign of the Four*, wrote:

Sherlock Holmes took his bottle from the corner of the mantel-piece and his hypodermic syringe from its neat Morocco case . . . "Which is it to-day?" I asked. "Morphine or cocaine?" He raised his eyes languidly from the old black-letter volume which he had opened. "It's cocaine," he said; "a seven percent solution. Would you care to try it?" "No, indeed," I answered brusquely. He smiled at my vehemence. "Perhaps you are right, Watson," he said. "I suppose the influence is physically a bad one. I find it, however, so transcen-dently stimulating and clarifying to the mind that its secondary action is a matter of small moment."

"But consider!" I said earnestly. "Count the cost! Your brain may, as you say, be roused and excited, but it is a pathological and morbid process, which involves increased tissue-change, and may at least leave permanent weakness. You know, too, what a 'black' comes upon you. Surely the game is hardly worth the candle. Why should you, for a mere passing pleasure, risk the loss of those great powers with which you have been endowed?"

"But I abhor the dull routine of existence. I crave mental exalta-tion . . ."

Why do recovering drug addicts (Sherlock never recovered) and alco-holics switch to coffee, cigarettes, and carbohydrates? Well, a little caffeine and a little nicotine are certainly the hair of the dog that bit them, but why food? Most addicts who are successful staying drug-free find they are unable to control their weight after recovery. How does food—especially carbohydrates, judging by the weight gain—ameliorate withdrawal?

By the same mechanism alcohol and drugs themselves use, that's how.

Presiding over all neurotransmitter activity—and all hormones that act as neurotransmitters—is a matched pair of master receptors. These mas-ter controls are in charge of firing or not firing the neurons in your brain that control the quantum effect of "lights out." Electrical excitation of neurons is always referred to as "firing," and these two substances are in control of the juice. The "stop" switch is called a GABA receptor. The "go" switch is called a NMDA receptor.

GABA receptors are the key to the effects on consciousness of alcohol and carbohydrates. Alcohol pushes the "stop" button by bringing up GABA receptors. This literally shuts cells down, electrically. Shutdown induces a sense of calm. Barbiturates, anesthesia, carbohydrates, and fat burned as ketones work the same way. Carbohydrates do it through insulin, which brings up GABA receptors just as alcohol does.

The problem occurs when GABA receptors are "up" too long or too pervasively. Remember the board on a log. While GABA is up, NMDA is down. Down, but not out.

NMDA receptors actually increase in proportion to GABA's sustained high.

Dr. Ronald Ruden, in his book *The Craving Brain*, uses the metaphor that while the lights are out, your brain is replacing all the bulbs with brighter ones. By increasing the number and intensity of NMDA receptors while GABA is up, the brain is "balancing." The you-know-what hits the fan when you stop the alcohol, drugs, or sugar, and GABA goes down, because then the NMDA goes up at least twice as high as before. Since there are twice as many "go" switches compared to normal, the noise and light are deafening. Twice as much synaptic and electrical activity is way too much. You have no option but to go back to whatever the stuff was that brought the calm in the first place. Now you can consider yourself hooked. Every time you attempt withdrawal, it just gets worse. Unless you are asleep. Melatonin brings up GABA receptors for the ultimate "lights out."

In our modern-life scenario, you're hooked on a Hershey's Kiss, a glass of wine in the evening, or a low-fat bran muffin with jam for lunch. You're certainly hooked if you consume all three in one day, every day, all year long, year in and year out. Thanks to insulin from your carbohydrate consumption, and GABA's response to insulin directly, we junk-food monkeys have the same potential to "jones" seen in alcoholics.

There are some people who can have just *one* drink *once* in a while. But the majority of us can't stop with just one glass of beer or one Coke, or one french fry, or even just one rice cake.

It's all the same thing.

WITHDRAWAL

Consider the scenario described by J. Madeleine Nash, writing in the May 5, 1997, issue of *Time:*

> Imagine you are taking a slug of whiskey. A puff of a cigarette. A toke of marijuana. A snort of cocaine. A shot of heroin. Put aside

whether or not these drugs are legal or illegal. Concentrate, for now, on the chemistry. The moment you take that slug, that puff, that toke, that snort, that shot, trillions of potent molecules surge through your bloodstream and in your brain. Once there, they set off a cascade of chemical and electrical events, a kind of neurological chain reaction that ricochets around the skull and rearranges the interior reality of the mind.

We'd like to add to that litany of addictive substances "a mouthful of any carbohydrate," or, in the "street lingo" of that notorious pusher Mary Poppins, "a spoonful of sugar."

The molecules Ms. Nash refers to in her acutely accurate description are dopamine. Dopamine stays high in the light, normally, because it lays in reward pathways in the limbic system of the brain by creating a sense of euphoria that is memorable. The limbic system connects the key survival parts of the brain with the cerebral cortex, the part from which thought emanates and the part that will make you remember how good it all felt.

Dopamine activates a reward system that brings the limbic information to the area of the brain that makes you act. That's why dopamine is also a major player in Parkinson's disease. You must activate motor function to act.

The limbic system with dopamine on board sorts and tags gazillions of bits of sensory input as emotionally "hot" or "cold." Dr. Kotulak, in *Inside the Brain*, describes it thus:

> Hot things are to be remembered and they are spritzed with pleasurable sensations ranging from the thrill of sex to the glow from a good deed. Cold sensory inputs receive no emotional tag and they drift away to be forgotten.

Reward pathways are very important to the basic premise of evolution.

The act of evolving is based on the ability to continue to exist, which is based on adapting, which is based on learning and *remembering*. This is the foundation of the mechanism of addiction. Dopamine drives experiences directly to the hippocampus. The hippocampus itself is the processor of long- and short-term contextual memories. The hippocampus is in play when the hearing of clinking ice cubes in a glass or the smell of coffee makes you crave a cigarette, even though you stopped smoking five years ago.

We part-time addicts who are only twenty to thirty pounds overweight on sweetened, processed foods are sent down a one-way path of self-destruction in fast forward when the AMA and the American Heart Association tells us to remove the protein and fat from our diets and live on nothing but sugar in the form of a low-fat, all-carbohydrate diet.

When alcoholics drink, they are taking in concentrated, refined carbohydrates, just as you are when you eat bread, pasta, or chocolate cake. When you drink, alcohol usually attaches to and activates serotonin receptors, not dopamine receptors, which is the reason some of us drink, make melatonin, and fall asleep. In other people, the activation of the serotonin receptor causes a release of *dopamine.*

Remember nature.

Remember that in order to be adaptive, your responses must be capable of infinite variety in terms of combinational strategies. Therefore, hormonal, immune, and neurotransmitter activity is really a lot like a pinball game; you can hit a post over here and a light will blink on over there. A hit to one receptor can actually produce another's product. It's a series of checks and balances, of compensatory actions that are meant to restore you to homeostasis, no matter what life throws at you.

The people who respond to alcohol with an uncharacteristic dopamine release get hooked. After the first drink, they are out of serotonin because their receptor responded with dopamine. Low serotonin means that wearing a lamp shade on your head seems reasonable. Most true drunks are completely uninhibited because they have no serotonin for impulse control. These are also mean drunks because they are aggressive. With each drink, their serotonin drops further and their dopamine climbs higher, causing a euphoria that is laid into memory pathways. These are the people who remember the experience and drink again and again. They become alcoholics.

Liquor in our time is hard enough to handle, since we're already chronically exhausted and depressed. But imagine that you're the new kid on the block, genetically. Adaptation, you now know, takes time. How you are affected by an evolutionary speed bump, or change, rests in large measure on how long your genetic group has been exposed to an environmental change, such as the availability of carbohydrates and how long they've had to adapt to the artificial time scale of the constant light. If you want to know what being a newcomer to our culture actually feels like, all you have to do is focus on, ironically, the *oldest* group of Americans known on this continent, the Native Americans.

THE CIGARETTE-SMOKING MAN

The following story is remarkable because it exemplifies the combination of journalistic and medical ineptitude that misinforms all of us and, simultaneously, it shines a light on wholesale cultural extinction in the person of one Britton KillsRight, a once proud Native American made famous by *The New York Times,* who has, instead, become the poster boy for the light-induced disease in all of us.

Britton KillsRight is the star of a very confusing article in *The New York Times* that was published on December 23, 1997, which ostensibly looks into the suffering of Native Americans in the grip of alcoholism. The article starts off with the statistic that although men in the U.S. live to an average of 71.66 years of age, Native American men only live to the age of 56 and Native American women die at least fourteen years sooner than their men.

To explain this statistic, the article offers that "diabetes is common on the reservation." Then, as though somehow it explains the connection between diabetes and alcoholism, the article concludes that "some people live almost an hour's drive from the hospital."

The wording leaves us wondering whether diabetes or alcoholism kills them on the way to the hospital. The reason the wording is murky is that the journalist is fishing through the facts and evidence he has. He is fishing for something currently "relevant" (read: trendy) to relate to those facts. So next, without ever actually connecting any dots, he drives home his point (?) by declaring: "It seems the vast majority smoke cigarettes." Okay, we see the relevance, but if you hadn't read this book, would you?

Next, the author describes "the traffic jams on the two-lane road to the closest liquor store." What? At least now we're back to alcoholism. Is he insinuating that these people are dying from smoking in closed cars while waiting in line to buy a bottle of liquor on their way to the hospital, so they can drive home drunk and get in a car crash, when their diabetes was the big clue all along? Of course these people drink and smoke and eat their way to diabetes. But genetically these are people who have no tolerance for sleep loss and the sugar craving or the depression that follows.

They are living in an alien environment for their group genetics.
Our environment.

They show all the same signs we do of light toxicity, coupled with extraordinary stress. Obesity, heart disease, hypertension, alcoholism, suicide from depression, and, eventually, infertility are all in their future.

Smoking is the least of their problems.

KILLS RIGHT

Genetics and lifestyle weigh equally in the Native Americans' predicament when you remember "Change the environment and the environment will change you." Predictably, without the genetic adaptation to deal with the toxic change in their environment, they are all going to die. In fact, at this point in time, only the Native Americans missing their "normal" genetic complement will survive.

At the moment, they're stuck on the same evolutionary "speed bump" that we faced about eight thousand years ago with the advent of agriculture, *plus* our newest cross to bear, light toxicity, resulting in sleep deprivation, the same cross that makes us eat ourselves to death. The biggest difference for them, in our time, is their socioeconomic status. Our cultural hegemony only adds insult to injury in every possible instance. A people under constant stress, with no grace period for genetic adaptation, when offered the opportunity to self-medicate at every turn, naturally become addicts. The truth of the matter comes together in the portrait of Britton KillsRight in the *New York Times* piece.

In the following quote from the article, Mr. KillsRight is discussing The Red Road, a new approach to alcoholic recovery being tested on reservations. The Red Road refers to the ancient belief among tribes that there are only two choices for native peoples: the Black Road, which leads to despair and death, and the Red Road, which leads to peace and harmony.

This oozing-cultural-awareness, pseudo-twelve-step program calls for the alcoholic Native American to "live in a Red Day." No easy task. Like most of the participants in the program, Mr. KillsRight has lived in a world driven by abandonment, addiction, and violence. You can bet his experiences have become his biology.

He began drinking at the age of six, when he saw a white man push his mother out a window. At the age of twelve, he acquired a tattoo that reads "More Beer." At the age of twenty-two, he was unemployed and living in government housing while reassessing his short life. In his interview, he attributed his past failure to kick alcohol to the treatment methods used by the white man.

"I had been to the White Man's alcohol treatment center at 16," said Mr. KillsRight, his jet black hair pulled back into a ponytail, his gaze intense and his fists clenched. "They had us do things like dance to Richard Simmons videos. They had us exercise to the songs I didn't know—'Sweating to the Oldies'—that's what they called it."

He should have called the Bureau of Indian Affairs.

The punchline is: One short week after leaving the "Deal-a-Meal" approach to abstinence, he was drinking again.

We wonder why he waited *that* long.

The New York Times ran a picture (fig. 4) of Mr. KillsRight during his recovery in his housetrailer, proudly displaying his "More Beer" tattoo under the unremitting glare of a fluorescent ceiling light with the TV on in the background. Notice the open, half-empty, two-liter bottle of Pepsi in front of him and the ashtray overflowing with butts.

We think this picture says it all.

Mr. KillsRight has just switched seats on the Titanic.

If his luck holds out, some well-intentioned social worker from the Indian clinic near the diabetes treatment center will get him a Prozac prescription and maybe some Zyban for his smoking. When it's discovered that he has coronary artery disease and diabetes at thirty-six, the doctors will blame it on smoking or the nearness of the liquor store, never realizing that a lifetime of incomparable stress and twelve years of Prozac to ease the torment created a "panic state" of high serotonin so unbearable his heart is about to stop.

SEVEN

THE BEST PLACE TO HIDE A LIE IS BETWEEN TWO TRUTHS:

How the Biggest Clock in Your Body Stops

Our own heartbeat reassures us that we're well. We dread its one day stopping, we dread the heart-silence of those we love. How are you feeling . . . deep in your heart, we ask. My heart is broken, we answer, as if it were a block of chalk hit by a sledgehammer.

—Diane Ackerman,
A Natural History of the Senses

The hidden truth buried at the bottom of the syndrome of antidepressant use is that the "sleepless" phenomenon that creates the higher-than-normal serotonin brain levels responsible for the depression we're all experiencing *simultaneously causes heart disease.*

The media, doctors, and researchers will all tell you that fat people are more likely to have heart attacks because they have high cholesterol and high blood pressure—from being fat. And everybody knows that fat people are fat because they eat fatty foods. Fat people do have high cholesterol and high blood pressure that lead to heart attacks, but eating high-fat food has nothing to do with it. That's the lie they're hiding.

Fat people just get too tired to live.

Sleep controls your appetite for carbohydrates, the consumption of which controls water retention (to change your blood pressure) and insulin production (which facilitates cholesterol production). No sleep, no control. And serotonin builds up. When you don't sleep and you eat carbohydrates all day, week, month, year, decade, you swim in chronically high serotonin because it never gets to turn into melatonin. That's where the depression comes in, and the actual heart disease.

It's common knowledge that sad people have broken hearts, and people with broken hearts are really sad.

117

Depressed people have more heart attacks, and people with heart disease are always depressed. Scientists know that depression and cardiovascular disease go hand in hand.

It's the American public that has no idea.

NAVAJO CODE

We have delineated the effect of no sleep—more carbohydrates, more cortisol, and less melatonin—on appetite and the metabolism of sugars and fats in the bloodstream. We concluded that when you fail to undergo famine, or hibernate, for a good portion of one planetary trip around the sun, all of the sugar and carbohydrate you consume "out of season" causes obesity, depression, and eventually Type II (non-insulin-dependent) diabetes. This happens because insulin exists to facilitate the "use" of the sugars as blood glucose only for a while, and after that normal evolutionary time frame—a few months or so—different climate change adaptations are triggered.

We can handle the intense stress of mating season and hibernation preparation for only a few months out of twelve. The rest of the year, all our systems require a respite to gear up for our next shot at the brass ring, when summer comes around again.

The stress of mating is unique. In nature, when the light is long, a man will spend his days trying to mate—which means continual fighting with other males, which means, for the most part, continual bleeding. A woman, with men trying to mate with her, feels excessive stress.

Serotonin (which rises in response to the stress of fear when you eat carbohydrates) controls vasoconstriction and platelet aggregation for a real reason in the natural world. You would never be in a panic state unless the thing that's panicked you might just bite your leg off or hit you with a club and cause you to bleed to death. The major chain of events in cardiovascular disease—high blood pressure, blood vessel constriction, increased clotting factors, high cholesterol, and lax calcium channels—mirrors all of the symptoms of prolonged prehibernation syndrome. All of these symptoms are reversible with adequate sleep, which raises melatonin and quells your appetite for carbohydrates.

You must stop eating sugar for more than half of the year to avoid heart disease because the higher-than-normal serotonin levels brought about by the insulin you're swimming in not only create a depressive-paranoid state, they also kick in your *sympathetic nervous system,* which is the quantum *primitive overdrive that connects your heart and brain.* It controls the "fight or flight" response that can save you when you can't save yourself.

More important, the sympathetic nervous system runs on molecules called nerve growth factor (NGF), in your heart, and its doppelgänger in the brain, brain-derived neurotrophic factor (BDNF). BDNF is responsible for the growth of brain cells called neurons and their branchlike extensions, dendrites. The energy centers that power the growth of these neurons and dendrites are cells in your brain called glia.

In chronically depressed people, researchers find a dramatic loss of glial cells. Cells only die when they run out of fuel. We think this death is a result of localized insulin resistance in the brain, a precursor to the cerebral diabetes of schizophrenia. The glia cells normally thrive on blood sugar fed to them through insulin receptors. However, when insulin resistance (brought on by eating carbohydrates too long) hits the brain, the glia die and BDNF drops. The effect on consciousness is depression. It doesn't matter whether it's a serotonin/dopamine, GABA/NMDA, or insulin/cortisol imbalance or a lack of BDNF/NGF, because it's all one thing. All of the trillions of feedback loops of trillions of different molecules in your cells with trillions of different names do their job simultaneously to keep you adapting.

Ordinarily, one of the main evolutionary functions of BDNF on your neurons has been to adapt to changes in the environment by sprouting new growth (dendrites) to open up new pathways, so we can learn and remember new things. This ability allows us to change our behavior to adapt to new circumstances and survive. Without BDNF to enhance expansion along the serotonin and dopamine pathways and strengthen connections to the hippocampus, not only can't we cope or remember or learn, we die. We either kill ourselves or our hearts stop.

NGF (nerve growth factor) in the heart performs the same tasks of nerve growth that help your heart remember and cope, too. But insulin resistance in your heart muscle means no blood sugar to the cells providing NGF. When there is no NGF, the memory connections (synapses) weaken and the heart literally *forgets* to keep the beat. This failure affects the variability of beat that you need to cope with stressful situations. Your heart and mind are one.

By keeping the lights on to create endless summer, and having access to endless carbohydrates, all of our hormones are in summer mode, too. Not only our minds but our hearts live in the constant "panic" of mating season (competition for resources, high hormonal mood swings, and, ultimately, loss), which used to coincide with *real* summer. So day and night, year-round, decade after decade, our sex hormones are in high gear, and we're ready for a fight. This peak state of readiness is something we are only equipped to deal with five months out of twelve.

The low-fat lies of the 1970s, 1980s, and 1990s have only exacerbated an enormous evolutionary glitch by prescribing a diet of *more* carbohydrates and exercise, which induce cortisol and insulin highs that have never before been seen in humans. There's also the psychosis of a population mentally consumed by sex, but we won't even go there. Because the important thing for you to know, and know it in your bones, is that when you don't sleep, *your heart dies.*

Just like that.

CRAWLING AWAY TO DIE

What's happening to the biggest clock in your body when the light never sinks into the sunset? When the fuel that feeds your heart never varies and the panic perceived by your head never ends? So many things you can't even imagine.

And not one of them is good.

Your arteries actually "feel" the blood flowing through them. The sensors that read how hard your blood pushes and pulls as it rushes through you are called endothelial cells. These cells are alive in their own right. They change shape, move around, and switch a myriad of genes on or off in response to blood pressure and velocity, hormones and cytokines they detect in the blood, and photons brought into the blood by cells called cryptochromes. (Endothelial cells alone control the fluid dynamics of blood flow; that is, they spread out the forces to avoid dangerous extremes.)

Endothelial cells also control how fatty acids floating in your blood are metabolized. Fatty acids are what the doctor measures when he threatens you about your high cholesterol. The blood tests they take to measure your cholesterol look at different components of fatty acids in your blood, components with acronyms like VLDL, HDL, and LDL. Whether the LDLs (low density lipoproteins) are split from the VLDLs (*very* low density lipoproteins) that were made in your liver from the carbohydrates that you've eaten and become heavy, oxidized, smaller LDL particles is at the discretion of your endothelial cells.

Doctors tell you to fast before the test, not because a high-fat meal will skew the results but because a high-carbohydrate one will. Carbohydrates turn into triglycerides (body fat) to insulate and nourish you when there's no sugar left to eat. Carbohydrates simultaneously turn into these fatty acids (cholesterol), too, to patch your heart cells against leaks if you freeze and as nourishment for your heart muscle cells.

Your heart has a *seasonal* metabolism, just like your brain. Your summer heart runs on straight sugar (glucose) and your winter heart runs on free fatty acids. Because it's always summer in our hearts, our arteries never get a chance to use up all the cholesterol. In addition, your serotonin keeps building, leading to ultimate serotonin resistance, which gives you high blood pressure on the way to blood clots, and—as long as the lights shine—your cortisol stays up. And you know what chronic high *anything* means.

Cortisol resistance is a nasty thing.

Cortisol production is a coping mechanism in place to deal with episodic stress. Your heart lining loves cortisol, in small doses. The endothelial cells in your heart lining can't do all the jobs they do without small, usable measures of cortisol. Big hits, however, signal big danger to your endothelial cells. Big hits all day long, all week long, all year long for decades mean cortisol resistance.

And a bad temper, and no patience, and skewed time perception, and pervasive panic.

It doesn't matter if you eat saturated or unsaturated fat, good fats or bad fats; if the endothelial cells lining your heart are dead; so are you. The lining of every blood vessel in your body is a player in the larger scheme of the sensory organ known as your heart.

The rush of your blood, the push and the pull, is called shear stress on the walls of your arteries. Shear stress over a smooth patch of endothelial cell lining activates three very important genes: one that produces nitric oxide, which controls the clamping down of your blood vessels, which, in turn, controls the speed and volume of your blood pressure, and two other genes that inhibit blood clotting and smooth any muscle over-growth (lumpy bumps). Endothelial cells that read too much turbulence or, on the other hand, none at all, produce very little activation of these genes. This is a bad thing.

That means that while constant running on a treadmill produces too much turbulence, never moving away from the television or computer screen at all from day to day is just as bad. A *little* stress, episodically, is a good thing. Just like a little cortisol, episodically, keeps the rhythm and proves you're alive.

A lot of chronic stress, of course, means you're a loser to nature and should go away permanently. Just a little cortisol bath makes endothelial cells very happy. A lot of cortisol will drown them. Since your cortisol stays up as long as the lights are on, you're probably drowning. So just keeping the lights on late, year-round, will cause endothelial cell death. Any increase in blood pressure from your sympathetic nervous system or heavy carbohydrate intake in the wrong season will change blood pressure to create even more shear stress and kill your endothelial cells two ways. Remember, the ten pounds of water weight you carry on a high-carbohydrate diet is enough of a volume increase to account for the chronic subclinical high blood pressure seen in the majority of men more than thirty-five years old.

Any high blood pressure, no matter how slight, always means shear stress.

The other major killer of the endothelial cells in the lining of your heart is chronically high levels of endotoxin LPS. Remember that endotoxin LPS is the bacterial "sweat" coming from the four pounds of symbiotic bacteria in your gut that, as it rises, activates your immune system and interleukin-2, which puts you to sleep and pushes the number of bacteria down again. When you fight sleep instead, those levels rise and stay high.

That kills your heart.

The most obscure way to kill your endothelial cells by not sleeping is through high homocysteine. A man named Kilmer McCully realized about thirty years ago that children with a genetic disease called homo-cysteinuria always died of heart attacks from clogged arteries by the age of ten or eleven. Children with homocysteinuria genetically fail to make an enzyme that metabolizes homocysteine to remove it from the blood-stream. McCully was smart enough to realize that high levels of building homocysteine must be associated with coronary artery disease in adults, too. He was right.

Of course, no one took him seriously until scientists found that an increase in folic acid supplements would compensate for the missing enzyme in the elimination pathway for homocysteine. Once there was a treatment, suddenly there was a disease—a genetic folic acid deficiency. Oh, boy.

A widespread *genetic* folic acid deficiency in the majority of the aging male population is a virtual impossibility, so knowing that no one had really solved the puzzle, we investigated the pathways of homocysteine manufacture and metabolism. Sure enough, only a few feedback loops and cascades backward, a crucial enzyme for metabolizing methionine, the precursor to homocysteine, is knocked out by a cryptochrome carrying blue light. The amount of daylight you are exposed to, compounded by the amount of artificial light, controls the production of a minuscule, seemingly esoteric, high-up-in-the-cascade-of-other-hormones-and-functions thing *that can kill you.*

So.

Endothelial cells—which line your heart—control clotting, overgrowth, fat metabolism, and blood pressure. You can kill your endothelial cells four ways:

1. Chronic high cortisol (never-ending light)

2. High levels of endotoxin LPS (no sleep)

3. High homocysteine (too much light)

4. Shear stress (seasonal high blood pressure—along with carbohydrate "water weight," and serotonin and insulin resistance—that never ends)

Since 1, 2, and 3 are all the result of modern life, and 4—*the all-sugar-all-the-time diet*—is the direct result of 1, 2, and 3, it's safe to say that heart disease, which is a state of dead endothelial cells, is caused by no sleep and too much light, right?

NO ESCAPE

It's also the endothelial lining that controls the overgrowth of smooth muscle tissue (bumpy lumps) that is the major factor, along with cholesterol plaqueing, in arteriosclerosis (clogged arteries). A disturbed blood flow over bumpy terrain activates an altogether different set of genes in the endothelial cells. These other genes are set in motion to "correct" what the endothelial cells perceive to be a "flow" problem mimicked by the lumpy bumps.

Cholesterol plaque, in and of itself, does not make for bumpy terrain.

It's the immune "factors" released from the endothelial cells themselves, in a protective attempt to restore homeostasis and distribute the shear stress of the flow of blood, that cause the problem. A disturbed flow actually causes the shutdown of protective genes and provokes panic in the endothelial cells. After releasing the immune factors that clamp down, increasing your blood pressure by mistake, they begin to crawl around by extending pseudopodia (little feet) in an effort to escape from areas where shear stress has changed abruptly.

The migration of these cells lining your arteries leads to thinning of the artery wall. The gaps are filled by immune cells called leukocytes that make a scab sticky enough to attract cholesterol floating in your bloodstream, which makes a fat "Band-Aid" to strengthen the thinning artery wall. Now you have cholesterol plaque and overgrown smooth muscle and immune cells making what's known as foam cells.

Foam cells constitute a "lesion."

This new mess creates an excessively bumpy terrain and a remarkably disturbed flow, which panics your poor endothelial cells further. They run away and the artery wall thins and then your immune system tries to repair it, and it gets bumpier and bumpier and then, of course, your endothelial cells run away again, and the whole shooting match starts all over again. And again and again.

You get the picture, because you're not dead yet.

You probably have the occasional severe chest pain when you exercise, though. No doubt you're also finding it harder and harder to fight off the depression caused by all of the carbohydrates you've eaten and by the higher-than-normal serotonin that builds up because it has nowhere to go. Because when you never turn off the lights, the serotonin has no way to become melatonin. In fact, the light actually takes out the enzyme that would convert serotonin to melatonin. In addition to making you blue, these sky-high serotonin levels create serotonin resistance in blood platelets, which makes them even stickier than usual. That's important, because it's hard to have a heart attack without a blood clot, and it's hard to have a blood clot without sticky platelets.

You're tired, freaked out, miserable, addicted to either sugar or alcohol, maybe living on Prozac, and walking around with a dead heart lining held together by cholesterol supports.

You have heart disease.

You're probably going to die . . . soon.

VOODOO DEATH

Any physician reading the description above would tell you that you're going to have a heart attack and you're going to have it from the cholesterol plaque clogging your arteries. But that's not true. Oh, you'll likely have a heart attack, all right, but cholesterol is not to blame. It's actually the least of your problems. In fact, your doctor, the newspapers, and the TV are more likely to kill you than the cholesterol Band-Aids you're wearing.

We make that statement after going through volumes of cutting-edge research on the phenomenon of "heart attack." Heart *disease* is not heart attack. Heart disease can run the gamut from cardiovascular disease, with attendant high blood pressure and cholesterol plaqueing, to cardiomyopathy (tired or damaged heart muscle), which leads to congestive heart failure, with more than a few variations on the theme in between. Heart attack is when your heart clamps down in one last fatal beat and doesn't come back.

If it's not the cholesterol plaqueing, and it's not the sticky platelets, what is the cause of heart attack? To deduce the real origin of cardiac death, let's ask the question we have tacitly asked in every other chapter so far:

Where and how could the physical event that we're observing ever occur in nature?

Unless we can answer that question, we've got the "medicine" (read: science) wrong. It is an unbeatable technique that always brings us to the undeniable truth by uncovering the natural mechanism that has inadvertently been tripped by modern life. We unraveled obesity with a look at feast-or-famine metabolism. We can understand the metabolic premise behind Type II diabetes within the framework of hibernation. Mental illness can be understood as a product of food supply and fatigue that is threshold-dependent—that is, how much can you take before you snap?

So, once more, for the first time in regard to coronary artery disease, *when and under what circumstances does a heart attack occur in nature?*

The answer is: *only* in a state of panic.

Animals only experience sudden heart attack when they literally die of fright. Their hearts are turned to stone by their own body's fight-or-flight mechanism. The basis for the human experience of a heart attack must lie in the same mechanisms.

We looked at studies evaluating deaths occurring during earthquakes and missile attacks to find evidence for this premise. We looked at deaths in the 1994 Northridge earthquake near Los Angeles and the Iraqi missile strikes on Israel in 1991. We not only found that many deaths did not result from trauma, but that people without previous cardiac disease did, in fact, often die of fright.

There was, on average, a forty-percent increase in heart attacks on both days in question. Terror, in an otherwise healthy person, can cause a mix of chemicals so potent as to induce a cataclysmic influx of calcium into all your heart cells, causing your heart to contract so violently that it never relaxes again. The "fear state" from chronic higher-than-normal serotonin levels that we elaborated on earlier puts your mind and heart in perennial, almost permanent, *physiologic* panic.

In a remarkable paper published more than forty years ago in *American Anthropology*, Walter Bradford Cannon, a Harvard Medical School physiologist, described how, in many primitive cultures, a curse from an all-powerful wizard or medicine man was enough to kill a believer. Their hearts stopped dead.

As if that's not tragic enough, modern medicine adds to the fear, making it palpable. TV and print ads bombard us with news from the front about the "war on heart disease"—just in case you didn't realize your heart was trying to kill you. We are taught to hate our hearts. It's true that human beings have always been obsessed with their hearts in life, art, and literature. Now we are obsessed with the "health" of our hearts. We seem to be locked in codependent relationships with cardiologists, researchers, and exercise physiologists and in a food fight to the death against the whimsical independence of our hearts.

Thanks to the media in particular, and American paranoia in general, we are far more panicked, minute to minute, about our health than we've ever been before in history. We'd like to include in that assessment the 1914 flu epidemic that killed twenty million people worldwide. People are far more worried about heart disease now than they were worried about catching the flu then.

We live in truly strange times.

Add to that free-floating terror the twice yearly visit to the cardiologist, or a trip to the grocery store, for that matter, to buy "fat-free" juice, defatted turkey burgers, and low-fat freezer-burned pasta concoctions under overhead fluorescent lights that shine with the glare of ten thousand artificial suns.

No wonder we drink more than juice.

ALIEN INVADERS

If you're trying to live low-fat and exercising until you hurt everywhere, you'll probably have a heart attack. It will come under some unusual stress, emotional or physical, while your heart is beating just a tad faster than it normally does. One of those newly formed plaques will crack as your heart squeezes down hard, and the unmetabolized liquid cholesterol pooling in the center of the plaque will spill into your bloodstream, and within tens of seconds your immune system will try to compensate and seal the hole with a barrage of white cells and blood clots. It will be the lack of room in your narrowed artery, filled to the brim with immune actions, that stops the blood flow to the muscle and causes the cells to die.

Unless you get lucky and the neighbors need a place to crash.

An occluded heart clogged with cholesterol may not kill you if your immune system will tolerate symbiosis with one or more of the opportunistic life forms that will inevitably move into the plaque that lines your arteries. If you've followed the newspaper articles regarding the "new" theory that cites infection as the cause of heart disease, names like *H. pylori*, CMV virus, *Chlamydia pneumoniae*, and dental caries will be familiar. To a certain extent, these articles are correct. One or more of these cohabitors of the earth will infect the cholesterol plaque that formed when your endothelial cells abandoned you.

H. pylori is also called *Helicobacter pylori*. This is a common bacterium that usually infects most of us in childhood. In people with unhappy gut flora (bacteria), *H. pylori* can cause excessive acid production, which leads to ulcers. Tagamet and Zantac are both big-selling drugs that suppress the immune system's response to this unhappy state of affairs. Now most doctors have decided that a course of antibiotic therapy to kill *Hp*, and probably a few hundred other harmless bacteria in your gut, is the best way to handle stomach ulcers. After all, why use a handgun when a hydrogen bomb will do?

We feel that the heart disease connections to *Hp* are flimsy at best. They're based on blood work showing that a great number of people with coronary artery disease are also shown to be positive for *Hp,* and that treatment with antibiotics reduces the incidence of heart attack. It's not much of a connection. The evidence for cytomegalovirus (CMV) as an evolutionary tool is much stronger. And the story on chlamydia is downright fascinating. It seems that chlamydia does not so much infect as it *infarcts.* A heart attack is called a myocardial infarction by doctors. But it's not chlamydia itself that causes inflammation leading to heart attack.

It's a much older story.

Whenever and wherever a parasite invades, it would never make any sense for it to harm the host in any life-threatening way. Chlamydia follows this rule. The harm that befalls chlamydia's host happens through the human immune system and molecular mimicry. In nature, one of the oldest tricks in the book is a disguise. Insects called walking sticks look, predictably, like the sticks they walk on. Chlamydia effects a disguise by wearing a protein on its outside coat that allows it to slip through your immune system. Unfortunately, the protein looks exactly like one that exists normally in the heart muscle, too. If you're unlucky enough to have a really smart immune system that's not fooled by the molecular mimicry of chlamydia's fake protein coat, you're still knee-deep in irony because it will be your own immune system that takes you out when it recognizes the impostor and kills the heart cells infected with it.

Both *H. pylori* and chlamydia, along with endotoxin LPS, high cortisol, homocysteine, and subclinical high blood pressure, could all be eliminated by sleeping in sync with the seasons because your immune system would naturally hold up your end of the ecological tug-of-war.

Viruses, on the other hand, are a whole different animal, literally.

Viruses are not microbes or germs. Viruses are snippets of RNA or DNA that act as evolutionary tools. New DNA entering an organism at the level of the genome means, for the organism, symbiosis or death. The entering virus often confers some benefit that contributes to the overall fitness of the new *combined* organism, but sometimes not. Viruses are species-specific and usually prefer their chosen species. Herpes viruses, for example, live with primates, which include us.

Herpes is capable not only of joining to our DNA, but also of turning on and off growth-regulating genes like P53, causing many researchers to believe that CMV and MDV, both of the herpes family, are implicated in the overgrowth of the smooth muscle cells that ultimately contribute to the infamous foam cells.

We don't think so.

We think that a herpes virus can actually save your life. We come by our theory by the way of physics, evolutionary biology, biochemistry and, of course, cosmology. We cite an investigation by Joseph Zasadzinski at the University of California at Santa Barbara, who's working on drug delivery systems. He has been able to create a cell membrane with a single layer of lipids. Apparently, all that RNA or even DNA needs to make a home is a phospholipid shell. In fact, these ancient buckyballs of fat are exactly what we're made of.

Inside every tiny balloon of phospholipids that are all stuck together in us, is our DNA. This model is the model of all life. Now, the only reason that viruses reside in an ambiguous netherworld of the nonliving is because they aren't truly alive until they find a cell to move in to. DNA snippets just like those of CMV or MDV can create a home in the plaque in your heart. We've correlated that fact with the finding that ninety-two percent of all plaque examined upon autopsy *in non-cardiac-related deaths* has CMV proteins evident in it.

We propose that the reason cardiologists are in agreement that a twenty-percent occlusion will kill you far more often that an eighty-percent occlusion of coronary arteries is that the virus moves in and uses the lipids in the plaque to create a "cell" to live and reproduce in. By doing so, the virus stabilizes the plaque, making it able to withstand far more pressure and solidifying the dangerously immunoreactive soft center liquid.

It may give you the creeps, but it makes evolutionary sense.

We find more evidence in the work of H. Kaunitz published in *Medical Hypotheses* in 1995. He found that "studies on persons who had died with advanced stages of atherosclerosis showed [that they had] the highest life expectancy." He felt that there was evidence that "the inflammatory nature of viruses (especially the human herpes family) were involved in a protective effect."

In other words: What doesn't kill you makes you stronger.

IN A HEARTBEAT

Bump-bump, swish, lub-dub, lub-dub, bah-boom, bah-boom . . . however the act is interpreted verbally or on the written page, we all recognize a heartbeat or the lack of one. All the cells of our hearts, like little tuning forks, resonate together to beat.

That beat, provided by our "heartstrings," reverberates throughout the circulatory system. But we don't think about it very often unless a knocking comes from within—or worse, pain. Palpitations are absurdly alarming, pain is downright incapacitating emotionally and intellectually. Babies in utero are treated to a moving concert that sounds more like the wind and waves than anything else. The wind and the waves carry the same amount of force or "energy" that the heart is throbbing with on any given day, so the music is the same.

Tibetan, Chinese, and ayurvedic medicine all consider pulse sounds the major key to diagnosis. Eastern physicians study the rhythms of pulse for many years in order to qualify to practice medicine. By studying at least six different pulse points, they are able to discern many different rhythmic patterns or "songs." These human EKG machines believe that there are as many different rhythms as there are diseases. Each illness has its own song.

They hear the music *and the discord.*

Luckily, the number of heartbeats we are allotted is higher than most of us can count or we would hear and feel the terror of time ticking away. Most of us couldn't count to a billion if we had to. That's the magic number—one billion lub-dubs.

The biologists at the Santa Fe Institute, in their attempt to categorize scaling, or how the various characteristics of all living things, like pulse rate and life span, change according to body size, have decided we all get only a billion. From the smallest tree shrew to a blue whale, nobody gets more than a billion. But size does matter when it comes to *time* on this earth. The mouse uses its billion up faster than the elephant because of their respective metabolic rate. These scientists have a formula—a cat, one hundred times more massive than a mouse, lives one hundred to the quarter power, or about three times, longer than a mouse. Therefore, a cat's heart beats one third as fast as a mouse's.

The fluctuations on all time scales, the timing of a beat being fixed from the timings of the last few before it, really mean your heart is *not tuned to only one frequency. The New England Journal of Medicine* reported in an article in February of 1999 that the human heart shows an electrical response to a variety of radio frequencies. By responding to a range of frequencies, our heart protects the brain and itself from damage that could result from an overreaction to any one stimulus at any one frequency. The heart is made of what scientists call an excitable medium, that is, one that generates and conducts electricity. The oppositely polarized inside and outside of your heart cells always have an unequal distribution of ions inside and outside of the cell. The sympathetic nervous system communicates with the nerves all over your body and brain by initiating waves of change in the polarity inside and outside the membrane of neuronal cells like those in the heart. The pouring of positive and negative ions in and out through gates in your heart cells' membranes produces a "current" of electricity. The muscle cells of the heart are thrown into play by an electrical current that comes in polarized waves and that contracts and squeezes blood through two adjacent pumping chambers called the left and right ventricles. There's a special colony of cells at the top of the right side. These cells electrically "keep the beat."

The rush of electricity sweeps in a spiral around the entire heart, from the double-humped top to the pointy little bottom, making a complete circuit top to bottom, bottom to top, squeeze, top to bottom, bottom to top, squeeze. That's the whole deal.

HEARTBROKEN

Your heart and your immune system, far more than the gray matter that we think of as constituting the mind, are sentient in their own right. Your brain's growth and development are, in fact, completely maintained by cytokines originating in your heart. Evidence of your heart's active intelligent participation in your existence is found in studies of beat rhythms.

Your heart clenches and unclenches like a fist about sixty times a minute on average. The image of a constant, unwavering, orderly "ticker" beating away like clockwork is given to us as schoolchildren. We're taught that the terms "health" and "order" are synonymous. In fact, we refer to almost all diseases as *dis*-orders. But the truth is just the opposite. An *"ordered"* heart is one of slow, steady, unvarying beats. Every first-year med student knows that this is the tempo of a sick heart.

If you look at recordings of long series of heartbeats and calculate the lengths of the beat-to-beat intervals, it looks like they are spaced at longer and shorter intervals in a completely random and erratic manner. Not erratic in the fluctuating way in which your heart responds to your body's activity level, but genuinely wild, even during sleep. There are speedups and slowdowns, not just hourly, but minute-to-minute, too. Researchers monitored ten healthy volunteers and ten people with congestive heart failure. On first look, the heart rhythms appeared much the same in both groups, but the beat-to-beat rhythms of the healthy hearts were, in fact, far different from those of the brokenhearted.

In the healthy hearts, a sequence of two hundred steps up tends to be followed by two hundred steps down. On an EKG, this means that the period in which the heart slows down will be followed by a period in which it speeds up, sort of like a built-in mechanism that sets the beat long-range, so it fluctuates to a predetermined mathematical landscape. The healthy heart has long-term "memory." The timing of the next beat depends on the "beat history" of the distant past. Disease, by contrast, is really heart *amnesia*. In a broken heart, if a run of two hundred beats gets progressively slower, the next two hundred are just as likely to get slower as they are to get faster. By measuring longer and longer intervals, the scientists can find the extra information about the "average" hidden in the fluctuations.

This information is enough to illuminate the rhythmic differences between healthy and sick hearts. Over the last twenty years, mathematicians and physicists have realized that what looks random is not random at all. It's chaotic, and unpredictability is a hallmark of a chaotic system. Chaos differs from randomness in that chaotic behavior always arises from simple underlying causes. Chaos theory tells us so.

Irregular rhythms like sunspots or the oscillations of El Niño are examples of chaotic rhythms rather than random occurrences. Healthy heartbeats are highly chaotic, just like cosmic activity or the weather, because a chaotic system is more *adaptable*. A chaotic system is highly dynamic, always changing and fluctuating to maintain homeostasis. A chaotic system is always poised in a state that is incredibly sensitive to small influences. Since the physiology textbooks used in schools and by physicians have no insight into the origin of this complexity, we're all taught that slow and steady makes the beat go on, when really, a wildly fluctuating heart is a healthy one.

BOLT FROM THE BLUE

One of the most basic and universal laws of nature is cellular memory. Single-cell paramecia have no brains, yet they all remember how to swim, find food, mate, and recognize and evade predators. They are perfect evidence of cellular memory, or "memory of function," emanating from a single cell. The assumption that follows is this: If one cell can remember more than one function, many cells might hold enough "memories" to create whole pictures. At least that's what heart transplant recipients tell us.

Claire Sylvia's life was saved by a heart and lung transplant in 1988, after she was struck by a fatal disease. In *A Change of Heart*, she writes candidly of her transplant experience. She emerged from her ordeal a very different woman. Immediately after regaining consciousness, Ms. Sylvia remembers wishing for a beer, although she never drank beer before. Later that day she asked for Chicken McNuggets, something she had never even tasted.

New tastes and memories, far different from her own, and her recurring dreams, in which she saw a lanky young man named Tim, sent her on a search for the donor's family. Sylvia and a friend were smart enough to check the obituaries for the day of and the day before her transplant. She found in an obituary the story of a young man who had died the day of her transplant. His name was Timothy Lasalle and he was eighteen years old. He was killed in a motorcycle accident on his way home from a trip to McDonald's for lunch; the McNuggets were in the pocket of his motorcycle jacket when they undressed him in the emergency room.

Stories like Claire Sylvia's abound in transplant literature. It is a common phenomenon for heart recipients to acquire tastes and personality traits of the donor. Given all of the references that we humans have made to the qualities and properties of "heart" from antiquity to the present, there is no doubt that we know in our hearts that the essence of personality resides there, and that we always knew it. But memories? Why not? One of the key substances in the processing of memory is acetylcholine, which is extremely active in heart tissue. We know that molecules of acetylcholine are at issue in the degeneration of Alzheimer's patients. Then there's the issue of the real stuff memories are made of—electricity and RNA.

In an incredible experiment performed at UCLA way back in 1966 and published in the journal *Nature*, a group of British scientists proved that they could transfer the memories of one organism to another just by transferring RNA. Four hundred teeny tiny worms were divided into two groups of two hundred each. One group of two hundred was "conditioned" (tortured) to find glucose or sugar by its association with the stimulus of paired light and shock. That means that in order to get food, they came to the end of their glass dish at the urging of the paired light and shock. The other half of the group was left in blissful ignorance.

The educated worms were "extinguished" (murdered). Snippets of RNA were extracted from them and injected into the happy dumb worms. Sure enough, the same sequence of lights and shocks brought the newly injected to the food end of the glass dish.

A very simple experiment that proves all of the transplant recipients' claims.

Memories are actually coded into sequences of RNA at the nuclei of your cells.

Just such a snippet of RNA as that which was transferred in the worm experiment could very well encode many memories, given the fact that it's all about electricity. Three billion years ago, when organic self-replicating molecules were formed, RNA was the very first. Later, RNA replication and joining became the DNA known in our present genome. In very recent findings, published in *Science* in 1997 and even newer information published in 1999, scientists have concluded that your DNA, and therefore your RNA, is as conductive as a coil of copper wire. In fact, entire genes can send electrical signals to one another along DNA circuits. Catherine Barton and her colleagues at the California Institute of Technology showed that a single electron can shoot far enough along a stretch of DNA to influence gene activity.

Electrons do this by hopping between the overlapping electron "clouds" of adjacent nucleotide bases, the molecular building blocks of DNA and RNA. Together the disk-shaped electron clouds form side-by-side stacks of memory chips in a "computer" that can transmit chemical information over long distances by switching genes on and off to produce proteins. Barton concluded, "There's no limit to the distances that signals could travel along DNA" wires. This news gives new meaning to the phrase "the body *electric.*" It also gives scientists a place to start an investigation of Eastern concepts and practices such as Qi and acupuncture. The electricity that sings along our DNA is proof of the "life force" that ancients insisted configures our soul. The fact that the most powerful generator of electricity in your body is your heart also makes perfect sense.

The "body electric" is real.

Where there's electrical smoke, there's fire. And where there's electricity and electromagnetic fields, there can be communication, vibration, and magnetism. There's no question that highly energized, polarized tissue such as cardiac muscle should be capable of emitting radio-wave frequencies. Radio waves received by the heart are used in certain medical treatments of degenerated muscle tissue.

Your heart has an electromagnetic field of five thousand millivolts, as compared to the brain, which emits only 140 millivolts. Remember, when Voyager transmitted signals from Saturn to Earth it used only a ten-millivolt battery. If Saturn to Earth only takes ten millivolts, then with five thousand to work with, heart-to-brain communication, or communication from your heart to that of another person, should actually be a "no-brainer."

We believe the heart *talks* to the brain through an electromagnetic field as well as electrochemically, through a feedback loop of something called ANP (atrial naturetic peptide). ANP is the chemical communication between the heart and brain through the pineal gland, where melatonin is made. Patients with coronary artery disease produce less melatonin when they sleep than healthy controls. The question remains—do sad people have broken hearts or does a broken heart really keep you up nights?

Corroborating evidence is also found in statistics measuring nighttime melatonin levels in the presence of low-frequency electromagnetic fields. Melatonin is uncharacteristically low in humans and animals exposed to EMF (electromagnetic fields). Low melatonin is already known to cause cancer; it's also well known that long-term exposure to excessive EMF correlates with increased cardiovascular death, as well as brain tumors and leukemias in electric utility workers.

So move the head of your bed away from the aquarium.

REMOTE VIEWING

The "frequency" theory of heart-to-brain communications and the fact of cellular memory could account for stories of donor memories and likes and dislikes crossing the transplantation barrier. It also could explain other anecdotal phenomena, like the legendary experiment in which one beating heart cell was placed in a medium in a petri dish and then, when another cell from a different biopsy specimen was added, the second cell picked up the beat of the first. With not a synapse or body to connect them, they fell into rhythmic unison.

This must be the way the fetal heart starts in utero, picking up the beat from Mom. A heart removed from its body still "remembers" how to beat. Even when a person is declared "brain dead," and lung and limbs give up without input from the brain, the heart beats on.

In the 1970s, a group of Japanese anthropologists created an observatory on a few small islands in the north of Japan to study the habits of small colonies of Japanese macaques, or snow monkeys. Two of the most remarkable observations to come out of the study were instances of nonlocal communication.

The first example was food washing.

A young female named Ima started dunking her sweet potatoes in the lake to remove the dirt. She was observed teaching this new idea to several other monkeys. After one hundred monkeys had learned this technique, all of the monkeys, in all of the colonies, on all of the islands, *simultaneously* knew Ima's technique. The same thing was observed in winter, when another young female took a dip in one of the island's volcanic hot springs.

The macaques are out all winter, often with icy snow covering their faces and extremities, but none of them has ever made an attempt to warm itself other than by huddling with other macaques for body heat. All of that changed after one hundred of them had taken a dip in the hot springs. Now they all routinely bathe in the hot springs all winter.

The premise of nonlocality is also known as Bell's theorem. This law of quantum physics dictates that *objects once connected affect each other forever, no matter where they are.* We think heart cells probably talk to the brain and the rest of the body through nonlocality, too.

There are other findings as well, like the treadmill experiment in which a group of biopsied heart cells taken from a runner were seen to beat faster and faster in their petri dish as the donor exercised on a treadmill across town from the lab. Or an experiment involving salivary cells from inside the cheeks of subjects later subjected to visual violence, in which the cells in the test tube two rooms away from the violent display produced increased electrical output.

Are these experiments spooky science-fiction fodder, or is the quantum law of nonlocality really evidence of quantum entanglement on the human and animal levels? Could this be how prayer works? Of course, as of yet, there's no *scientific* proof. But does that mean there's no proof?

Nonlocality? Quantum entanglement? We may be talking about the physics of love here. How ridiculous is that?

Not so ridiculous.

No one doubts the wind. It's invisible and has no taste or smell of its own, yet we believe it's there because we can see and feel its effects.

In Carl Sagan's novel *Contact,* a young scientist argues the notion of "faith" with an up-and-coming religious leader, insisting that she can't fathom his unwavering belief in God given that there is no scientific proof of God's existence.

He responds by asking her the simple question, "Did you love your father?"

She sputters, "Yes, of course, I did."

He challenges her. "Prove it."

This dialogue is an acutely accurate metaphor for the belief in something tangible but invisible and unprovable by science.

Science isn't big on faith in anything but science.

EIGHT

TEN SECONDS TO SELF-DESTRUCT:

In the Evolutionary Scheme of Things, Cancer Is Just the New You

So I traveled, stopping ever and again, in great strides of a thousand years or more, drawn by the mystery of earth's fate, watching with a strange fascination the sun grow larger and duller in the westward sky, and the life of the old earth ebb away.
— H. G. Wells,
The Time Machine

When you eat too much carbohydrate for too many months of the year, never empty your storage sugar, or burn fat to imitate famine, insulin, produced by your pancreas day and night in response to all of the sugar, causes rebound addictions and substance abuse through the production of serotonin and dopamine, bipolar behavior (ultimately), and maybe even schizophrenia in your tired brain.

And that's just *from the neck up.*

Below the neck, results of excess insulin due to light toxicity include high blood pressure from the water retention caused by eating too many carbohydrates for too long, and the storage of the surplus carbohydrate in the form of body fat and cholesterol to keep you from starving and freezing. But since neither starving nor freezing is on the horizon in your "virtual" future, you'll become diabetic. In addition, heavy LDLs will stick in your heart because you've killed the cells lining your heart three or four different ways by now.

And then there's cancer.

Everyone agrees that the biggest killers—breast, colon, and prostate cancer—are all strongly linked to obesity. We cannot disagree with the facts.

We *can* disagree with the logic.

Obesity, according to common wisdom, points to a high-fat diet. But fat consumption, whether saturated or unsaturated, causes no release of insulin. There's no possibility of storing fat in fat cells unless insulin opens the receptors, and only eating sugar can make that happen. That's why Type I diabetics who have no insulin die emaciated. *Obesity is simply a different symptom of the same syndrome that causes everything else that plagues modern man.*

Lack of sleep.

DARK SKIES

We know what you're thinking.

When it comes to obesity and Type II diabetes, it really does add up; too much light equals summer, summer comes before winter, so putting on a fat coat from an appetite controlled by the light, which indicates what season it is, makes sense. If you just continue that summer behavior, no matter what the real season is, because your global positioning system is confused by artificial lights and long days, inevitable Type II diabetes also seems reasonable to assume. But it's almost impossible to believe that you can avoid dying from cancer by doing something as simple as turning off the lights late at night. Everybody in this country and a good part of the world is sure that toxic waste, carcinogens (cancer causing chemical agents), and genetic susceptibility are the only ways you'll ever contract cancer. Genetic susceptibility means *it's your fault.*

You were born to get cancer.

Well, we've got some big news for you: Science and medicine don't understand cancer any better than they do obesity, diabetes, mental illness, or heart disease.

Bet that was a shock.

We're here to tell you that it's not in your genes—at least not the way you think it is. You are not going to get cancer because you are a victim of random mutations as you age, or because you are exposed to common carcinogens on a daily basis. Nature is much more organized than that. All cell growth or death is controlled by the promoter regions on genes. These genetic switches, which are thrown by hormones, react in response to environmental pressures so you can keep adapting, minute to minute or millennium to millennium.

The "regulatory genes" that are implicated in cancer are called oncogenes. All the hoopla that appears every so often in the news over a gene called P53 is about just such a regulatory gene that is active in almost all cancers. P53 is in every cell in everyone. P53 is one of the genes in control of growth, death, or the neutral state for repair. Medical research has decided that it must be "mutated" P53 genes that are responsible for most cancer. Mutated P53 gene research chews up billions of dollars every year to no avail, as does research on genes known as BRCA I and II (get it? BR—breast, CA—cancer). BRCA I and II, known as *the* breast cancer genes, are also common regulatory genes in men, too, and really have nothing to do with having breasts.

Scores of epidemiologists have looked at the possible mutation of BRCA I in "inbred" populations of descendants of Ashkenazic Jews on Long Island, where breast cancer is statistically through the roof. Their findings were released prematurely in a fragmented fashion. The hot news blaming one gene for the epidemic of breast cancer made all the national newspapers. Acting on this supposed link to "inherited breast cancer," Jewish women all over the world rushed to get gene testing. And subsequently, a great many of these women made a panicked decision, based on the research they believed to be airtight, to permanently mutilate themselves.

Many women had prophylactic mastectomies.

Women live in such terror of breast cancer and have such remarkable faith in science and medicine that thousands of them *voluntarily mutilated* themselves, believing their sacrifice would prevent their deaths from cancer.

Predictably, a little more than a year later, the scientists began to waver. It was only a matter of time before the evidence was recanted altogether. But for those women who acted on unclear, unfounded, premature reports, it was too late to change their minds.

Their breasts were gone forever.

That's how terrified we are.

Studies have linked three types of cancers—breast, colon, and prostate—to obesity. But way back in 1994, a study in the *Journal of the American Medical Association* admitted that there is *no association* between dietary intake of fat and breast cancer. Close on the heels of that mumbled retraction, *The New England Journal of Medicine* "indicated" that it is, in fact, not how much fat women eat, but *how fat women are* that affects their potential for breast cancer. We would call that a big clue if researchers understood *how* we get fat.

But it's a start. The authorities are now able to recognize obesity as a *symptom* (not a cause) of another disease. If there is a link between obesity and cancer, and obesity is directly caused by elevated insulin levels from sleep loss, *then insulin must be implicated in the rise of cancer.* If high-carbohydrate diets are responsible for consistently elevated insulin levels, then the coming of electric lights and processed foods should correspond perfectly with the increase of cancer. *It does.*

So much for genetics.

THE SHINING

Let's examine the role of carcinogens. Since we're telling you it's all in how you read the research, let's start with a very recent Johns Hopkins University study that says it all. Researchers injected mice with "known chemical carcinogens" *after altering their natural sleep patterns.*

The experiment was simple: Give these brave little mice "short mouse nights" and "long mouse nights," and then one by one add carcinogens to their unsuspecting systems.

Please note that these carcinogens were not viruses or obscure xeno-estrogens, but man-made poisons like Windex and plastic from your water bottle and the components of antiperspirant.

The short-night mice began developing tumors at such a rapid rate that the researchers couldn't tell which substances were responsible; but in the long-night mice—many, many carcinogens down the line—they couldn't *give* them cancer.

Even the researchers admitted that it was the presence of more melatonin in the long-night mice that made them impervious to carcinogens.

Mice are mammals.

So are you.

The scientists commented only that, "oddly enough, short-night mice also became withdrawn and paranoid."

Well, duh.

There are two possible reasons why.

Either:

(a)They had a feeling that they would get cancer and were really bummed, or

(b)The hormonal changes in their immune systems caused by sleep deprivation actually caused simultaneous mental shifts in neurotransmitters as well.

Unless the mice decide to confide in someone, we're going bet that, after reading this far, you'll go with (b).

Even if you're not overweight or a cardiac patient, if you don't sleep, you, too, can get cancer and go crazy just like tired mice.

We can prove it.

The NIH research we've cited concludes that six hours of prolactin production in the dark is the minimum necessary to maintain immune function like T cell and beneficial killer-cell production. But you can't get six hours of prolactin secretion on six hours of sleep a night; it takes *at least three and a half hours of melatonin secretion before you ever even see prolactin.*

In terms of cancer: If the lack of prolactin at night doesn't get you, the lack of melatonin ultimately will. Melatonin is the most potent antioxidant known. Less melatonin and more free radicals mean faster aging even *without* chronic high insulin racking up a "clock time" of four years for every one you live.

The insulin is as big a player in your ongoing existence as melatonin is. Forget all you've been told about cancer and environmental pollutants, cancer and genetics. Cancer is not a horrible, painful, rotting, de-evolving state *except on the personal level.* In the larger scheme of things, it is an evolutionary strategy and a proven mathematical function in physics.

Cancer is simply *life,* finding a way.

When the character of dotty old John Hammond in Jurassic Park describes with egomaniacal glee how he intends to keep raptors sterile, Jeff Goldblum's character, Dr. Malcolm, offers him this crumb of reality. "Life finds a way."

Life always finds a way around any and all environmental pressures. Unfortunately for all suffering cancer victims, there is no cure coming because there is no cure but to *live right.*

We just wish the doctors and the scientists would start to try to "think out of the box," so to speak. Creative science, like creative thinking, just means asking the right questions. Questions like:

- Why is there no cancer in nature?

- Why do only humans and their pets get cancer?

- Why do women have more cancer than men?

- Why does cancer most often strike after forty?

- Where and when else, in the body, are oncogenes actively turned on?

- If there is a time they're turned on, what turns them off?

- Why do diabetics have more heart disease and cancer than the rest of the population?

We asked ourselves all these questions. Since we're sharing the answers we've found, now you're going to ask them, too—of your doctor, we hope. We think things are going to change.

There's a revolution coming.

THE FORCE OF TRUTH

At the time Ovid was writing his seminal work, the *Metamorphosis,* Christ was born within the existing structure of the Roman Empire. Christ and Rome had very little in common, but the clashes between these two "cultures" at the end of *their millennium* made for great changes—as it will for us in the year 2000, particularly in our relationships to doctors and medicine. Ted Hughes, in his classic translation *Tales From Ovid,* portrays these times in images that feel very familiar:

"*The Greek/Roman pantheon had fallen in on men's heads.*
"*The obsolete paraphernalia of the old official religion were lying in heaps, like the old masks in the lumber room of a theater.*
"*The mythic plane, so to speak, had been de-frocked.*
"*At the same time, perhaps one could say as a result, the Empire was flooded with ecstatic cults.*
"*For all of its Augustan stability, Rome was at sea in hysteria and despair, at one extreme wallowing in the bottomless appetites and suffering of the gladiatorial arena, and at the other searching higher and higher for spiritual transcendence.*
"*Ovid's tales establish a rough register of what it feels like to live in the psychological gulf that opens at the end of an era.*"

Ovid, man, we feel your pain.

These ideas, our conclusions, do fly in the face of conventional medicine at every turn, especially when it comes to cancer. Conventional medicine believes in surgery, chemotherapy, radiation, and now selective estrogen receptor modifiers (SERMs).

Practitioners of these treatments all claim to make cancer survivable.

They're lying.

A review article in the *Journal of Clinical Oncology* in October of 1998 compiled the results of a twenty-two-year study following 31,510 women with breast cancer. Their overall conclusion was that over the course of twenty-two years of reviewing twelve different therapeutic regimens in various combinations, the cancer therapies only provided "a modest improvement in survival rates."

If the paper is read carefully and the truth is told, the "modest improvement" amounts to *three months.*

Three months of extra suffering.

Thirty-one thousand, five hundred ten women, twelve different possible combinations of therapy over twenty-two years. Think about those staggering numbers.

Could the outcome in other forms of cancer really be any different?

No.

We bet that as little as you know about cancer, doctors and researchers know even less. They really can't tell you what it is or where it comes from. They only know bits and pieces of information and have no real *understanding* of the entity itself, because they, for the most part, are not acquainted with life.

BACK TO THE BEGINNING

The most salient fact about cancer that never makes it into the feature articles in the health sections of your local newspaper is that the *onco-genes* give cancerous tissue all the *unstoppable growth properties* of fetal tissue. All of the regulatory genes that are known to be active in cancer growth, with names like P53, P21, and survivin, are *only* otherwise ever active in fetal tissue.

They are never found switched on in a child or adult without cancer.

This is a big deal and a big clue.

An even bigger clue is that these genes are only really active in the first nine weeks of fetal life, when the complement of genes you have will certainly predict whether or not you are male or female but you haven't become one or the other yet. In a sense, "the jury's still out." Depending on the environmental pressures that control the hormones your mother's body makes during her pregnancy—estrogen, testosterone, cortisol, insulin, etc, and their ratio to each other—you will become boy or girl or somewhere in between.

Remember that the environment, through light, food, and stress, flips the switches on genes to produce hormones, which in turn flip other genes—for growth, death, or repair—on and off. When cancer does strike, it is really a phenomenon of reorganization to a self-similar state. The self-similar state is fetal in the human case because in the first nine weeks we are neither female nor male, we are running through the evolutionary stages of development. Those beautiful Lennart Nilsson photos of babies in the womb show us stages of human development when fetuses resemble embryonic fish and a variety of mammals and birds. We are barely differentiated from other species, let alone a male or female human, before the ninth week of pregnancy.

The first weeks of fetal development are a human "critical state" hallmarked by self-similar organization to a neutral, not male and not female, undifferentiated state seen in the embryonic development of all species. We reenter a critical state when we live so long that our sex hormones are out of balance and we eat too much (carbohydrates): Our sex hormones, now deranged, just keep pouring. Every animal in nature, except us and our pets, dies when its reproductive duties end.

Because when we cease to be what we are, we must become something else. The perfect order of quantum physics demands it.

But we never disappear without reappearing as something else.

EVERYTHING IS ONE

Just as Type II diabetes is the end product of perennial adaptation to coming famine or cold, cancer is the end product of the largest chaotic scheme in nature—universality. The principle of universality contends that at a critical point of transformation there is a kind of universal reorganization in which the details of the particular organism are obliterated.

This principle is at the heart of chaos theory. Whether it's cell biology, oncology, mathematics, financial markets, or the dynamics of ecosystems, dissecting the behavioral dynamics underlying the interactions of individuals that make up cooperative systems, like flocks of birds, colonies of bacteria, or even tumor cells, shows us what really controls physical systems.

The onset of chaos is really a *threshold,* or what physicists call a phase transition or critical state. Much like the formation of a tornado or a tidal wave or an earthquake, the appearance of cancer is just a manifestation of transformation during a critical state.

In Ovid's epic the *Metamorphosis* he elucidates how from the beginning of the world right up until his own time, bodies, from stellar to human to microbe, had been magically changed by the power of the gods into other bodies.

Critical states are ones in which ordinary matter is transformed into something quite different under the influence of heat or light. The rules of universality theory are evident in the magical transformation of liquids to solids. Water, when it is transformed to glassy ice or the evanescent vapor of steam, is the most familiar example of this magic. A more exotic illustration would be the cooling of a piece of ordinary tin to three degrees Kelvin. The deep cold turns tin into a superconductor. Somewhere in the middle is the phenomenon that occurs when heat demagnetizes a magnetic piece of iron.

A piece of iron is made up of microscopic "domains," each maybe the size of a grain of sand, and each one, on its own, a tiny magnet. At room temperature, all of these rod-shaped domains are lined up in rows next to each other. It is their *cooperation* that makes the iron magnetic; but at high temperatures, the thermal "noise" disrupts the cooperation of the domains and the iron becomes nonmagnetic. At 175 degrees Fahrenheit, the iron is on the edge between magnetic and nonmagnetic. Some of the domains still manage to clump together, but they do so only in localized clumps that point in different directions.

While this looks random, *it is not.*

If you cut out a small piece of the magnet at this point and magnify it, you'll see an image that is an exact replica of the bigger piece. This phenomenon is called self-similar organization on a fractal level. Self-similarity is the defining property of a critical state. Water on its way to steam, tin on the edge of becoming superconductive, and crystals under pressure as they collapse from one molecular structure to another all show *mathematically* identical critical states. That means atoms, molecules, magnets or the spin of electrons, it doesn't matter what's interacting, *at the point of phase shift,* all materials everywhere are *mathematically* identical to one another.

At critical phase, order spreads across the system just like a fungus spreads across an orchard. The component parts of these systems are as different as they could be, but their critical states are indistinguishable from each other. It's too hard to visualize the math; take our word for it— *so are ours.*

Cancer is the critical-phase phenomenon that is the by-product of transformation. The transformation is one of she to she-male and he to fe-man at menopause and andropause. When hormonal falloff occurs during peri-menopause in women, their ratio of estrogen to testosterone shifts until, when they are postmenopausal, progesterone is nil and estrogen is all but gone. It's testosterone that lingers. Old women, for all intents and purposes, are men on the inside after menopause.

That's when they begin to get cancer.

Men, at andropause, lose muscle mass as testosterone wanes, then glucose has nowhere to go except into fat-pad expansion. Those fat pads make estrone (estrogen), and by their late fifties or sixties, with low testosterone and high estrogen, men have begun to turn into women.

That's when men begin to get cancer.

These phase shifts into a self-similar organization at critical state are always collateral to temperature fluctuations (hot flashes), just as water turns to vapor at the boiling point, or water turns to ice at the freezing point. In us, the temperature change probably starts when we fail to go dormant at night or in the winter. The phase-shift threshold could be as simple as heating up the furnaces called mitochondria in your cells with excess carbohydrate energy that gets transformed to ATP energy. The oxidation or burn rate of carbohydrates is 1.0 and only .07 for fats. Maybe, like the rest of the planet, we're supposed to heat up all the way down to our cells in the summer. Winter is a time of shutdown for all things in the absence of the sun's energy.

That means something.

Oxidation is a chemical reaction that uses oxygen to burn with food and release energy (ATP). Its by-products are called free radicals. Free radicals are really loose cannons made up of loose electrons that bounce around in your mitochondrial DNA like balls in a pinball machine. Mitochondria are infinitesimal bean-shaped energy generators in each cell that you inherit directly from your mother's egg. They have been passed down from mother to child for forever. These inherited maps reside in your mitochondria only. Each of your cells has about 10,000 of them.

The double-helix DNA in the nucleus of each cell in your body is an amalgamation of both parents' DNA. This nucleic DNA has a repair mechanism consisting of enzymes that troll up and down the rungs of the ladder of the helix looking for breaks to fix. This is not so for your mito-chondria. Every hit and bing from a free radical makes breaks in the DNA there, unless you have enough melatonin. That's why the health-food stores sell melatonin as an antioxidant.

The falloff of athletic prowess, the decline of intellectual abilities, and the legendary failing eyesight of middle age are directly attributable to mitochondrial death. As the mitochondria die, the cells lose power. This slow death of cells is *not* the catalyst for critical phase. More likely, the trigger for a critical-phase shift would be a lack of "temperature rhythm."

If you are meant to be hot, hot, hot in the spring and summer, filled with sugar, insulin, and estrogen, up all hours in the warm sun, then, in famine or winter, when the carbohydrates are gone, insulin and estrogen fall off, too, as well as a good part of the sunlight, which drops your body temperature. With furnaces and air conditioners, we remain "climate con-trolled." In nature, longer nights of famine would also cool you off for more hours at a time. Just like perishable food, the meat that is you lasts longer in the cooler. When we never sleep, we never experience enough "shutdown" time. We have too little melatonin and too much heat from too much light.

One of the reasons melatonin is known to be such a glorious antioxi-dant is because of its property of nightly temperature reduction. That's the reason you need some sort of cover while you sleep. What happens to you, cancer-wise, when you stay up late? You have no melatonin because your night starts three to seven hours late, and because your body thinks it's summer, you have high insulin to make high estrogen.

INTO THE DARK

Almost any adult woman in the Western world, whether she's considered having hormone replacement therapy or not, can tell you the party line: Estrogen causes cancer. Both men and women produce estrogen in three variations at varying levels throughout their lives. Estrogen is part of the healthy normal reproductive phase of life in all mammals.

In the case of breast cancer, current opinion indicts estrogen on the basis of its properties as a growth factor. Since fat women produce more estrogen than thin women, and because you can also produce a variant of it from your fat base, the assumption is that being fat puts you at greater risk for breast cancer.

Unscientific, but true, assumption.

However, in reality, the same factor that made you fat is causing cancer via estrogen.

High insulin.

Let's start with the assuption that if estrogen was the sole cause of cancer, all young women would be dead.

So it's probably not *just* the estrogen.

That said, let's look at the fact that pregnant women have sky-high estrogen levels in order to grow the fetus. Pregnant women rarely suffer from cancer, especially breast cancer. In fact, all science agrees that having borne and nursed children decreases the risk for breast cancer. So how can young and/or pregnant women be drowning in estrogen and be cancer-free, if breast cancer is only fed by high estrogen levels?

Well, in reality, just because estrogen is in the bloodstream doesn't mean it's available to tissues all over the body. Sex hormones in your bloodstream are not all "active" all the time. Some are bound to a protein molecule made in the liver. There is an estrogen-binding protein called sex hormone binding globulin (SHBG) that binds estrogen and testosterone, making them unavailable to latch on to receptor sites in the body, such as breast or prostate tissue. This is another regulatory mechanism to ensure time-release action. More than a few studies show clearly that—you guessed it—high levels of insulin down-regulate the production of this control protein, leaving excess amounts of enormous growth factors like estrogen circulating *to ensure reproductive capability when the carbohydrate food supply is high.* This is not a good thing in the modern world.

In our world, the insulin/estrogen synergy stimulates tumor production.

The reason the whole of Western medicine believes that estrogen alone causes cancer rests in the Nobel prize–winning work of Charles Brenton Huggins, done in the 1950s at the University of Chicago. He proved that sex hormones like estrogen and testosterone are the controllers of proliferation by means of an experiment in which he removed all the steroid-producing organs and glands in mice and watched their tumors shrink. This new knowledge was such a breakthrough during a period when cancer deaths were skyrocketing that medical science embraced the evidence and ran with it.

The problem is, they ran *the wrong way.*

COLONIZATION

Always remember: In nature, there is duality—day/night, man/woman, hot/cold, sun/moon, up/down, in/out, growth/death. Instead of realizing that if sex hormones can control proliferation, they can probably control apoptosis (or preprogrammed cell death), too, the researchers saw only "tumori*genesis*." Almost immediately, the premier treatment for cancer became hysterectomy and castration, soon to be followed by the invention of site-specific hormone receptor blockers like Tamoxifen and enzyme blockers like Proscar.

What a mistake.

Insulin and estrogen do fuel new growth. That's the way it was meant to be. But estrogen on its own is no more the cause of cancer than cholesterol is of coronary artery disease. Only insulin can make estrogen receptors, and estrogen, in turn, gives insulin a second door in—in the form of IGF-I (insulin-like growth factor 1) receptors. New growth, or neoplasm, is the form of life found in garden-variety breast lumps and BHP, or benign hypertrophy of the prostate, in men. "Benign" is the key word here.

Neoplasm is not cancer.

If you remove or block the production of estrogen and testosterone, there is a minor regression in tumor growth, but the lull is always followed by a storm, a virulent period of rapid unchecked metastases. Hysterectomy or vasectomy only exacerbates the environmental pressure that has already started to occur—*aging.* Cancer happens predominantly after forty. The hallmark of aging—the single highest risk factor for cancer—is being hormoneless. Charles Brenton Huggins was right in citing hormones as the controllers of growth.

What he failed to see was that sex steroids are also the controllers of cell *death.*

He never looked for the homeostatic relationship.

He overlooked the *point of balance.*

Hormonal decline is the hallmark of aging. Sleep loss is the ultimate culprit in cancer because chronic carbohydrate consumption causes *accel-*

erated aging, meaning you hit menopause or andropause sooner. Menopause and andropause are both states of hormonal depletion. It's well known that at age forty, Type II diabetics often have the joints and organs of at least an eighty-year-old.

OUT OF TIME

It is universally agreed by scientists and doctors that the biggest risk for cancer is aging. So any act that will increase your rate of aging can be said to give you cancer, even by their definitions.

Now, work what you've learned about insulin into this equation. You've learned that sleep (melatonin and prolactin) controls appetite for carbohydrates (insulin), meaning that insulin, in nature, would be high for maybe four months out of the year, only in the summer. But we live with high insulin twelve months out of the year, because the lights are always on and the sugar is always available.

Therefore, we age about four times as fast in our world.

How did the low-fat liars sell us on this premature version of "the golden years"?

In the beginning, the story goes, we evolved in a tropical garden continuously full of a veritable cornucopia of ripe fruit. Naked and naive, we stumbled through one low-fat meal after another, reproducing like rabbits.

What a *crock.*

In reality, fruit abundance varies greatly on this earth, even if temperature varies little. Even in the tropics on either side of the equator, seasons exist. Take Borneo, for example, located pretty much *right on the equator,* halfway around the world, just north of Australia.

Periods of high fruit production happen there about every seven years, when all the indigenous species of fruit come into season together. Alternatively, smaller crops of various fruits flourish every year at the same time. Cheryl Knott, a Harvard anthropologist, chose the fruiting season to visit the orangutans in the wild there. She spent more than 15,000 hours observing them. Her mission was to observe how changes in food abundance (read: carbohydrates) influenced orangutan reproduction. Dr. Knott spread plastic sheets beneath the orangutans sleeping in their tree nests to collect their morning urine and analyze its hormone content. A dirty little job, but we're sure glad she did it.

As with humans, orangutans *store fat only when fruit is abundant.* By measuring the insulin in their urine she proved the same points we make about "feast-or-famine" metabolism: that reproduction is only possible when carbohydrates are abundant. In the season when the trees flower instead of fruit, the insulin levels in the urine of the orangutans is low—because they are living on twigs, grasses, termites, ants, and the occasional murder of another primate. During carbohydrate shortage, when the trees are flowering, the orangutans' urine always contains ketones from the normal fat burning characteristic of a period of famine.

The remarkable finding in Dr. Knott's work concerns estrogen. Dr. Knott's urine samples prove that in orangutans, as in humans, estrogen is high when insulin is high. It was reassuring for us to find that half a world away, in the tropics below the equator, in not a marmot or ground squirrel *but a primate like us,* there is evidence of seasonal breeding in sync with the food supply. There was no Ice Age in Borneo to cause genetic changes to make the orangutans into energy savers. Their metabolic response to even minor changes in the light keeps them reproducing in sync with the food supply as a result of the synergy between insulin and estrogen.

Because all God's creatures *must have a carbohydrate source in order to reproduce.*

That's how leaving the lights on too late controls your appetite to raise your insulin and your estrogen and ultimately cause cancer.

Unless you and the orangutans eat carbohydrates, estrogen is never kicked into play. No estrogen, no lining for the egg to implant, no pregnancy. At puberty, the whole shooting match begins when kids about eleven or twelve years old start refusing to go to bed and their appetites soar. It is so ingrained in the public consciousness that teenagers stay up late and then can't get up for school that more than one state has proposed rescheduling junior high and high school to start later in the morning to assure better grades. This tedious and aberrant teenage behavior is preprogrammed.

By shortening their melatonin phase at the beginning of the night, teenagers not only throw the hibernation switch to change the timing of prolactin and leptin production, they decrease melatonin levels, which normally would suppress estrogen and testosterone, so they're up all night eating and mating or fantasizing about eating and mating. At any rate, just staying up late is enough to make their appetites soar, which is another common teenage phenomenon.

This timed phase shift at puberty is meant to increase "energy" for reproduction. The more carbohydrates teenagers consume, the higher their insulin and leptin. The insulin is making estrogen receptors and filling fat cells. The leptin is pouring into their brains from the new sexually placed fat pads. The leptin from expanding fat cells stimulates a response from pituitary hormones like FSH (follicle stimulating hormone) and LH (lutinizing hormone) and signals that there is enough energy stored to reproduce. At that point, ovulation or spermatogenesis begins. In anorexic teens or athletes with lean body mass, the process never begins or becomes stalled for lack of a fat base.

In the orangutans, copulation and conception take place.

For most teenagers, copulation takes place, and sometimes conception.

It is this self-limiting feedback loop that keeps all God's creatures in sync with the food supply and now causes cancer.

EVERYTHING MUST DIE

Estrogen and testosterone may foster growth in a young vital state, but estrogen's counterpart, progesterone, the result of ovulation in women, and testosterone's secondary form, dihydrotestosterone (or DHT) in men, bring closure to growth by fostering creative destruction (death) in accordance with normal sun-moon rhythms.

Always listen for the music.

A menstrual cycle, when represented by a graph, has a peak of estrogen in the first two weeks and then bottoms out at day fourteen, as progesterone starts to peak. If pregnancy doesn't occur, progesterone diminishes, and after menses, estrogen starts to rise again.

Since the male's hormonal patterns mimics their breeding partner's, as it does in birds, as women age and run out of eggs, both women *and men* lose the beat.

Every menstrual cycle, women ripen about 150 eggs, but usually only one ever surfaces to pop and vie for fertilization. A declining egg base in the ovary means less and less estrogen is thrown off from "nurse cells" around the eggs. Estrogen must peak to reach a feedback loop in the pituitary with lutinizing hormone, or LH. When your pituitary reads the estrogen peak, LH feeds back to the ovary and pops the egg at the surface.

The rush of progesterone from the dissolving egg sac peaks in the middle of the next two weeks.

It's a song sung by all species.

Estrogen up, then down, then progesterone up, then down, no pregnancy . . . menstrual period . . . then estrogen up, then down, and so on and so on until all of those cycles of 150 or so eggs being expended over and over again every month reduce the number of eggs significantly. As time passes, with very few or no pregnancies to call a moratorium on egg loss, estrogen production declines.

No estrogen peak, no feedback of LH.

No LH feedback, no popped egg.

No popped egg, no progesterone.

All of the cells that were grown in preparation for pregnancy in the uterine lining and breast and brain, and God knows where else, just keep growing because there's no progesterone to cause genetically programmed cell death in all of the cells that estrogen and insulin have created.

In effect, the fat lady never sings.

DEATH IS JUST THE BEGINNING

This single mistake in the music, allowing estrogen-created cells to live, causes a keylike substance, or ligand, called CD44 to rise. CD44, which is sent out from all cells when they multiply, is normally an expression of your immune system during wound healing. In order to make new skin, one cell must let go of another to reproduce. The appearance of CD44 is the activator of that process. It is the increase of CD44 and another product called hyaluronic acid from multiplying cells that gives this new growth of cancer cells the wheels to travel across (cut through) tissue that the cancer would otherwise never make it through. Given its new attributes, this new cell growth looks and acts like an immune cell, and with keys (CD44) to unlock functions for immune actions, it heads for home.

Your closest immune factory site is home.

That would be your lymph system.

Later, the cancer will find the ultimate immune factory, your bone marrow.

Once in your lymph nodes, the new growth takes on even more immune functions as it continues to evolve into *the new you*. It picks up other keys to cellular functions, like FAS ligands, to turn off your natural germ-killing cells and T cells, which would normally destroy any mutant life in you. That means it can turn off your own original immune system with keys it has acquired in the lymph system, and in effect, take its place.

CLONING

Cancer has become the more successful life form. It has replaced you because it can reproduce and you can't, because you're too old. You didn't pop an egg, there was no progesterone to lock on to the promoter regions of death-causing genes in the cell. The cells in your breast or ovary or prostate just kept multiplying to make more cell surfaces to make more receptors to "hear" the death song sung by the missing hormone—progesterone in women, DHT in men. In no time at all, the new growth that began as neoplasm turns into cancer, because it becomes metastatic. Metastases are simply cells that have evolved to the state in which they can look for food.

In essence, the new you now has the keys to the car and *it's hungry.*

IT CAME FROM WITHIN

We're going to tell you that under "nutritional" stress, hypermutation occurs in every organism from the *E. coli* bacterium to us. Hypermutation is a global function in nature essential to Darwinian success. That means your genes actually *panic* when they suspect they will be deprived of food. If your genes suspect a hostile environment, they mutate in an effort to find a better game plan. "Spontaneous mutation" is not a term from the Sci-Fi Channel, it is a legitimate phenomenon that occurs in all species undergoing starvation.

An article in the journal *Nature* from June 5, 1997, said:

> When a population [of DNA] is unable to grow because nutrients are exhausted or cannot be used, it makes sense for [the DNA of the] individuals in that population to experiment with genomic response to overcome the deficiency.

"Cannot be used," in this case, means insulin resistance. When insulin receptors have "gone down" or closed up shop to insulin's action, the tumor cells *starve* for glucose. In lay terms: They're *real* hungry, and they're looking for a way to solve their problem.

The article continued;

One approach would be for the population to start mutating vigorously at random in the hope that this hyper-mutation would cause to rise a mutation that would enable growth to begin again. It is now clear that mutations may arise at an unexpectedly high rate during nutritional stress [insulin resistance].

What the man said was: Their genes start to mutate to get smarter to find food. So if you stay up too late and take in too much carbohydrate energy for too long, your systems read:

1. It's summer, so you eat sugar

2. Your chronic high insulin levels make you insulin resistant for fat accumulation during the winter that is expected to follow

3. Just being insulin resistant means that your estrogen, which has been up as long as your insulin has, has created neoplastic growths (new cells), particularly at reproductive sites that are very estrogen-stimulated

4. These neoplastic cell sites will inevitably get hungry enough to mutate to find a way (life finds a way) around the nutritional dilemma created by your insulin resistance

Know that none of this usually matters if you're truly young.

It only matters if you're out of progesterone or DHT.

The apes, the classification to which orangutans belong, and most other primates, including us, live to the ripe old age of forty, at most fifty. Through antibiotics and surgery, we have, just in the last eighty years, extended our life expectancy from fifty-five years in 1920 to seventy-five years in 1990. The apes don't have the advantage of surgery to repair wounds and deficits or antibiotics to keep them alive, plague-free and post-op. In nature, we would have the same life expectancy they have.

We did at the turn of the last century.

There is a natural population-control mechanism built into the system. It's called reproductive competition and stress. We would barely have lived past reproductive age in nature. Now we live too long and eat too much.

And the men are supposed to die first.

In those *National Geographic* specials, when two bucking antelope or moose go antler-to-antler over a nearby furry damsel in estrus, they are fighting over the right to her egg. Whether it's territory, resources, or hierarchical power, one or more of these items will win the prize.

The prize in this case, the egg, translates to immortality.

During the battle, the cortisol or stress levels in both of the studs is through the roof. However, when the fight is over, the cortisol level in the winner drops like a stone because the stress is gone; but in the loser it stays as high as it was during the fight . . . because he's a *loser*.

If this pattern of defeat goes on for our loser two or three more times, his cortisol levels, never having dropped, will have so suppressed his immune system that any wandering virus or itinerant bacteria can take him out. Or he will be so depressed by his plummeting status that he might stop eating or walk in front of a tiger. No matter how death comes, it is ordained. Survival of the fittest is the law. Our loser is not *fit* to live, because he didn't win the right to reproduce. His stress levels alerted Mother Nature to his stature as a big-time loser.

He is expendable.

In nature, it only takes one male to "service" many, many females.

In our time, a man's body reads the stress of being cut off on the highway or jockeying for a parking space or just receiving a bad memo from his boss as the *only* stress and he begins to die. Men die of heart disease or Type II diabetes via obesity and sleep loss long before cancer can strike them. The ones who do live long enough to get cancer, usually prostate or bladder cancer, are in their sixties and have phase-shifted.

Chronic high insulin, year in and year out, is the reason men die first. The cortisol bath they swim in from misreading cues in everyday skirmishes constantly mobilizes blood sugars—that's cortisol's raison d'être. So even if men are living on a high-quality protein like steak, as nature intended, their insulin still stays high because of cortisol's role as a blood sugar mobilizer. Add sleep loss to increase their appetite for beer and potato chips and increase their levels of endotoxin LPS, and you have the recipe for obesity, heart disease, and depression.

From the long view of evolution, it's even simpler: Men with chronic high levels of insulin have *eaten too much* of the planet. Males who take too many resources have violated a prime directive: Never compete for the food supply with the offspring and reproductive females.

Nature hates that.

DENOUEMENT

For hundreds of years, science has proceeded on the notion that things can always be understood—and can *only* be understood—by breaking them down into smaller pieces, and by knowing those pieces completely.

The medicine men are always looking down the wrong end of the telescope.

Universality theory mathematically attests to the reality that there is in this world and surely the rest of the cosmos a universal organization in which the details slip away. Mathematically speaking, if the rules are independent of the original function, then the application of the rules does not require that we understand the function. That means that alternative therapies, chemo, and radiation won't buy you time if nature targets you for transformation.

The truth is, if you use hormone replacement therapy correctly and sleep and eat in sync with the seasons, there is no cancer.

PART IV

ONLY THE PARANOID SURVIVE

NINE

DAMAGE CONTROL:

The Rhythm Method of Eating to Sidestep Extinction

*Fitzroy longed with all of his heart for simplicities, but his mind was
committed to precision. And precisely, the line he might have reproduced from simple looking turned out not to exist in any continuous
way, but became manifold . . .*

*The obvious concavity of the cove became a multitude of ins and
outs, set within the greater simpler shape, as coming closer, the outlines
of the many rock formations of which it was made up were defined.
Then, moving closer still into shallower water, a myriad of individual
pebbles on the shoreline grew visible and undulated away all remaining hope of smooth simplicity. Finally, wading on to land, his heart
pounding, desperation thudding in his head, Fitzroy sank to his knees
on the beach, to the alarm of his men, examining the shingle and even
grains of sand, each minute one of which, of course, also had an outline
of its own—and so many, too many ever to hope to give an account of
the pattern they made.*

—Jenny Diski,
Monkey's Uncle

This is the "prescriptive chapter." We felt a recap was necessary. If you've
read and absorbed every word so far, you can skip to Step 1.

It's the carbohydrate content of food that drives the chemical reactions
that turn the proteins and fats you eat into steroid (sex) hormones, muscle tissue, cytokines in your immune system, and neurotransmitters in
your brain and body. Fats called triglycerides can fuel *all* of the same
chemical reactions that carbohydrates do. Remember that even your heart
has a summer and a winter metabolism—in the summer your heart uses
glucose and in the winter it's meant to run on free fatty acids. In other

words, *you are designed to live on both carbohydrates and fats, depending on the landscape and season.*

There is *no* scientific evidence that you were ever meant to live solely on carbohydrates. Carbohydrates are converted and stored to see you through lean times. Protein and fat in the form of other living things would be available *wherever* you were living, no matter what the season—unlike carbohydrates, which would grow and be available only during the warm-weather growing season. So summer eating—carbohydrate consumption driven by the number of hours of light—is a physical imperative to secure sugar storage for famine, and it's driven by the timing of the light.

THE DARK STORY

In times of actual famine, not just when your side of the planet went dormant (winter), only those of us with stored carbohydrate got to live. Those of us who didn't have any stores died. Our DNA hates that. So an acute insulin response to eating carbohydrates became genetically entrenched over millennia for survival.

Through the miracle of technology, we have lost the famine period. *The famine period emptied the stored sugar in your muscles and liver and, more important, from your accumulation of body fat.* The next summer, feasting filled it again. That means that episodic high insulin was our salvation. For four or five months out of twelve, insulin levels were elevated to make use of the feast-before-famine period. *Continuously* elevated insulin meant only one thing for mammals.

Winter was on the way.

If that day of need never comes, you just keep storing as long as there are long hours of light.

Now you are in deep trouble with Mother Nature.

Research and common sense would indicate that being overfed, in the grand scheme of things, is asking for it. In the "food web," every species must stay in balance or all bets are off.

Since the stakes are so high, the rules are pretty strict.

Light-and-dark cycles control insulin through carbohydrate craving but also, more directly, through your stress mechanisms. Remember, when the lights are on, your cortisol stays up because it's a blood-sugar *mobilizer*—and it helps you to be ready instantly to run or fight. *Continu-*

ously high levels of cortisol—which are mobilizing your blood sugar—means insulin stays up, too, to disperse that blood sugar to your muscles. *So just watching TV late into the normal sleep period keeps your insulin up longer than nature wants it to be,* causing insulin resistance—and you know what that means.

You get fat just by *smelling* a cookie.

For Paleolithic man, long days meant the end of summer and the approaching end of the food supply. The short sleep cycles of long days translated into an increased need for carbohydrates to store fat and to turn serotonin into melatonin for the part of the year when he would sleep more in order to reduce metabolic functions to save energy when it was scarce; so carbo-craving is a precursor to sleep, and modern man still responds to instinctive behaviors led by hibernation drives.

As a result, we crave carbohydrates only when we're tired, not when we need food.

STEP 1: FOR ALL PEOPLE

We suggest that you start to plug the leaks in your psyche by dealing with reality.

Needing food, protein, and fat—being hungry for *food*—is very different from being hungry for sleep, and we're so eternally hungry for sleep that we've destroyed the trip switch for normal appetite. As far as breakfast, lunch, and dinner are concerned, figure out what season it is and try to eat in sync.

Don't run, StairMaster, or aerobicize. Lift weights or try Pilates instead and learn to meditate. Go buy a teach-yourself-yoga tape or find a yoga class. That act alone will buy you an extra ten or fifteen years of life.

In winter, eat meat and green stuff and very little carbohydrate, 25 to 45 grams per day. When designing your food plan for winter, the first thing to do is choose your carbohydrates. Your body does not discriminate among carbohydrates. The complex carbohydrate of vegetables and grains, and the simple sugars in fruits and candy, are all registered as sugar by the body.

And for God's sake, lose the pasta and fruit and all the whole-grain bread unless it's June, July, August, or September. Any bread is still fake food. Just don't eat it. There are no bread trees or pasta bushes. Bread and pasta do not occur in nature.

Eat more cheese and eggs instead. Have some organ meat, eat liver or pâté. And drink a cup of coffee; it's full of antioxidants.

If you want to control your appetite, you must sleep as many hours as you would in nature according to seasonal light exposure. That means for six to seven months out of the year you need a minimum of 9.5 hours in total darkness every night to keep your hormones from switching to summer mode. Up to fourteen hours a night is normal in winter for animals in nature.

During summer, you can live on margaritas and stay up late and have sex all day and all night.

But as fall comes, say, the middle of September:

- Go to bed earlier, incrementally.

- Turn off the TV after 9:00 P.M.

- Better yet, take it out of the bedroom.

- Sleep as many hours as you can without getting fired or divorced.

- Always get up as close to dawn as possible.

If you can't go cold turkey, read for fifteen or twenty minutes. Reading will put you to sleep faster than late-night television anyway. Bottom line: The pulsing light of the TV screen after dusk erodes melatonin secretion over the long haul by frying your pineal gland, which is as bad as it sounds.

Your new mantra: Nine and a half hours of solid sleep at least seven months out of the year is the minimum required to beat cancer, diabetes, heart disease, and depression, sayeth the National Institutes of Health.

Strive for a steady pushing forward of bedtime until 9.5 hours of sleep is a habit at least seven months of the year. *Once it happens, you'll wake up without an alarm clock and you won't be able to stay awake any later than 9:30 or 10:00 P.M.* Will this affect your social life?

Yes, but so will obesity and cancer.

Your immune system will thank you for it by keeping you alive.

- Keep lights in the house at low levels of intensity after dark. Pretend it's romantic. There's really no reason to have your kitchen or living room lit up like Yankee Stadium during a night game. Besides, the money you save on your electric bill and your shrink will pay for the supplements we're going to suggest.

- If you're going to a movie or watching TV after 9:00 P.M., wear rose-colored glasses to block green light. In a small clinical trial, just wearing red glasses after sundown increased melatonin secretion by seventy percent. It doesn't look *that* goofy.
- Once you do make it to bed, be sure you sleep in utter darkness in a fairly cool room. Think cave.
- Hang heavy drapes. Remember that the University of Chicago did a study proving that shining the light from a fiber-optic tube behind the knee of a subject who was completely covered still stopped melatonin production. This means all skin cells read light to your pineal gland. Any part of your whole body will register *any* light leaks in your bedroom.
- For God's sake, put tape over all lit-up, blinking, digital anythings.

STEP 2: FOR FAT, SICK PEOPLE

If you can accomplish Step 1, you will lose weight naturally and pretty fast. It happens because when you're rested, you're able to resist carbohydrates. It should be much easier than ever before to stop eating sugar, drinking, or smoking. If you're more than twenty pounds overweight, now would be the time to cut carbohydrates down to no more than 45 grams a day and no less than 25.

If you're so lost when it comes to food that you can't even pick out your own lunch, you can buy a copy of *Dr. Atkins' Diet Revolution* or *Sugar Busters!*, or you can go to the back of this book to choose carbohydrates and vegetables. Buy some Ketostix and Advil. Look for ketones in your urine about five or six days after your first low-carbohydrate day. You'll probably have a headache for a few days from the drop in serotonin, but the day you see ketones, the headaches will stop. Remember, if it's spring or summer, eat, drink, and be merry. Party hearty. Stay up as late as you want.

However, if it's past September or you're overweight now, consider every day a snow day.

SOYLENT GREEN IS PEOPLE

Protein is essential. Eat it every day, at every meal. Remember: No protein, no neurotransmitters or immune function. Vegetarianism is morally laudable, but it's impossible to get enough protein. Even monkeys murder for meat.

Fats are essential. They are necessary for all cellular function. No fat, no hormones—and that means cancer. Don't eat any fat that didn't start out alive—make sure it's from a plant or an animal.

Don't eat packaged or processed foods. This includes highly refined or hydrogenated oils, anything shrink-wrapped (just think "s" for sugared), or anything with a proper name or a capital letter. Capital letters, as in Oreos, mean that the substance was invented, not grown. Eat a lot of real butter.

Don't eat anything labeled "low-fat" or "nonfat." These foods contain sugar and other chemicals as additives to fool your palate into believing that they have fat in them.

Only eat as many carbohydrates as you need in a day, in season. If you are going to a place where food is scarce, or you intend to sleep through the winter in your own locale, feel free to eat all of the *natural* carbohydrates you want. Otherwise, summer is an all-you-can-eat proposition, and winter is *no more than 45 grams a day.*

Eat only fresh fruits and vegetables. Canned fruits and vegetables are *processed.* Frozen fruits and vegetables would be a rare accident in nature; treat them the same way in your own life.

Drink a decent amount of plain water, the original beverage. You don't have to drown yourself, but living on high protein, it's a good idea to drink at least five eight-ounce glasses of water a day. Do not drink bottled liquid sugar, especially drinks sweetened with fructose or artificial sweeteners. If you must, go with saccharine; it will kill you more slowly than NutraSweet, and cane sugar is better than corn sugar.

RAW MATERIALS

Atoms make up molecules and molecules make up chemical structures ranging from simple neurotransmitters like serotonin to high-molecular weight compounds like the human genome. Carbon, in living things, forms a myriad of very stable chemical compounds.

These compounds are like Tinkertoys.

The "sticks and wheels" deconstruct and then reconstruct into the physical world of which you are a part.

Carbon and water make up carbo-hydrates.

Energy is released or burned as ATP when the carbohydrate molecules split apart. The water molecules (the hydrate parts) are dispensed with when you sweat, cry, or urinate; the leftover two-carbon molecules are stored as body fat to be relit later, like charcoal. This reburned, recycled energy is called ketones—carbohydrate charcoal. They are the product of already ignited carbohydrate that has spent some of its energy. Just as the charcoal in your grill was once wood and has been burned already, ketones can be ignited again to produce more energy. Since a ketone burns hotter than fresh sugar and is pure energy, it cannot be stored again; therefore, no insulin, like that needed to change sugar to fat, is necessary.

When human beings eat any of the possible compounds of sugars, proteins, and fats—food—available to us in nature, energy is released from these sources. Science measures this energy release in the form of heat loss. We call these measurements of energy calories, because in Latin the word for hot is *calor.*

A calorie isn't a *calorie,* per se.

According to the popular definition of a calorie, a calorie is really a carbohydrate, not ever a fat or a protein. Popular confusion is fueled by the medical profession's dedication to numbers. Any dietitian or "nutritionist" will enthusiastically tell you that fat has nine calories per gram while carbohydrate has only 4.5. Protein, although it can be turned into glucose during extreme starvation, causes little or no release of insulin and cannot be stored as body fat. But dietary fat, eaten all by itself, can never be stored as body fat, because it never causes an insulin response.

Carbohydrates are the only foods that can turn into cholesterol in your blood. That's why a rice cake will become body fat or up your cholesterol number before a pork chop will.

You break the chemical bonds in carbohydrates to release energy to drive chemical reactions. You can store the energy, either in the short term in your muscles or liver or in the long term as body fat. The release of the energy of carbohydrates starts with their breakdown under the heat of cooking. Then the saliva in your mouth, using an enzyme called amylase, continues the breakdown process. Finally, carbohydrates are broken down into simple sugars by water and more enzymes during digestion. The final product is *glucose,* or *sugar.* The minute glucose is evident in your bloodstream, your pancreas sends insulin to open the doors for the sugar to enter your liver and muscles for storage.

Once the sugar is in storage in your liver or muscles, it is called glycogen.

Carbohydrates stored long-term are called body fat.

Storage is completely controlled by the light you are exposed to and the attendant insulin resistance.

The way we live now, we store fat continuously month after month, season after season, year in and year out, because our stored sugar (glycogen) is *never* depleted by winter or famine. All athletes know the most successful way to "carbo-load" for a race is to exercise while following a high-fat and high-protein diet for a day or two, then to have a carbohydrate-rich day or two. In clinical studies following the athletes' premise, stored-sugar saturation was reached in only four days. Past that point, respiratory quotient measurements indicated that fat was being produced. And cholesterol production was up tenfold.

That's the big deal.

Nature meant you to empty your stores in between heavy feedings.

Therein lies the premise of a feast-or-famine metabolism. It's impossible to empty those glycogen reservoirs on a low-fat, high-carbohydrate diet. The high-carbohydrate regimen of a low-fat diet only results in weight loss because you lose muscle and bone mass. After your glycogen stores stop accepting sugar, your muscles become unresponsive and insulin resistant, too. That's why the longer you're on a low-fat diet, the *harder* you have to exercise to lose weight.

THE HARD STUFF

Not just the amount, but the *kind* of carbohydrate you eat matters a great deal. Refined sugar (sucrose) was not ever considered a foodstuff until the common era. In fact, it was unknown to mankind until sometime after A.D. 600. Until that time, only sugarcane was traded as a rare and expensive luxury.

The University of Djondisapour in the very center of what was once the Persian Empire is credited with developing a process for solidifying and refining the juice of the sugarcane into a form that would not ferment. It was referred to as "stone honey" and considered a rare and precious miracle drug. This "medicine" was used sparingly because of its remarkable effect on the body. It is clear from a review of history and common sense that refined sugar never formed any part of the human diet for our first couple of million years.

Even the Greeks, post-Persia, still had no name for any such substance. A Roman around the time of Nero gave it its name—*saccharum*. Refined sugarcane was the Roman *saccharum*. Note that the only artificial sweetener on the market today that *doesn't* cause a reaction in the body, as a carbohydrate would (insulin spike), is called saccharine and marketed under the name Sweet'n Low.

Sugar beets became the sugar of *our* childhoods. The contemporary heir to the throne is a substance called high fructose corn syrup. It has replaced sucrose (cane or beet sugar) as the sweetener in soft drinks. Processed from corn, it's an additive found in almost all processed foods, especially low-fat products. The calorie content of low-fat processed foods comes mostly from high fructose corn syrup. It is highly concentrated, so very small amounts will do the same job sucrose used to do, and for much less money. Its effect on your system is even more disastrous, because again, it is a substance that never occurs in nature and *you are part of nature*. If you remember our discussion of GABA receptors, this gives you a clue why products like *Snapple* and it newest competitor, Fruitopia, are so addictive, and why Snapple's spokeswoman, Wendy, looks so happy.

SCIENCE FICTION FOOD

Unrefined carbohydrates qualify as whole foods; refined carbohydrates do not. These include white flour and refined sugars of any kind. These foods are more like drugs. Refined sugar, in fact, may not be food at all. It probably should be listed as a chemical additive. In 1973, it was declared to be an *anti*-nutrient by the same Senate committee that shut down Dr. Atkins. There's irony for you. Atkins attributed obesity and heart disease to the overconsumption of carbohydrates. The committee declared Atkins a quack and refined sugar an anti-nutrient all in the same month. Here's the laugh: An anti-nutrient is defined as *any substance or drug with properties that are in some way antagonistic to nutrients, interfering in some way with their use or metabolism.* Atkins was right.

All carbohydrates are burned with the aid of enzymes that contain a myriad of B vitamins. So it follows that the more carbohydrates you eat, the more B vitamins you need. Real and whole carbohydrates such as vegetables, whole grains, and fruit all contain B vitamins and minerals in their outside husks as sort of a package deal. White flour, the husk of which is thrown out during refinement, is the only kind used in processed foods and is packageless, vitamin- and mineral-wise. When you throw away the chewy stuff on the outside, you're left with pure sugars.

Without the cane or without beet fibers, refined sugar is the same kind of incomplete food. When you try to digest refined sugar or white flour, not only are you denied the vitamins they were stripped of during the refining process, but you must contribute your own B vitamins to the process in order for digestion to happen. The same process of refinement removes the germ (seed) and bran from whole grains (complex carbohydrates), leaving the meal, which is the powdered product we know as flour. That's why we tell you that the beavers aren't eating Danish, and bread and pasta do not exist in nature.

Both bread and pasta are as refined *as a candy bar.*

Ten thousand years ago, grain was ground between stones. This process expended as much *or more* energy than would be taken in (eaten) when the job was finished. So, like the original farmers, pulling your own plow compensated in energy expenditure for the increased consumption of carbohydrates. Later on, mill operations on a grander scale that fed masses of people were still driven by human energy. Eventually, stones were exchanged for steel rollers, and water and then steam for manpower.

The sociopolitical history of refined sugar is completely economic and has as its high points the rise of Islam, the fall of Islam (it was all about sugar and the Crusades), Columbus's voyage, the rise of the British Empire (refined beet sugar, as a cheaper source than cane, funded the rise), the Revolutionary War, slavery in the New World, and, by distant relation, booze (the Whiskey Rebellion and rumrunners), the ensuing Prohibition, and the organized crime Prohibition spawned. Bottom line: Refined sugar is really bad for people, but especially good for the governments and enterprises who sell it. They're our dealers, man.

How addictive is sugar?

How much do we consume?

Who is making money feeding our habit?

It is not a pretty picture.

The U.S. Department of Agriculture tells us that, as of 1993, the average American consumed 150 pounds of sugar and other natural sweeteners a year. That's an increase of twenty percent over 1983 statistics. In 1993, we were eating about two and a half pounds a week per person. One and a half of those pounds came from the high fructose corn sweeteners in processed foods. It bears mentioning here that high fructose corn syrup is six times as sweet as sugar, but that doesn't mean we eat one-sixth as much. Who is making the big bucks?

The world price for raw sugar is one half the domestic price, about twelve cents a pound, compared to the artificially elevated twenty-two cents a pound at home. Quotas severely limit imports. The quotas and price supports that keep the cheaper imported sugar out of the U.S. actually cost about $3 billion per year. All processed foods, especially low-fat foods, are full of high fructose corn syrup. And all low-fat food is expensive, especially low-fat *fast* food. Between 1994 and 1999, the marketplace exploded with low-fat fast food. In 1999 alone, the processed food industry produced more than 3,500 new low- or no-fat products. We get almost two-thirds of our sugar from processed foods. Getting the sordid picture?

All of America's factories and food manufacturers have literally retooled to produce food made with fake fats and more sugar. Analysts estimate the new Healthy Choice products alone may be worth as much as $100 million in annual sales. That's just the *new* products. Since 1988, Healthy Choice has consistently grown. Healthy Choice is owned by ConAgra, the second-largest food processor in America after Kraft. Its annual sales from the Healthy Choice line hover at $1.3 billion. It licensed Healthy Choice to Nabisco, the creator of SnackWell's no-fat cookie. Nabisco generated 32 percent of its total sales volume from low- and no-fat products in 1998. The cookies alone were worth half a million dollars.

Manufacturers will tell you they've done this only in response to public demand. What they won't tell you is that high fructose corn syrup is a cheap ingredient that will do more to improve moisture content, add a chewy texture, and extend shelf life than any sort of fat or oil. And believe us, once you take the fat out of baked goods and cold cuts, nobody is going to eat them unless the sugar content is doubled. Once the sugar content is doubled, the manufacturers and the fructose guys make out like bandits.

This news item ran in the January 6, 1995, issue of *The New York Times:*

RANGERS KILLING DEER ADDICTED TO SNACKS
Grand Canyon National Park, Ariz. (AP)—Park rangers are killing off more than two dozen mule deer that have become addicted to junk food left by visitors. Thirteen animals have been shot to death since early December. The Rangers plan to kill twelve more by the end of the week. The deer have been hooked on snack food and candy, losing their ability to digest vegetation. The chief of resource management for Grand Canyon National Park, David Haskell, called junk food "the crack cocaine of the deer world." "They've become in extremely poor health, almost starving to death," he said. Mr. Haskell said that the muscles of all the deer have atrophied and that the animals are so tame they walk right up to the rangers who shoot them.

ARTIFICIAL LIFE FORM

A lot of us just fill the void in our diets with fakes. Americans consume 26 million pounds of fake sugar every year, about half of the world's annual production. Three-quarters of that figure is in the form of diet soft drinks. These sales are worth $1 billion to the makers of the stuff. All of them except saccharine affect the body as a carbohydrate. Saccharine is known as Sweet'n Low, and has the smallest market. It's made by a Brooklyn company called Cumberland Packing Corporation and is the oldest sugar substitute on the market. Monsanto, the maker of aspartame, controls 70 percent of the market. Aspartame is sold under the names Equal and NutraSweet.

Artificial sweeteners are like all other overprocessed, man-made, lab-created, mad-scientist "foods"—no more than two molecules away from plastic, literally. Artificial sweeteners are not food. Silly Putty has more in common with actual food than artificial sweeteners do.

THE CARBOHYDRATE CHOICE

In the winter, it matters which carbohydrates you eat because only root vegetables and bark, along with dried herbs and grasses, would have been available to you in prehistoric times. In our time, those choices would translate to carrots and potatoes sautéed in onions and thyme with an aspirin for dessert (bark).

An important term to understand is glycemic index, which is a measure of how the body digests carbohydrates and how fast digested sugar gets into the body and is met by insulin. The glycemic index of any food can be altered by combining it with fats. Remember, the higher the glycemic index, the faster the sugar enters your system and the higher the insulin response. Conversely, the lower the glycemic index, the lower and slower the insulin response.

Green vegetables also slow down the transit time through the digestive tract and will thus lower the glycemic index. This works with proteins and non-starchy vegetables, too. You can change the glycemic index of any food by adding a fat to any carbohydrate. Add butter or sour cream to a baked potato and you even slow down the enzyme activity in the mouth. Grease your enzymes prophylactically. Think of fat as a condom for your carbs.

- **If you need to lose weight, no matter what season it is, eat foods with lower glycemic indexes.**

- **Carbohydrates are the only foods you ever need to count out.** Refer to the carbohydrate list and seasonal availability choices in the Appendix.

- **When you eat carbohydrates in summer, enjoy.** But remember that carbohydrate junk food will kill you nine ways to Sunday.

- **Read labels.** "Sugar-free?" *Never.* This is a very sneaky label. Usually, all "sugar-free" means is that the product doesn't contain sucrose (cane or beet sugar). Many "food products" (that's right, "food products" are not real food) that are labeled "sugar-free" contain other sweeteners that will raise your blood sugar and spike your insulin just as real sugar would.

- **Try checking the list of ingredients for the amount of carbohydrates and sugar per serving.** If this information is not there, *they must be hiding something.*

- **Don't drink milk.** You're an adult.

EAT GREEN VEGETABLES

- **Green vegetables are important.** Their fibrous content slows down the digestive process, which lowers the glycemic index of your entire meal. Although they are not converted into vital structures, they do have value as vitamins, minerals, and fiber.

- **There is no nutrient or vitamin found in fruit that is not also found in vegetables.**

- **Don't take those weird vegetable pills instead of eating vegetables unless you're an astronaut.** It isn't the same thing.

- **Eat vegetables in season.** A good rule of thumb is that if it's grown *underground* (except for the onion family, which consist of real sugar), it's *starchy,* which means it has more carbohydrates. That's why you'd be rewarded with them in the winter, when the rest of the planet's carbohydrates have gone dormant. If it's grown *above* ground (except for peas, corn, and beans), it's non-starchy.

DEAD MEAT

It's late September. Most of what you've raised outside your door has played itself out. Some late-harvest green vegetables are still to come, but the fruit has been gone for a while, unless you live in apple country. Your meal is mainly animal protein and some green stuff this time of year.

If you lived in the pastoral setting we've just described, how would your body react to the change in the light, the available food, and the weather?

Your body would react by losing weight.

Because you'd be living on less carbohydrate, fewer green vegetables, and more protein, you'd be beginning to burn your own accumulated fat to sustain the energy required for internal processes. Even your heart would be starting to run on free fatty acids instead of straight glucose. Remember, body fat can replace carbohydrate energy for every metabolic process. That's how bears survive hibernation. And that's why there are no essential carbohydrates, only essential fats and proteins.

The proteins you're eating more of now are turned into enzymes that serve both as materials and as the tools that do the job. When proteins reach the stomach, they have not been partially predigested the way carbohydrates have. Cooking and the amylase in your saliva have no affect on them the way they do on carbohydrates. Proteins wait to undergo a slow process of breakdown in the stomach. The hydrochloric acid in your stomach activates an enzyme called pepsin, which is a protease enzyme that cuts up other proteins. Proteases turn proteins back into amino acids, which are absorbed into the bloodstream to become neurotransmitters, clotting factors, and a part of cell membranes.

The amino acids cause your small intestine to send signals of "satisfaction" to your brain through the hormone cholecystokinin, or CCK. This tells your brain you're not hungry anymore. If CCK is *over*produced, it causes pain and nausea. This means you can't overeat proteins. You have built-in regulatory controls that tell your body when to stop eating protein.

By living on protein and fat for a while, you actually give your heart a rest from all of the free radical production, too. In a 1971 *Lancet* study, "Plasma Lipid and Lipoprotein Pattern in Greenlandic West-Coast Eskimos," conducted by a group of Danish researchers, 130 Eskimos, consuming a predominantly meat-and-blubber diet, were found to have a markedly lower cholesterol and triglyceride count than the non-Eskimo citizens of Denmark. These findings corroborate the known "paradox" that there is no heart disease and no diabetes among Eskimo populations. The study summed up the dietary habits of these Greenlanders with an insensitive footnote: "Their dietary habits are very like those of carnivorous animals."

Remember, this was twenty-nine years before this book was written.

Political correctness was in its infancy.

They also included in their peer-review paper the definition of the word "Eskimo," just to douse any debate. They said, "The word 'Eskimo' is of Red Indian origin and means 'people eating raw meat.' "

Don't try cultural relativism like that in the year 2000.

THE REAL MEAT OF THE ISSUE

- **Do not buy packaged meat products.** They'll always be filled with preservatives, and some, such as nitrates, are known carcinogens. Packaged meat products will also have a lot of salt and sugar. The deli section of the supermarket contains prepared foods that are all laced with additives. Ask the counterman to read you the ingredients on the package label before you buy it.

- **Buy fresh meat every day.** Humans, even though we are carrion eaters, aren't meant to eat old food. Two-day-old cooked chicken in your refrigerator has already begun to oxidize. This approach will necessitate shopping more often. Pretend you are in Europe. (French women have the lowest death rate in the world from all causes, including heart disease, and they look really swank with their little shopping bags picking things up for dinner.)

- **Vary your selection of protein.** Include eggs, nuts, cheeses, and tofu in your diet. It's good to eat red meat, just don't do it three times a day. Eat fish, chicken, and other poultry. In the natural world, you wouldn't necessarily catch the same prey for every meal. And don't cook it to death. It's already dead. (The average serving of barbecued or burned meat imparts to you an amount of cancer-causing particles equivalent to what you would get from smoking 250 cigarettes.)

VEGETARIANS, WE HAVE A PROBLEM

The big question is: Are you a fat-free vegan with an active lifestyle and a cellular phone who loves animals and networking on the Internet? We bet you're not alone. In this sad, ass-backwards world, many people have been convinced by factions of medicine and certainly the media that the moral and physiological high road leads not only to political correctness, but also to social attractiveness and good health.

Not even.

Why do we buy this bizarre reverse take on real life?

We're media hounds on the one hand, and on the other, we still need Mom to tell us what to do, but she's in a meeting. The lack of cohesive tribal and cultural wisdom leaves the average American lost, always latching on to the next cool thing.

If you are a vegetarian, the thin, lighter-than-air body that you have or aspire to have on your starch-and-fruit diet may be visually appealing; but the way you're eating to achieve it is like pouring sugar in your gas tank, physiologically. The result to your metabolism is exactly the same. You may look like a supermodel, but there are all sorts of nasty processes going on inside. You will grind to a halt, probably sooner than later.

Your vehicle may not be a car, but it is a bioengineered machine, a mini-machine, just a cog in the mega-machine. In the larger picture, we are, in fact, a linchpin in the biosphere. Man is a part of the food chain. Since we're part of a larger scheme—just like everything else alive, from the smallest one-celled organism to your dog—respiration, excretion, and reproduction are the laws of life that hold true for us, too. This would logically include the laws of feeding and diet.

Imagine how long your dog would last on coffee and a low-fat bran muffin for breakfast every day.

You are both mammals.

Since we're mammals, in order to keep muscles reacting to those stress triggers, we must take in protein and fat. The massive carbohydrates of a low-fat diet are pure energy, not structural materials. Remember, structurally, proteins and fats form all the chemicals needed for survival in the form of hormones, enzymes, and neurotransmitters. Without hormones, neurotransmitters, and an immune system, you can't react and adapt to the environment.

When you can't adapt, nature replaces you.

History tells us that mankind has made it through many a winter without fruits and plant materials (during the Ice Age, for example), but *never without protein and fat.* The fact that fat and cholesterol are so necessary to the human organism that they make the difference between life and death is a well established scientific fact.

Vegetarians, beware:

- **Tofu is an almost-complete protein.** The only essential amino acid that tofu does not contain enough of is methionine. Eat the firm type, not soft tofu. It has twice the protein per serving size.
- **Rice and beans together only make a complete protein if you eat like Godzilla.** Size does matter, when it comes to carbohydrates. The bad news is that one cup of brown rice has 5 grams of protein and 46 grams of carbohydrate and a cup of kidney beans has 15 grams of protein and 40 grams of carbohydrates. That makes 20 grams of protein and 86 grams of carbohydrates, but who's counting? *This doesn't even include the tortilla.* To stay under 87 grams of carbohydrate, you must eat it out of your hand. (That was a joke.)

- **Legumes (beans) and grains (rice) both contain a lot of carbohydrates.** This food combination will make your insulin soar. Still, it's better to eat legumes and grains together than to eat pasta and salad. But you'll lose more weight on a tofu-based regimen.

OUT OF THE FIRE AND INTO THE FRYING PAN

Some time after the first human carried a burning ember away from a lightning strike, we started to cook, literally and figuratively. Literally, because a mammal or bird, maybe even one of us, fell into the fire. Rather than waste such a precious resource, we ate the burned flesh and found that the fire had taken a lot of the work out of chewing and digestion. The more meat we ate, the more obvious it became that the fire burned brighter when there was fat in it. When the fat bound up in that roasting flesh caught fire, so did our imaginations.

It was just such a grease fire that lit the way to artistic enlightenment. Early humans solved knotty social and emotional conundrums through their art in dark, dank caves by the light of burning animal fat. (Fifty thousand years later, the very same tallow became the candles that made Paris the City of Light.) Before our memory created history, our whole day as humans was directed toward the acquisition of meat to get at the fat when sugar was unavailable.

Homer's heroes ate only roasted meat. Throughout all of antiquity, religious rites and gods have been dedicated to fat and fat sources. The Aztecs had corn oil as a fat source, the Greeks had olives, and the Chinese had the soybean.

Pungent fragrances are absorbed by fats. The real flavors of fruits and vegetables are in contained droplets of oil. Because oils and fats in cooking can be heated hotter than water, they produce the intense flavors we love that accompany browning reactions.

Harold McGee, a phenomenal food writer, in his *On Food and Cooking*, said that the Egyptians were frying foods in fat and using it for perfume at least 3,500 years ago. The lure of fat has greased the skids for economies and romance as long as there have been both. Maybe fried food and sex have always gone hand in hand on a hot date. The flavor and the "mouth appeal" are the seduction factors. Health is the payoff. Animal fat, ours and theirs, has always been invaluable in human evolution to keep the lights on inside and out.

Fats, like protein, begin being digested in the stomach and end up as amino acids in the small intestine, where they are broken down into fatty acids and glycerol. Fatty acids and dietary cholesterol are absorbed into the small-intestine wall, where they are repackaged together into protein-coated droplets called chylomicrons. (Chylomicrons never become VLDLs, and they can never stick in your heart.) These can only be stored as body fat if you also eat sugar, which—all together now—releases insulin. Since nothing can be processed for storage without insulin around, don't eat cookies, which provide the sugar that gets the insulin going. Butter can't get processed into fat on its own.

Some of the largest quantities of structural fats in the body are found in nerve membranes, especially in the brain. Fats are the major components of the myelin sheath, a fat membrane that wraps around fast-conducting nerve fibers, like insulation on electrical wires, speeding the nerve impulse. Without the brain, there is no operations control; without the body constantly processing dietary fats into fatty acids and cholesterol, there is no brain function to control operations.

As a nutrient, fat solves the human energy dilemma between feedings by encompassing both structure and storage. Carbohydrate energy can be turned into "storage energy" (body fat) in the liver, but cannot replace the need for essential fatty acids that go directly to the structure of cells, bones, and blood. Therefore, we must eat protein to acquire the attendant fat.

DEATH AS A DIET AID

As we've said before, there are no essential carbohydrates, only essential proteins and fats. These essential proteins and fats are so termed because your body can't make them internally from any other foodstuff and must have them for structural repair and system functionality.

The *essential* fatty acids for humans are linoleic and linolenic. They can't be synthesized anywhere in the body from anything else already in the body. You must acquire them directly from the foods that you eat. Linoleic acid is found in most foods. Eggs, proteins, vegetables, and grains all have varying amounts.

Linolenic acid is found abundantly in flaxseeds, meat fats, and, in small amounts, green leafy vegetables. Our first food on the outside, breast milk, contains both of these acids and one more, gamma-linolenic acid

(GLA). GLA is found almost nowhere else except in human breast milk, and, in trace amounts, in raw oatmeal and really esoteric oils such as borage, black currant, gooseberry, and evening primrose. GLA is made in the second step in the fatty-acid metabolism of linoleic acid, so you're going to get it anyway.

Newborn nursing also serves another purpose beyond nutrition. It actually keeps babies warm. Newborns contain a specialized, metabolically active, heat-producing tissue called brown fat. Its thermogenic action smoothes out the rough transition from a hot womb to a cold world. Brown fat is highly metabolically active and there is evidence that brown fat, which is brown as a result of an abundance of mitochondria, is responsive to GLA and other fatty acids.

It seems that temperature is really the key in adults, too. Remember Ice Age conditions. Breast milk, after all, is a whole and complete food comprised of protein, fat, and carbohydrate: exactly what you need to eat to thrive as adults. It's become common knowledge that formula-fed babies are fatter and, in a multitude of ways, unhealthier than breast-fed babies.

Get your fats from nuts, olives, avocados, and anywhere else you would find them in nature. *If you can step on it and it makes a grease spot under your foot, it's okay to eat.* Think about the world we're really from. There were no machines, and therefore there was no corn oil. This premise is hereafter referred to as the step-on-it rule.

Now that you know that the pervasive use of an anti-nutrient like refined sugar in the last century has undermined normal health, and that the current trend of low-fat living has added fuel to the fire, it's pretty easy to see why Americans are sick and dying. *If your insulin was already up thanks to the invention of cheap artificial lights and packaged processed foods, where is it now that you've removed all the fat and replaced it with more sugar?*

Barry Sears called fat a "control rod" for digestion of carbohydrates. We *wish* that that was its most important job. Fat doesn't just slow down the glycemic index of foods. Essential fatty acids and cholesterol control the health and well-being of every cell you've got.

What's in a fat? Would a fat by any other name do the job? *No.* Especially not if it's hydrogenated or it's called olestra, a.k.a. Olean. Hydrogenated fats are not only biologically detrimental to the body, but they also stick in your cells' power plants (mitochondria) and age you prematurely. Olestra, besides being a bizarre idea, is an anti-nutrient like sugar.

It removes fat-soluble vitamins A, D, E, and K from your body because these vitamins usually hitch a ride into your system by fat transport. These vitamins have no idea that olestra is an impostor, and they hop on. But since it's not real fat, they end up coming out the other end with the undigested fat molecules.

So Procter & Gamble has fortified olestra with synthetic versions of those vitamins. You are now on your way to being one hundred percent artificial. The problem is, how do their vitamins know they should jump off when ours don't?

These are not minor vitamins we're losing. Vitamin A deficiency is characterized by macular degeneration (blindness). Vitamin D is a vitamin/hormone that's activated in the kidneys to control calcium absorption for bone strength. Vitamin E's major role is in preventing oxidation and degradation of fatty acids and includes the formation of red blood cells. Do we need to lose any more antioxidants? Vitamin K prevents hemorrhaging.

Needless to say, this is the short list.

The big flap about olestra concentrates on anal leakage and fecal urgency. We wonder if it's truly a coincidence that Procter & Gamble owns the patent on both olestra and Depends. There's urgency all right, but it's about your life and health, not your underwear.

The other fats that you encounter in processed foods, such as mayonnaise and anything fried, will be *hydrogenated.* Hippolyte Mege-Mouries won the prize offered by Napoleon III for the creation of an edible synthetic fat. His goal was to make a liquid into a semisoft solid. He accomplished this feat by artificially saturating the oils of plants during exposure to hydrogen gas at high temperatures. All naturally occurring saturated fats are semisolid at room temperature, too. Otherwise, spreading butter couldn't happen. It's the mixture of different triglycerides in a given fat that causes gradual softening. As the temperature changes from the friction of the knife, each faction of triglyceride melts at its own rate, causing the gradual softening.

Partial hydrogenation produces the same effect. As a fat replacement, hydrogenated oils extend shelf life and impart moisture better than butter. They also prevent rancidity due to oxidation. The problem with this rocket science is, of course, that it has created something that does not occur in nature—solid plant fats. You, as part of the food chain, have a system that can't handle futuristic, man-made, not-part-of-nature substances. To your body, it's akin to birds on the bottom of the ocean; it does not compute.

During the hydrogenation process, the actual shape of the fatty acid is altered. Plant oils naturally occur in a molecular shape known as the cis configuration; on the carbon chain, the hydrogens stick out on one side of the molecule. During hydrogenation, the groups may rotate so that they are on both sides of the bond, in the trans position, hence the name trans-fatty acids. Everyone finally agrees that trans is bad acid. This shift effectively makes the most essential fatty acid, linoleic acid, biologically damaging.

It's not just useless. It's dangerous.

Hydrogenated soy oil or palm oil is in virtually every packaged food you buy and has been for most of your life. To your cells, hydrogenated oils are "virtual reality" fats. That means your body seems to experience fat, but cannot really interact with it.

Cyber-dining.

This modification contributes to your demise because the cell sends these misshapen, impotent molecules to the mitochondria, where they lodge and cause dysfunction and general slowdown of cell metabolism by reducing the activity of enzymes that process fatty acids. When you consider the fragile system of checks and balances going on in the cell, how could you possibly be healthy eating a thirty-four percent *dead fat* diet?

Once you add sugared, processed, and low-fat foods to your already fat-deprived diet, you can kiss yourself good-bye.

Again, government-regulated science is responsible for this nutritional disaster. Back in 1905, hydrogenation never had to wait twenty-five years for FDA approval to enter the marketplace, as olestra did. In fact, hydrogenation's point of origin was Germany, not the United States. The era had something to do with it, too. It was the good old days of real freedom. No driver's licenses or income taxes existed; why, you could tell anybody to eat anything and he would.

Not like today.

It was really about money back then, too. This quote from Mark Twain's *Life on the Mississippi* is reported as a conversation overheard between two businessmen aboard the riverboat *Cincinnati*:

Why we are turning out oleomargarine now, by the thousands of tons. And we can sell it so dirt-cheap that the whole country has got to take it—can't get around it, you see. Butter don't stand any show—There ain't any chance for competition.

These same sentiments are circulating at the water cooler at Procter & Gamble right now. After all, P&G has already invested more than $200 million developing olestra. Preying on the fear and ignorance of the American population, something like 3,000 new low-fat products were proffered to the confused public in 1999. Now make that 3,001. Here comes the most dangerous idea the snake-oil salesmen have come up with so far.

Take an already weakened population, convince them that fat is killing them, and then offer them a nonfat, two-molecules-away-from-plastic solution that will leach all the vitamins out of their systems. That premise should cause slow painful death, and it won't be cheap.

Olestra, marketed under the brand name Olean, is a man-made fat molecule that is too big to be digested. It almost confuses the tongue, but not the body. Your tongue will register a slight aftertaste; your body doesn't respond at all. This molecule will pass through you undetected as fat by everything in your body except the fat-soluble vitamins A, D, E, and K. They will jump off the other foods you've eaten and onto olestra, looking for transport into the cells. They will, however, roll out the other end of you without ever reaching their destination, because eating olestra, on the molecular level, is like eating teeny-tiny Styrofoam peanuts.

After twenty-five years of deliberation, the FDA finally pulled the plug on public health and approved olestra for snack foods. Limiting it to snack foods was their attempt at a cautious, conservative stance. That move was a thinly veiled marketing ploy.

Americans in 2000 subsist almost solely on low-fat foods. American children do exist completely on packaged snack foods. If they had added it to the water supply, it wouldn't reach as many people. Most food additives, except high fructose corn syrup and hydrogenated oil, are eaten by the milligram. The FDA bases its reviews on that premise. Olestra is a macronutrient, not a micronutrient. People will eat it by the gram. That's a thousand times more "pretend fat" per bite than most toxic substances. Olestra will account for about one-third, by weight, of every potato chip.

Ordinarily, the FDA would do a toxicology test. But that would mean feeding to rats one hundred times as much olestra as humans would eat. Since humans will eat enormous quantities, the rats' entire diet would be olestra. This would kill them by simple malnutrition because olestra has no food value. Besides, you could watch the eating habits of dying rats for twenty-five years and never learn anything. Maybe that's what the FDA has been doing for all those years in between the first P&G petition and the approval. Apparently, the FDA never turns anybody down; they just make them wait twenty-five years.

P&G tried reclassifying olestra as an anti-obesity drug, but "it didn't do a good enough job to qualify as a medicine," according to the January 8, 1997, issue of *Time.* Now we know that's because fat can't make you fat, so removing fat can't cure obesity. Anyway, drugs have to produce evidence of benefit, but food additives don't.

So olestra went back to being a food additive.

Since the FDA has no money to do its own studies, it depends on the petitioners, like P&G, to provide the research proof. That's rich. The question is, if petitioners provide their own evidence to support their claims, how really, *really* bad for you might olestra be? In twenty-five years, P&G's longest trial was thirty-nine weeks—on pigs.

And this is just the beginning.

Now that olestra has its metaphorical foot in the door with snack foods, it will soon permeate the market, that market being all fats in all processed foods. Between its promise and its price and its potential to be hydrogenated, it will put all other fat merchants out of business. If eighty percent of the fat in the diets of 200 million Americans is indigestible, what will control the glycemic index of foods? Where will we get the fatty acids for cell function? We'll really be running on empty. We are, after all, not what we eat, but what we digest.

The FDA mandate stated that its only mission was to make *reasonably* certain that olestra was harmless. What kind of dangerous precedent does that set? "Harmless" does not seem well defined. Unless a thirty-nine-week trial of all additives becomes the standard for how long it takes the body to become "harmed," we know nothing. And, frankly, vitamin deficiency and dehydration from diarrhea can kill you. And the word "reasonably" seems eerily familiar.

Reminiscent of an O. J. moment.

Olestra was discovered when P&G rocket scientists lucked out as they were trying to—*what else?*—improve baby formula. They were working toward an understanding of what kinds of fats premature infants could digest more easily. One wonders why they didn't consider breast milk.

Fats belong to a class of compounds called *esters*. Esters are fatty-acid molecules attached to alcohol molecules. In nature, of course, they are attached in threes to the alcohol spine (triglycerides).

The researchers started at one fatty acid attachment and kept adding more and checking the digestibility. Of course, as soon as they added the fourth fatty acid, digestibility decreased. Five and then six fatty acids eventually made it completely indigestible. Oh, boy, what a find. Actually, the real find was a compound called sucrose polyester (yes, it does sound like something you'd wear, not eat) that has eight fatty acids around the alcohol ring attached to another ring of sucrose molecules.

Your enzymes can't cut these monsters down to size to fit through the wall of your intestine. If they can't fit, you get no essential fatty acids, even if olestra does qualify chemically as a fat on some planet.

Here's what you do:

- **Eat real fat.** Fats become useless when they are accompanied by sugar, or when their chemical structure is changed. Chemical processes used in the packaging and processing of food can damage the structure of fat.
- **Do not eat fats that have been invented.** Do not eat anything made with margarine, hydrogenated oil, or trans-fatty acids, or anything labeled Olean or olestra, ever, not even if you're starving.
- **Eat unprocessed cheese.** Heating, hydrogenating, or chemically manipulating fats in cheese alters the nutritional quality that makes it possible for your body to use them. Read the label.
- **Always put unwhipped heavy whipping cream in your coffee.**

Here's what you don't do:

- **Margarine is one of the most toxic substances you can put in your body.** The processing of margarine involves gathering natural plant oils, which are always in liquid form, and rearranging the chemical bonds to make the oils solid at room temperature, mimicking saturated fats, like butter. This is what gives margarine a butter-like quality, sort of like the way vinyl resembles leather, but it also means that it can't be broken down by your body in its not-occurring-on-this-planet state.

- **Polyunsaturated oils are also highly unstable.** That means that heating changes them further into those damaging trans oils.
- **Try to use cold-processed, expelled, pressed oils above all others.** These oils have not in any way been chemically altered. Remember the step-on-it rule.
- **All forms of heating change oils to some degree.** High-temperature cooking, such as frying, damages the naturally occurring cis molecular configuration of the oils by changing them to the trans configuration. The lower the temperature, the less the damage. Keep in mind that saturated and monounsaturated oils have more stability under heat than polyunsaturated oils.
- **Danger ! Danger!** Fast-food chain restaurants have switched over to cooking with polyunsaturated fats; some even use olestra, the ultimate poison. Just stay away from them. Remember, the words "fast" and "food" do not occur together in nature, either.

These products will kill you:

- Sucrose (white sugar)

- Added fructose

- Maltose

- Dextrose

- Polydextrose

- Corn syrup

- Molasses

- Sorbitol (this is really, really bad stuff)

- Maltodextrin

- High fructose corn syrup (worse than sorbitol, a poisonous, mad-scientist creation)

- Margarine

- Hydrogenated oil

- Olean or olestra

EXERCISE

- On our planet, to get food, you have to walk somewhere before every meal, as animals did way back when, or even as people do in 2000 in most countries except ours. If you were a hunter-gatherer, you would have to chase it.
- If you didn't have a car and a big refrigerator in which to store a day's worth of food, you would fetch, touch, and smell food three or more times a day. Every day.
- In this country, if you drive up to a grocery store or 7-Eleven and pop something shrink-wrapped into the microwave and pretend it's nourishment, you have short-circuited all responses and processes in your body and brain that make you part of the natural world. *Don't do it.*
- If you haven't moved for a while or you're tired, start slowly. Five minutes three times a day will do.
- Keep adding time in increments of five minutes until you are up to fifteen to twenty minutes three times a day. Extended periods of chronic extreme exertion raise your cortisol levels and make nature think you're a loser.

STEP 3:

You can take a pill, or a few pills:
- 200 milligrams of alphalipoic acid every day with an equal amount of evening primrose oil completely reverses insulin resistance, *if* you cut back on the sugar and get some sleep.
- 2,500 milligrams of vitamin B_5 will burn fat faster *once you reach ketosis,* and so will l-carnitine.
- 400 micrograms of selenium before bed can actually rejuvenate T cells for immune function.
- 150 milligrams of zinc morning and afternoon blocks prolactin at the pituitary origin to reset your internal clock for appetite control. Take it with coffee to enhance dopamine, which also blocks prolactin.
- Kava kava (with 30 percent active kavalactones), tyrosine, or Tylenol PM before bed will all make you sleepy, but you still must have nine and a half hours of darkness to reset your clock. On airplanes, take

one of the sleep aids listed above and cover all exposed skin while wearing one of those weird sleep masks.

- If you still can't sleep through the night, women can buy natural progesterone cream (Emerita's Pro-Gest) and use it in sync with their menstrual cycles; and men can ask their doctors for testosterone or use some of their wife's progesterone. It will cascade into testosterone.
- Take the "keep-refrigerated" kind of acidophilus. Take a lot of it. All the time. Those bacteria own you.
- Take 2,000 or 3,000 milligrams of L-glutamine to reline your gut and make your new friends—the bacteria you've just swallowed—happy.
- And, finally, have a drink or a cigar *once in a while;* and remember, unless it makes you jumpy, coffee's good for you.
- **Important:** Do *not* use bad over-the-counter products like melatonin supplements, which actually down-regulate your own production of the hormone, "natural" or unnatural sleeping pills, *valerian, hops, NoDoz,* diet pills, or a lot of herbal and Chinese remedies like *ma huang* and *dong quai.*

THE TRUTH WAS ALWAYS OUT THERE

Here are the diet books that recommend a low- or no-carbohydrate approach to permanent weight loss. Some of them may even predate some of our readers:

- *Eat Fat and Grow Slim,* Richard MacKarness, M.D., 1957

- *Calories Don't Count,* Herman Taller, M.D., 1961

- *The Doctor's Quick Weight Loss Diet,* Irwin Maxwell Stillman and Samm Sinclair Baker, 1967

- *Dr. Atkins' Diet Revolution,* Robert C. Atkins, M.D., 1972 (he recently wrote a sequel, called *Dr. Atkins' New Diet Revolution*)

- *The Carbohydrate Addict's Diet,* Rachael F. Heller, M.D., and Richard F. Heller, M.D., 1991

- *Enter the Zone,* Barry Sears, Ph.D., 1995 (these have two sequels, called *Mastering the Zone* and *The Anti-Aging Zone*)

- *Protein Power,* Michael R. Eades, M.D., and Mary Dan Eades, M.D., 1996 (their first book, published in 1976, was called *Thin So Fast*)

- *Sugar Busters!,* H. Leighton Steward, M.D., and Morrison C. Bethea, M.D., 1995

All these were best-sellers and are based on volumes of actual scientific research reported in peer-reviewed papers and books. Although some people remember the Stillman "water diet," you'd be hard-pressed to find someone who could name Dr. Taller or Dr. MacKarness.

In 1944, here in America at a New York City hospital, a Dr. Pennington treated diabetics with a diet of twenty-four ounces of fatty meat a day. All the patients lost enormous amounts of weight and were virtually cured, but it was wartime and the idea of curing people with vast amounts of rationed meat didn't fly.

In England, in 1956, two researchers named Keckwick and Pawan published the results of a clinical trial of a Dr. Harvey's one-hundred-year-old diet. Besides proving that Dr. Harvey's success was real, they concluded that "from 20 to 30% of weight loss is derived from total body water and the remaining 50 to 70% from the body fat."

It is our conclusion that a constant high-carbohydrate diet also causes excessive water retention in preparation for hibernation. No food, no water, right? Kekwick and Pawan also proved that daily intake of "under 60 grams of carbohydrate is compatible with extreme weight loss." The next year, MacKarness wrote his book based on their findings.

In America, Pennington's 1944 attempt was the last high-fat blip on the weight-loss radar screen until Dr. Atkins made a ripple twenty-nine years later, in 1973, with his *Diet Revolution.* Dr. Atkins is probably the most memorable weight-loss guru to baby boomers. He is the American granddaddy of the "quick results" high-protein diet.

His book sold six million copies. He's our idol because he had enough of the courage of his conclusions to actually address the Senate Subcommittee on Nutrition and Human Needs about the "truth of metabolism." We are going a few steps further to unravel the truth about weight gain.

SYNDROME X FILES

While Dr. Atkins was fighting the good fight in the late 1970s on the East Coast, two scientific hotshots named Gerald Reavens and Gerald Olefsky at Stanford University in California were proving Dr. Atkins's contentions and calling them Syndrome X. We're willing to bet the only place you've ever seen Reavens and Olefsky mentioned is in this chapter. Today, their work is legendary *among scientists.*

Since no one knew about Reavens and Olefsky, the very same magazines and newspapers that had, five months earlier, run excerpts of Dr. Atkins's *Diet Revolution* said that various medical groups were declaring the diet dangerous. They mounted an attack, calling him a quack, a faddist, and a charlatan. Even the chairman of the Senate committee that Atkins had addressed declared that Dr. Atkins would be "one of the first diet 'frauds' to be investigated," *before they even investigated him.* The attack was led by the American Medical Association's Council on Food and Nutrition.

Their biggest complaint was that the Atkins "diet," as detailed in his *Diet Revolution,* was, "for the most part, unscientific." These same people approved amphetamines and five-hundred-calorie diets for the treatment of obesity. And they called Dr. Atkins unscientific. These are also the people who brought you Fen-Phen and Mevacor. The political and professional medical climate of the time had a great deal to do with Dr. Atkins's public discreditation. On April 12, 1973, the American government had one more chance to determine the truth of it all when they examined Dr. Atkins's testimony before they issued the misleading 1977 Surgeon General's Committee Report. In 1972, Atkins testified that he had successfully treated more than 10,000 patients. As Atkins told the subcommittee, "Medical literature of the '50s and '60s was replete with studies and anecdotal evidence proving that carbohydrate restriction provided predictably successful results."

He was referring to, among other things, the famous British study of the 1950s conducted by Kekwick and Pawan. MacKarness used it in 1957; Barry Sears cites this study today in *Enter the Zone.* The British study used a very low-calorie, high-fat approach to weight reduction. The researchers studied people on a 1,000-calorie-per-day diet that was ninety percent fat. All the patients lost an extraordinary amount of weight in a very short time. When these same people were put on a ninety-percent-carbohydrate diet, there was *no* weight loss.

The question is, why didn't they listen?

While the Senate was rolling over Dr. Atkins in Washington, Reavens and Olefsky at Stanford in California already had the studies to back up his suspicions. Too bad they never teamed up with Dr. Atkins. So many lives wouldn't have been lost.

SO NEAR AND YET SO FAR

In 1991, a garden-variety diet book finally brought to light the notion of hyperinsulinemia (chronic high insulin levels) and insulin resistance (reduced insulin response activity). Not since Dr. Atkins in 1972 had anybody directly connected obesity with the high consumption of carbohydrates. All the scientific work of the British in the 1950s had been forgotten in the twenty years after Dr. Atkins, until *The Carbohydrate Addict's Diet* by Doctors Rachael and Richard Heller was published. Unfortunately, not very many people in the medical world took the Hellers very seriously.

The title was probably part of the problem.

The book described carbohydrate craving in the common vernacular of drug lingo. This approach was, unfortunately, too accurate for public acceptance.

In *Enter the Zone*, Barry Sears, Ph.D., draws conclusions from his work with athletes and from research done by his friends the Eadeses in Arkansas. His message is "eat protein, control hormones." The hormones Dr. Sears is talking about are a subclass called *eicosanoids*. They are hard to pronounce and even harder to understand. The diet is ridiculously low-fat for a high-protein diet. *Protein Power* and *Sugar Busters!*, on the other hand, both continue the work Dr. Atkins has done since 1972.

And that's the state of research and advice, pop culture and otherwise, in these United States in the year 2000. Still, *in twenty-five years' time*, no one has ever asked any pertinent questions.

Why hasn't anybody ever asked *why* people crave carbohydrates and why eating fat *never made anyone sick until the late 1950s?* Or why science and medicine keep insisting that lowering the fat in our diets and exercising until we drop will turn the tide of disease, *when neither of these strategies is effective?*

PEOPLE ACCEPT THE REALITY WITH WHICH THEY ARE PRESENTED

In America, we believe that the altar of television brings truth, not fantasy. To hold our jaded interest, television must bring drama, too. Our ancient perception that truth is more memorable or palatable in the dramatic form further skews modern-day reality.

Drama's hallmarks since time began are the contest of good over evil and the struggle for life over death. There are always heroes and villains. Science and medicine have a natural appeal. TV and medicine have been in love with each other since Dr. Kildare met Ben Casey in the ER.

Real, cutting-edge, slow-as-molasses analytical science is too dull to pull ratings and money, and besides, it takes too long to prove anything. As television, it would be canceled before the Nielsens were in. You can't hold the interest of the television viewing audience with close-ups of mold growing. The short attention span we've all acquired via the electronic medium has contributed to the lack of understanding the public displays in regard to nutrition, too. The information itself lacks cohesion, and people are used to being spoon-fed the news about everything in small sound bites, a bad combination. Overlay this form of education with the ever-present herd mentality and you've got the low-fat movement rolling full steam. Americans have always had a deep and abiding need to be part of the newest and the latest and the greatest of *whatever* is going down. We love trends and fads and movements. We love to be in the know, on the ball, first at bat.

In this case, we get to be the first to die.

The beginning of this disaster was the cholesterol-and-heart-disease association that was made in the late 1950s. Some rocket scientist concluded that the cholesterol on your plate had the same chemical constituents as the plaque in your heart. It never occurred to the willing believers to find out *how* it could get there. If they'd done basic research into the biochemistry, they'd have found out that it can't. The fat of another animal on your plate can't become the cholesterol found in your blood. It doesn't work like that. It never did.

Television pounds you day in, day out, hour after hour, year after year, with the idea that low-fat living and exercise will save your life. Eating fruits and vegetables and starches exclusively should solve all of the problems caused by a high-fat diet and yield weight loss in the bargain. For almost three decades, it's been cool, hip, the only way to go. It's been Health Gospel.

But the Gospel according to whom?

Thirty-five years is a long time. By the time *Sleeper* hit the theaters in 1973, the Woodman could count on getting a laugh with that little bit of dialogue referring to fat and meat as "health food." That means that by 1973, the low-fat lie was already ingrained in the public consciousness. Magazines, TV, the newspaper, and definitely your doctor all bought into the lie. But where did these eminent authorities derive their outlooks?

It was from the *government.*

Did the government ever really tell us what to eat?

Yes, it did.

Its goals recommend reduction in the percentage of calories ingested as fat by the United States public from 42 percent to 30 percent, which should consist of less than 10 percent saturated fats and 20 percent mono- and polyunsaturated fats. At least 12 percent of total calories should be ingested as protein, and total calories from carbohydrates should be *increased* from 40 percent to 58 percent. This recommendation was like a gift to a population already light-poisoned and desperate for any carbohydrates they could get.

This was to include an increase in complex carbohydrates and naturally occurring sugars (fruit) from 28 to 48 of the recommended 58 percent. In addition, we were told to restrict our intake of dietary cholesterol to 300 milligrams per day and of sodium to three grams per day.

Wow, that's almost low-fat living.

These recommendations are still excessively high in fat by today's standards. Television commercials still say that thirty percent will kill you. You can't possibly count on hearing "happy birthday" from Willard unless you consume less than twenty percent on any given day.

BUILD IT AND THEY WILL COME

There you have it. American doctors trust the people who decide for the Top Doc. Americans, in turn, trust their own personal physicians and the media to report the bottom-line research to us.

We don't trust anyone. So we checked the records.

The actual beginning of the end of real food in America goes back to the early 1950s. That's when Dwight D. Eisenhower had a heart attack.

His physician, the renowned Paul Dudley White, who was in his eighties at the time, told the press that when he attended medical school before the turn of the century there was no such condition identified as "cardiovascular disease." He and his peer group very rarely saw arterial occlusion. We'll tell you that was because sleep loss was just beginning to kill the first generation truly exposed to it. It was Eisenhower's second heart attack that got researchers on the job trying to figure out the lowdown on heart disease; otherwise, the government might never have gotten involved so early.

For the next ten to fifteen years, scientists at major research institutions fished around for an answer, but could only relate heart disease to Type II non-insulin-dependent diabetes, the kind that strikes middle-age overweight Americans most.

Those people are the baby boomers.

THE FIRST WAVE

As *Happy Days* turned into *The Wonder Years,* we all began to dance to a different drummer. Actually, any drummer would do, as long as it wasn't one that our parents listened to. This blanket rejection of all that came before extended to our nutrition, too. Anti-war, anti-violence sentiments spilled over into our diets and many of us were ready to embrace vegetarianism by the mid-1960s—a wrong turn that laid the foundation for ever-increasing carbohydrate consumption.

By 1967, the early fruits-and-grains diet movement, now referred to as the Mediterranean inverted pyramid diet, turned up in the legendary work of Ancel Keys, who conducted his *Seven Countries* study back in the 1950s. In it, he compared diet and rates of heart disease in seven different countries. Keys found that the least amount of heart disease was on the island of Crete, where the predominantly rural population ate a huge amount of meat. The balance of their caloric intake consisted of grain, fruit, and vegetables, along with a *staggering* amount of olive oil—it accounted for forty percent of their diets.

For the farmers there, it was literally a beverage. They actually drank it for breakfast.

Our government took Keys's study and, of course, completely misinterpreted it. They ignored the enormous meat consumption and focused on the olive-oil intake.

They also ignored the fact that the Cretans had no processed or packaged foods, no electricity, and no stress compared to the postwar Americans in pursuit of the American Dream. They ate *real* food, walked a lot, went to bed when it got dark, got up when it was light, took care of their own children, and didn't worry a great deal about "keeping up with the Stovropopouloses." The comparison between them and us was meaningless.

The newspapers, via the Associated Press, picked up every government release and made sure it hit every corner of America. Once embedded in our consciousness, the "lower-your-fat-and-cholesterol-intake" mantra matured in the heads of the maturing boomers. By 1985, America believed that it was perfectly reasonable to take nutritional advice from Geraldo. Cable TV, too, has changed all our lives, but mostly it's changed the lives of all of the cheap grifters trying to make a buck on confused sick people.

Also, let us not forget that President Kennedy's physical fitness "movement" was into its second decade by the early 1980s. The low-fat movement actually found an already-in-motion vehicle to hitch a ride with in the fitness movement, where there were already more than a few opportunists in place to take advantage of a nutritional plan that required extraordinary amounts of exercise to show results.

But then, suffering is a big part of absolution.

AMEN, SISTER

Now we Americans, as long-standing members of The Church of Low-Fat, worship daily together in the market, in our doctors' offices, and in front of the television, where "media docs" still lead us in prayer and Oprah sings in the choir. In this real religion of abstention, almsgiving takes the form of paying through the nose for defatted products; and the fasting is constant, not just on high holidays. Our faith in medicine, too, is ever-constant. It is symbolized by our semiannual pilgrimage to the cardiologist.

We have increased our consumption of processed, chemically enhanced, sugar- or salt-preserved foods. In our time, soups are labeled "Skinny Soups," ice creams are "guilt-free," once they've been through low-fat analysis, and even the Girl Scouts of America make a fat-free cookie. Boy, oh, boy . . . what a racket.

The food manufacturers fall into line with numbers on their chests, too. The advertising they put forth has always been based on the premise that "if you buy this product you will be pretty, smart, thin, datable." Now they can add the weighted-by-medicine word "healthy" to the list. When the National Growers Association says that the American Cancer Society says that you must have at least two glasses of orange juice a day to stay "healthy," "healthy" is really a thinly veiled euphemism for "alive."

Just think of all the publishers and authors alone raking in the cash: *366 Low-Fat Brand-Name Recipes in Minutes, Thin for Life,* all the *Lowfat and Fabulous* whatevers, the Jim Fixx exercise and nutrition books, and everybody who's ever worked for Oprah or Kirstie Alley. If Jim Fixx was before your time, know that he was the carbo-loading, low-fat runner who died of a heart attack while jogging.

BE AFRAID, BE VERY AFRAID:

We Are a Species in Peril

It is an intolerable thought that he and all other sentient beings are doomed to complete annihilation after such a long-continued slow progress.

—The Autobiography of
Charles Darwin 1809–1822

In chapter one, we discovered that there was never really any scientific basis for the low-fat movement, only a financial one. And the exercise imperative that they handed us just further altered our brain chemistry and left baby boomers with broken knees.

In chapters two, three, four, and five we examined our world and found that when it comes to obesity, diabetes, heart disease, cancer, and depression, everything we believe is a *lie*.

We know now that the truth is that America in the 1940s and 1950s was already dying in fast forward from fast-food products preserved with sugar, and from its changing lifestyle thanks to the light. Longer working hours, cheaper electricity, and television kept people up later at night, and death followed.

The biggest truth is: When the government got on the case to investigate, they blew it. For the feds, the work of Ancel Keys was the beginning and the end of their nutritional investigation. They told us to stop eating meat and fat, which left us with nothing in our already corrupted diets but more sugar to add to the refined chemical waste of the burgeoning fast-food market.

The saddest truth is, thanks to less than rigorous scientific principle and some very suspicious motives, many Americans have already lost their lives.

Using metaphors, examples, and sometimes outright farce, we've tried to make plain in *Lights Out* who you really are and where you really live. By telling you about the God module, Woody Allen, and Daisy World, and through imaginary concepts like horizontal gene transfer, genetic music, and "standing on the board on the log," we've tried to make the mechanics of life here on earth and beyond much clearer. Other blatant metaphors for disease like the bugs, the Ice Age, frozen frogs, passive-aggressive salamanders, and Britton KillsRight all embody, each in its own way, the misconceptions and mistreatment we've suffered at the hands of the experts.

Through the undetectable communication of snow monkeys, orang-utans in heat, the universal physiological and psychological responses to panic, as well as the complex aspects of chaos and universality theory, we tried to illustrate that there are invisible laws in nature that we are subject to, just as we must breathe air. While all this power, beauty, and wisdom governs our lives, we "live" oblivious to it in a world of addicted deers and hopscotching vitamins.

TIME TRAX

The elders of our tribe used to think of time as cyclic, just like the shape of the sun and the moon or the faces of clocks before they went digital.

The moon spins in space, spitting the light of the sun back at us, one month at a time, as the earth wobbles like a singing top—itself spinning around the sun once every 365 days. All of these whirling Dervishes circle the sun as old Sol pinwheels around the Milky Way every 225 million years. The galaxy, too, revolves around the universe, which probably spins around God knows what.

When you stay up with the lights on out of season, you're screwing up all the plates that are spinning all at once on tall sticks in the universe that is inside of you.

You're jacking around with *time.*

When you stay up too late in artificial light, you begin to live in fast forward with every fiber of your being.

We live on Prozac and our children live on Ritalin because life and time perception, too, is governed by the spin cycle of the planets and the sun. With our serotonin so high and dopamine so low, we all become Parkinsonian. It's no accident that cigars have become chic again. Cigars pack a much bigger wallop than cigarettes because they have higher concentrations of nicotine, which is absorbed through the tissues of the mouth and nose, just like cocaine. The sales of cigars increased for the first time in twenty-four years in 1994, when two billion cigars reached ten million smokers. Sales continued to rise, by twenty-five percent in 1995 and then by one hundred percent in 1996—and there's no sign of a slowdown.

THE KILLER CONNECTION

So our time perception is off, our blood pressure's up, we live with diabetes and heart disease, cancer can't be cured, and our waists are ever-expanding—*and the medical profession hasn't got a clue why.* Neither do the researchers. An editorial piece called "Fat Rats and Carcinogenesis Screening" that appeared in the "Commentary" section of the journal *Nature* in July of 1997 just about says it all. The author criticizes toxicologists for using "inappropriate strains of rodents, in badly designed experiments, for the screening of the safety of noxious chemicals."

In other words, the guys who paint dangerous chemical carcinogens on the backs and bellies of mice and then see how long it takes them to get cancer are doing very sloppy work.

When we examine the issues more closely, it's easy to see that it's not really their fault. You see, toxicology studies in these experiments on carcinogens always use just *one* strain of mice, known for its longevity. The author of this commentary is wagging an accusing finger at these irresponsible, lame toxicologists because more and more of their experiments are ending up *useless.* These mice, known for their longevity, have begun to die earlier and earlier, before the experiments are ever finished.

We quote from the commentary: "Toxicologists are now in trouble. Their laboratory mice and rats are *fat, frail and dying young,* sometimes before the tests for long-term toxicity are completed. The problems arise from *improved diets and environments* [italics ours]."

Improved diet, in this case, means more *concentrated refined carbohydrate content.* Wow—vitamin-fortified, highly refined "mouse chow" (think corn flakes, Cheerios, Special K, shredded wheat). We understand what the problem is, but according to the author, it's not what we think at all. The real problem for science is that carcinogenesis screening experiments probably cost the U.S. $250 million a year and involve 70,000 animals. There's the money again.

He continues, "The final step [in testing] involves an 18–24-month death watch." At least fifty percent of the animals must survive the "death watch" to the end of the test period for the study to be considered acceptable. But improvement in diet and animal-house environment, as well as the elimination of infection, have resulted in fatter rats with more heart disease and, of course, a shorter life span.

So just to review, it seems that if you experiment with mammals and eliminate infection, contagious disease, add a cushy lifestyle, and complete the picture with a chronically high-carbohydrate diet, the food and lifestyle will kill them long before they could die from cancer, unless . . . you leave the lights on.

A second piece of evidence completes the picture we see. It is from the *Journal of Laboratory Animal Science,* and was published in 1997. It was performed at the Bassett Research Institute in Cooperstown, New York. This is the reprint of the abstract page, so we can all feel scientific.

LIGHT CONTAMINATION DURING THE DARK PHASE IN PHOTOPERIODICALLY CONTROLLED ANIMAL ROOMS: EFFECT ON TUMOR GROWTH AND METABO-LISM IN RATS

Abstract: Enhanced neoplastic growth and metabolism have been reported in animals maintained in a constant light environment. [Readers: this means tumors and higher insulin and blood sugars.] Results from this laboratory indicate that tumor growth is directly dependent upon increased ambient blood concentrations of arachidonic and linoleic acids, particularly linoleic acid. Tumor linoleic acid utilization and production of its putative mitogenic metabolite, 13-hydroxyoctadecadienoic acid, are suppressed by the circadian neurohormone melatonin, the production of which is itself regulated by light in all mammals.

This study was performed to determine whether *minimal* light contamination (0.2 lux) [that's less than a candle to you in the audience] in animal rooms during an otherwise normal dark phase may disrupt normal circadian production of melatonin and affect tumor growth and metabolism.

The results indicate that minimal light contamination of only 0.2

lux during an otherwise normal dark phase inhibits host melatonin secretion and increases the rate of tumor growth and lipid uptake and metabolism.

This data suggests that great care must be taken to prevent light leaks in animal rooms during the dark phase of a day–night cycle, because such contamination may adversely affect the outcome of tumor growth investigations. We'd like to suggest that such "contamination" may adversely affect *your* life expectancy.

What these excerpts truly mean is that these bozos are acknowledging that *all investigations into cancer growth may be affected by light leaks*—but no one's investigating the light itself as the source of tumor growth. These cancer researchers can't see the forest for the trees. They even cite the light leak and subsequent lack of melatonin as the cause of tumor growth, but never respond reasonably with—oh, my God, it's the light that causes the cancer to grow in people, too!!

EVENT HORIZON

If the last two examples of short-sighted science leave you agape, a snapshot of tomorrow should leave you gasping. The potpourri of man-made disasters on the horizon that will affect our health is breathtaking. Cloning and genetically altered vegetables aside, newer, more devastatingly powerful antibiotics and targeted selective hormone and neurotransmitter blockers promise us a tomorrow filled with crazy mutant bacteria and more Alzheimer's and obscure cancers than would ever occur in nature. The good news is that these tragedies should be confined to the high-tech, overdeveloped nations of the Western hemisphere. The bad news is that our self-inflicted extinction-level event—sleep loss and light poisoning—is on its way to the other hemisphere. This news flash is straight from *Time* magazine: "Scientists from Russia intend to brighten the future of some of the darkest places on earth by launching into space an 82-foot in diameter disc-shaped mirror."

Oh, boy. More mad science. In November of 1999, the ever-ready cosmonauts of the continually crumbling Mir space station deployed this solar-reflecting satellite. Thank God we can always count on the predictably defective Russian craftmanship. If their attempt had succeeded, it would have been as illuminating as ten moons *all night long*. An enthusiastic and slightly giddy spokesman for the project said, "Young eyes . . . will be able to read by it!"

That's right, if the Russians eventually succeed, some very lucky earthlings will soon be hit by an eight-mile-wide spotlight from space shining in their windows all night. In the next round of experiments, The Russian consortium plans to create a constellation of even larger plastic mirrors capable of illuminating large areas of the world at night with constant *free* light aimed at replacing costly electrical lighting, especially within the Arctic Circle in Russia.

Now those poor people above the Arctic Circle with xeno-estrogens and PCBs from our pollution in their breast milk will be put out of their misery once and for all by Russia's penny-pinching. The most painful irony is that those Eskimos have never had to visit the cardiologist or suffer through chemotherapy. They eat right and worship the gods of nature, like the sun and the moon. So basically, they'll never even know what hit them.

Most cultures the world over, according to Roy Porter in *The Greatest Benefit to Mankind,* have, like the Eskimo, eternally construed life and death primarily in relation to the wider cosmos: the planets, stars, mountains, rivers, their spirits and ancestors, gods and demons, and, of course, the heavens and the underworld. Only in Western culture is disease itself an agent and natural force that creates its own narrative.

As another Roy (Cohn) once said, "Only in America, baby."

In the cultural milieu from which we so shamelessly borrow our motif for *Lights Outs*—American television—it is the science-fiction series *The X-Files* that bears witness to the fact that, even in a netherworld of free-floating angst inhabited by a guy called Flukeman, replete with extraterrestrials who snatch abductees from warm beds to probe *their* netherworlds, it's really the mundane and familiar that truly creeps us out. *MAMM* magazine, a monthly dedicated to informing women infected by the "epidemic" of breast cancer, even commented that when the writers of the series gave the character of FBI agent Scully brain cancer, it became apparent that even on *The X-Files* "nothing is scarier than real life."

Except that maybe "the very agencies charged with protecting our well-being are behind all the biological mayhem, in the first place."

The fact that almost *half* of the cutting-edge information in medicine comes from the hallowed halls of the National Institutes of Health in

Washington, D.C., displays the intimate relationship between science and the state envisioned in Huxley's *Brave New World*. This marriage of church and state, now that science is our new religion, is truly dangerous. Not only does it put the American public in the position of having its health and survival interests looked at by parties with primarily monetary concerns, it also means we are only privy to the breakthroughs and discoveries *they* deem appropriate.

AUTHENTICALLY ANXIOUS

In 1996, an asteroid three miles wide barely missed earth. It was as close as our moon. No one's ever heard about it. The reason you've never heard about it is *not* because it was discovered by an amateur astronomer. The reason it wasn't made public is because the asteroid was discovered only *four* days before it was due to whistle right by us.

Certainly it has crossed all our minds before a flight, as the stewardess runs tells us how to inflate our life jackets "in the event of a water landing" that no one of us would ever be able to pull the inflate cord, even if we weren't on fire, after falling five miles straight down out of the sky and head-butting the raging sea.

We are all just as well aware of the remote probability of NASA's ever coming to our rescue as a "near-earth object" comes screaming toward us. But the government somehow believes that we don't know this, or that we haven't already lost faith in them. Those misconceptions translate to government policy that would give us neither the time nor the opportunity for a heartfelt good-bye or even a Kodak moment, should we ever be so deeply impacted.

Believe us, the same paternalistic attitude most certainly extends to your health.

Asteroids and killer comets aside, snippets of declassified trivia easily found on the Internet, and which most Americans are unaware of, read like plots from dogeared paperback thrillers:

- On at least two separate occasions, the Pentagon decided that the best way to estimate how biological warfare might damage our largest cities was to simulate an attack. The Pentagon ordered the U.S. navy in 1950 to spray a cloud of "harmless" bacteria over San Francisco. The upsurge of pneumonia-like illnesses took at least one life, probably many more. In 1966, the Pentagon launched a similar attack on the New York City subway system. The details of that attack remain classified.

- Soon after the Soviets exploded their first nuclear bomb in August of 1949, the U.S., "to better understand the types of weapons its enemy was building," conducted the Green Run experiment at the Hanford nuclear plant. On December 2, 1949, the plant released three tons of irradiated uranium fuel that had been cooling only sixteen days. The exercise—aimed at duplicating pollution from a Soviet reactor—placed more than 7,800 curies of radioactive iodine, known to cause human thyroid cancer, into the air in the Pacific Northwest. Three Mile Island's "accident" released only fifteen curies.

DARK EVIDENCE

It ceases to be paranoia when they actually lie to you. Each of these chilling events really happened. The last two alone prove that no one is guarding your health and survival except you. To place your trust in press releases and media blurbs containing "low-fat advice and exercise tips," when no progress has been made in the last thirty-five years on cancer or heart disease, and as obesity and diabetes statistics continue to rise, is suicide. Most of the science and health news that reaches the American public is by way of the FDA, the surgeon general's office, or the more recently formed Department of Health and Human Services. None of these agencies even promises, let alone guarantees, you the truth.

We can. When it comes to our government, the truth is: *There is no truth.* And we all know it. The most recent piece of propaganda picked up by the paranoid is the news that JFK's casket surfaced last year from the depths of the ocean—nine thousand feet below the surface of the water.

The CIA says it was dumped at sea—the middle of the Atlantic, to be exact—because it was damaged in transit from Dallas to Washington, D.C., and after obtaining a new one for the late president, the Kennedy family asked the government to dispose of the damaged casket so that it wouldn't become a "curiosity."

Sure.

And if gray aliens with big black eyes are sytematically abducting the world's populations to gather DNA samples, it's not because they're infertile, it's because we are. Remember, William Burroughs said, "Paranoia is the highest form of consciousness."

If you, like many Americans these days, see conspiracies everywhere, just know that the *real* conspiracy is that while we continue to die, it's just "business as usual" for government researchers and scientists.

E N D N O T E S

PART I SECRETS AND LIES
Chapter One: We Want to Believe
Abate, N., et al., "Physico-Chemical Properties of Low Density Lipoproteins in Normolipidemic Asian Indian Men," *Horm Metab Res* 85, no. 7 (July 1995): 326–331.

American Heart Association Steering Committee, "Dietary Guidelines for Healthy American Adults," *Circulation* 74, no. 6 (December 1986): 1465A-1468A.

Anderson, Curt, "New Milk Labels Will Describe Fat Content More Accurately," *Santa Barbara News Press,* December 7, 1997, A8.

Barinaga, Marcia, "How Much Pain for Cardiac Gain?" *Science* 276 (May 30, 1997): 1324–1327.

Brody, Jane E., "Eating Fish Cited Anew As Good for the Heart," *The New York Times,* April 11, 1997, A12.

———, "Making Sense of Latest Twist on Fat in the Diet," *The New York Times,* November 25, 1997, B15.

———, "Study Sees No Growth Risks in Low-Fat Diet for Children," *The New York Times,* May 10, 1995, A12.

Buxton, Orfeu M., et al., "Roles of Intensity and Duration of Nocturnal Exercise in Causing Phase Delays of Human Circadian Rhythms," *American Journal of Physiology* 273 (1997): E536-E542.

Casti, John L., "Lighter than Air," *Nature* 382 (August 29, 1996): 769–770.

Demmelmair, H., et al., "Trans Fatty Acid Contents in Spreads and Cold Cuts Usually Consumed by Children," *Zeitschrift fur Ernahrungswissenschaft* 35, no. 3 (September 1996): 235–240.

Gavzer, Bernard, "Are the New Doctors Better?" *Parade,* June 8, 1997, 8.

Gegax, T. Trent, "Fast-Food Fast Tracker," *Newsweek,* May 26, 1997, 57.

Gilbert, Susan, "Should Babies Eat Less Fat?" *The New York Times,* February 26, 1997, B11.

Inder, W. J., et al., "Elevated Basal Adrenocorticotropin and Evidence for Increased Central Opioid Tone in Highly Trained Male Athletes," *Journal of Clinical Endocrinology and Metabolism* 80, no. 1 (1995): 244–248.

Jeppesen, Jorgen, et al., "Effects of Low-Fat, High-Carbohydrate Diets on Risk Factors for Ischemic Heart Disease in Postmenopausal Women," *American Journal of Clinical Nutrition* 65 (1997): 1027–1033.

Katan, Martijn B., et al., "Beyond Low-Fat Diets," *New England Journal of Medicine* 337, no. 8 (August 21, 1997): 563–566.

Key, T. J., et al., "Dietary Habits and Mortality in 11,000 Vegetarians and Health-Conscious People: Results of a 17-Year Follow-Up," *BMJ* 313, no. 7060 (September 28, 1996): 775–779.

Kraemer, W. J., et al., "Endogenous Anabolic Hormonal and Growth Factor Responses to Heavy Resistance Exercise in Males and Females," *Int J Sports Med* 12 (1991): 228–235.

Leddy, John, et al., "Effect of a High or a Low Fat Diet on Cardiovascular Risk Factors in Male and Female Runners," *Medicine and Science in Sports and Exercise* 29 (1997): 17–25.

Liebman, Bonnie, "Carbo-Phobia: Zoning Out on the New Diet Books," *Nutrition Action,* July/August 1996, 1–7.

Lowry, Brian, et al., "Chris Farley: Heavyweight 'Saturday Night Live' Film Comic," *Los Angeles Times,* December 19, 1997, A48.

Miller, Debra L., et al., "Effect of Fat-Free Potato Chips with and without Nutrition Labels on Fat and Energy Intakes," *American Journal of Clinical Nutrition* 68 (1998): 282–290.

Mirsky, Steve, "Chewing the Fat," *Scientific American,* January 1997, 31.

Morgan, S. A., et al., "A Low-Fat Diet Supplemented with Monosaturated Fat Results in Less HDL-C Lowering than a Very-Low-Fat diet," *Journal of the American Dietetic Association* 97, no. 2 (February 1997): 151–156.

Nelson, Gary J., et al., "Low-Fat Diets Do Not Lower Plasma Cholesterol Levels in Healthy Men Compared to High-Fat Diets with Similar Fatty Acid Composition at Constant Caloric Intake," *Lipids* 30, no. 11 (1995): 969–976.

Nemetz, Allison, "Get Slim 15 Times Faster," *Women's World,* April 21, 1998, 16–17.

Ochs, Ridgely, "The Skinny on Fat: It's Not All Bad," *Los Angeles Times,* March 2, 1998, S2.

Ornish, Dean, M.D., "Low-Fat Diets," *New England Journal of Medicine* 338, no. 2 (January 8, 1998): 127–129.

Rimm, E. B., et al., "Vegetable, Fruit, and Cereal Fiber Intake and Risk of Coronary Heart Disease among Men," *Journal of the American Medical Association* 275, no. 6 (February 14, 1996): 447–451.

Ritter, M. M., et al., "Effects of a Vegetarian Life Style on Health," *Fortschr Med* 113, no. 16 (June 10, 1995): 239–242.

Roberts, Paul, "The New Food Anxiety," *Psychology Today* 31, no. 2 (March/April 1998): 30–38; 74.

Shapiro, Laura, "Is Fat That Bad?" *Newsweek,* April 21, 1997, 56–64.

Venkatraman, Jaya T., et al., "Influence of the Level of Dietary Lipid Intake and Maximal Exercise on the Immune Status in Runners," *Medicine and Science in Sports and Exercise* 29 (1997): 333–344.

Walker, Alexander R. P., letter to the editor, *New England Journal of Medicine* 336, no. 8 (February 20, 1997): 584.

Chapter Two: Into the Dark

Alexander, R. McNeil, "Life and How to Define It," *New Scientist,* April 5, 1997, 46–47.

Amabile-Cuevas, Carlos F., et al., "Horizontal Gene Transfer," *American Scientist* 81 (July/August 1993): 332–341.

Artlett, Carol M., et al., "Identification of Fetal DNA and Cells in Skin Lesions from Women with Systematic Sclerosis," *New England Journal of Medicine* 338 (April 23, 1998): 1186–1191.

Bahcall, N. A., et al., "A Lightweight Universe?" *Proceedings of the National Academy of Sciences (USA)* 95, no. 11 (9 May 26, 1998): 5956–5959.

Barnes, Brian M., "Freeze Avoidance in a Mammal: Body Temperatures Below 0°C. in an Arctic Hibernator," *Science* 244 (June 30, 1989): 1593–1595.

Bigwood, R., et al., "The Vibrational Energy Flow Transition in Organic Molecules: Theory Meets Experiment," *Chemistry* 95, no. 11 (May 26, 1998): 5960–5964.

Blakeslee, Sandra, "Surprising Theory on the Body Clock: Illuminate the Knee," *The New York Times*, January 16, 1998, A1.

Bogomolni, R. A., et al., "The Photochemical reactions of bacterial sensory rhodopsin-I. Flash photolysis study in the one microsecond to eight second time window." *The Journal of Biophysics*. Volume 52. Number 6. (December 1987): 1071–1075.

Broadway, J., et al., "Bright Light Phase Shifts the Human Melatonin Rhythm during the Antarctic Winter," *Neuroscience Letters* 79 (1987): 185–189.

Brody, Jane E., "Americans Gamble on Herbs As Medicine," *The New York Times*, February 9, 1999, D1.

Brookes, Martin, "The Species Enigma: Disappearing Life Going Extinct," *New Scientist*, June 13, 1998, 1–2.

Brown, S., et al., "Desiccation Resistance and Contamination as Mechanisms of Gaia," *BioSystems* 17, no. 4 (1985): 337–360.

Coleman, Richard M., "Sleep-Wake Disorders Based on a Polysomnographic Diagnosis," *Journal of the American Medical Association* 247, no. 7 (1982): 997–1003.

Conrad, Michael, "Origin of Life and the Underlying Physics of the Universe," *BioSystems* 42 (1997): 177–190.

Cose, Ellis, "Forgive and Forget?" *Newsweek*, April 21, 1997, 45.

Dorit, Robert, "Molecular Evolution and Scientific Inquiry, Misperceived," *American Scientist* 85 (September/October 1997): 474–475.

Duncan, David Ewing, "Counting the Days," *New Scientist*, August 22, 1998, 45.

Dunlap, Jay, "An End in the Beginning," *Science*, June 5, 1998, 1548–1603.

"Evolution: The Dissent of Darwin," *Psychology Today*, January/February 1997, 56–63.

Fletcher, Suzanne W., M.D., "Whither Scientific Deliberation in Health Policy Recommendations?" *New England Journal of Medicine* 336 (April 17, 1997): 1180–1183.

Fankhauser, C., et al., "Light Control of Plant Development," *Ann Rev Cell Dev Biol* 13 (1997): 203–229.

Gellert, George A., et al., "Health and Climate Change: Modelling the Impacts of Global Warming and Ozone Depletion," *Nature* 393 (June 11, 1998): 534.

Gibbons, Ann, "Calibrating the Mitochondrial Clock," *Science* 279 (January 2, 1998): 28–29.

Gould, Stephen Jay, "As the Worm Turns," *Natural History*, February 1997, 24–27; 68–73.

Grady, Denise, "Reactions to Prescribed Drugs Kill Thousands Annually, Study Says," *The New York Times*, April 15, 1998, A1.

Holmes, Bob, "Heads in the Clouds," *New Scientist,* May 8, 1999, 32–36.

Ings, Simon, "Chance Is a Fine Thing," *New Scientist,* May 23, 1998, 50.

Jackson, F. R. et al, "Oscillating Molecules and Circadian Clock Output Mechanisms," *Molecular Psychiatry* 3 (1998): 381–385.

Jenkins, Mark, "The Secret Garden," *Men's Health,* October 1997, 143–155.

Jibrin, Janis, "Gene Defying Diets," *American Health,* April 1998, 70–74.

Knott, Cheryl, "Orangutans in the Wild," *National Geographic,* August 1998, 28–56.

Krieg, Arthur M., "Human Endogenous Retroviruses," *Science and Medicine,* March/April 1997, 34–43.

Lazarou, Jason, et al., "Incidence of Adverse Drug Reactions in Hospitalized Patients," *Journal of the American Medical Association* 279, no. 15 (April 15, 1998): 1200–1205.

Lelkes, P. I., et al., "Microgravity Decreases Tyrosine Hydroxylase Expression in Rat Adrenals," *FASEB J* 8, no. 14 (November 1994): 1177–1182.

Lenton, Timothy M., "Gaia and Natural Selection," *Nature* 394 (July 30, 1998): 439–447.

Lin, C., et al., "Enhancement of Blue-Light Sensitivity of Arabidopsis Seedlings by a Blue Light Receptor Cryptochrome 2," *Proceedings of the National Academy of Sciences (USA)* 95, no. 5 (March 3, 1998): 2686–2690.

Markos, Anton, "The Ontogeny of Gaia: The Role of Microorganisms in Planetary Information Network," *J Theor Biol* 176 (1995): 175–180.

McMillen, I. C., et al., "Melatonin and the Development of Circadian and Seasonal Rhythmicity," *J Reprod Fertil Suppl* 49 (1995): 137–146.

Mitchell, Alison, "Polarized Flight," *Nature* 394 (July 30, 1998): 425.

Miyamoto, Y., et al., "Vitamin B_2-Based Blue-Light Photoreceptors in the Retinohypothalamic Tract As the Photoactive Pigments for Setting the Circadian Clock in Mammals," *Proceedings of the National Academy of Sciences (USA)* 95, no. 11 (May 26, 1998): 6097–6102.

Morell, Virginia, "Are Pathogens Felling Frogs?" *Science* 284 (April 30, 1999): 728–731.

Morris, Kelly, "New Day Down for Research on Circadian Rhythms," *The Lancet* 353 (March 20, 1999): 990.

Muller-Enoch, D., "Blue Light Mediated Photoreduction of the Flavoprotein NADPH-Cytochrome P450 Reductase: A Forster-Type Energy Transfer," *Z Naturforsch* 52, nos. 9–10 (September 1997): 605–614.

Munoz-Hoyos, A., et al., "Absence of Plasma Melatonin Circadian Rhythm during the First 72 Hours of Life in Human Infants," *Journal of Clinical Endocrinology and Metabolism* 77, no. 3 (1993): 699–703.

Oren, Dan A., et al., "Restoration of Detectable Melatonin After Entrainment to a 24-Hour Schedule in a 'Free-Running' Man," *Psychoneuroendocrinology* 22, no. 1 (1997): 39–52.

Reppert, S. M., et al., "Forward Genetic Approach Strikes Gold: Cloning of a Mammalian Clock Gene," *Cell* 89, no. 4 (May 16, 1997): 487–490.

Roach, Mary, "My Quest for Qi," *Health,* March 1997, 97–104.

Sassone-Corsi, Paolo, "Molecular Clocks: Mastering Time by Gene Regulation," *Nature* 392 (April 30, 1998): 871–874.

Schoch, Deborah, "Two Frog Studies Link Parasite to Deformities," *Los Angeles Times,* April 30, 1999, A1.

"A Smoking Gun?" *New Scientist,* March 21, 1998, 13.

Song, Zhiwei, et al., "DCP-1, a Drosophila Cell Death Protease Essential for Development," *Science* 275 (January 24, 1997): 536–540.

Sternberg, Esther M., "The Mind-Body Interaction in Disease," *Mysteries of the Mind,* 8–15.

Sternberg, E. M., "Neural-immune interactions in health and disease." *The Journal of Clinical Investigation* 100. no. 11. (December 1, 1997): 2641–2647.

Stolberg, Cheryl Gay, "Gifts to Science Researchers Have Strings, Study Finds," *The New York Times,* April 1, 1998, A13.

Teran-Santos, J., M.D., et al., "The Association between Sleep Apnea and the Risk of Traffic Accidents," *New England Journal of Medicine* 340, no. 1 (1999): 847–851.

Vines, Gail, "Into the Dark: Does the Strange Decline of Amphibian Populations Hold a Sinister Message for Us All?" *New Scientist,* June 13, 1998, 48.

Vodovnik, L., et al., "Treatment of chronic wounds by means of electric and electromagnetic fields. Part 1. Literature review," *The Journal of Medical Biological Engineering and Computation* 30, no. 3. (May 1992): 257, 266.

Wade, Nicholas, "Can Social Behavior of Man Be Glimpsed in a Lowly Worm?" *The New York Times,* September 8, 1998, B9.

Wechsler, Pat, "A Shot in the Dark," *New York,* November 11, 1996, 38–43; 85.

Zuger, Abigail, "Drug Companies' Sales Pitch: 'Ask Your Doctor,' " *The New York Times,* August 5, 1997, B9.

PART II WE ARE NOT ALONE
Chapter Three: Earthling Autopsy

Acheson, Kevin J., et al., "Glycogen Storage Capacity and De Novo Lipogenesis during Massive Carbohydrate Overfeeding in Man," *American Journal of Clinical Nutrition* 48 (1988): 240–247.

Ahmed, S. Ansar, et al., "Genetic Regulation of Testosterone-Induced Immune Suppression," *Cellular Immunology* 104 (1987): 91–98.

Alexander, R. McNeil, "Life and How to Define It," *New Scientist,* April 5, 1997, 46–47.

Arendt, J., "Biological Rhythms: The Science of Chronobiology," *Journal of Royal College of Physicians* 32, no. 1 (January 1998): 27–35.

Assmann, S. M., "Electrifying Symbiosis," *Proceedings of the National Academy of Sciences (USA)* 92, no. 6 (March 14, 1995): 1795–1796.

Bauman, W. A., et al., "Pancreatic Hormones in the Nonhibernating and Hibernating Golden Mantled Ground Squirrel," *Comparative Biochemistry and Physiology* 86, no. 2 (1987): 241–244.

Bazan, J. Fernando, et al., "Structural Design and Molecular Evolution of a Cytokine Receptor Superfamily," *Proceedings of the National Academy of Sciences (USA)* 87 (September 1990): 6934–6938.

Bigwood, R., et al., "The Vibrational Energy Flow Transition in Organic Molecules: Theory Meets Experiment," *Chemistry* 95, no. 11 (May 26, 1998): 5960–5964.

Blakeslee, Sandra, "Some Biologists Ask 'Are Genes Everything?' " *The New York Times,* September 2, 1997, B7.

———, "Surprising Theory on the Body Clock: Illuminate the Knee," *The New York Times,* January 16, 1998, A1.

Blazer, Ivonne, et al., "Photoperiodism and Effects of Indoleamines in a Unicellular Alga, Gonyaulax polyedra," *Science* 253 (August 16, 1991): 795–797.

Born, Jan, et al., "Effects of Sleep and Circadian Rhythm on Human Circulating Immune Cells," *Journal of Immunology* 158 (1997): 4454–4464.

Bray, George A., "The Nutrient Balance Hypothesis: Peptides, Sympathetic Activity, and Food Intake," *Annals of the New York Academy of Sciences* 676 (March 15 1993): 223–241.

Bry, L., et al., "A Model of Host-Microbial Interactions in an Open Mammalian Ecosystem," *Science* 273, no. 5280 (September 6, 1996): 1380–1383.

Brzezinski, Amnon, "Melatonin in Humans," *New England Journal of Medicine* 336, no. 3 (January 16, 1997): 186–195.

Buxton, Orfeu M., et al., "Roles of Intensity and Duration of Nocturnal Exercise in Causing Phase Delays of Human Circadian Rhythms," *American Journal of Physiology* 273 (1997): E536-E542.

Campbell, Scott S., et al., "Extraocular Circadian Phototransduction in Humans," *Science* 279, no. 5349 (January 16, 1998): 396–399.

Cannon, B., et al., "The Biochemistry of an Inefficient Tissue: Brown Adipose Tissue," *Essays in Biochemistry* 20 (1985): 110–164.

Castex, C., et al., "Glucose Oxidation by Adipose Tissue of the Edible Dormouse (Glis glis) during Hibernation and Arousal: Effect of Insulin," *Comparative Biochemistry and Physiology* 88, no. 1 (1987): 33–36.

———, "Regulation of Endocrine Pancreas Secretions (Insulin and Glucagon) during the Periodic Lethargy-Waking Cycle of the Hibernating Mammal," *Diabete et Metabolisme* 13, no. 3 (June 1987): 176–181.

———, "Insulin Secretion in the Hibernating Edible Dormouse (Glis glis): In Vivo and In Vitro Studies," *Comparative Biochemistry and Physiology* 79, no. 1 (1984): 179–183.

Chentao, Lin, et al., "Expression of an Arabidopsis Cryptochrome Gene in Transgenic Tobacco Results in Hypersensitivity to Blue, UV-A, and Green Light," *Proceedings of the National Academy of Sciences (USA)* 92 (August 1995): 8423–8427.

Coghlan, Andy, "Shared Roots: Hormones Took Control Long Before Plants and Animals Went Their Separate Ways," *New Scientist,* February 28, 1998, 6.

Conrad, Michael, "Origin of Life and the Underlying Physics of the Universe," *BioSystems* 42 (1997): 177–190.

De Lonlay-Debeney, P., "Clinical Features of 52 Neonates with Hyperinsulinism," *New England Journal of Medicine* 340, no. 15 (April 15, 1999): 1169–1175.

Dhurandhar, N. V., et al., "Association of Adenovirus Infection with Human Obesity," *Obesity Res* 5, no. 5 (September 1997): 464–469.

Diamond, Michael, et al., "Suppression of Counterregulatory Hormone Response to Hypoglycemia by Insulin," *Journal of Clinical Endocrinology and Metabolism* 72, no. 6 (1990): 1388–1390.

Ehrhard, P. B., et al., "Expression of Nerve Growth Factor and Nerve Growth Factor Receptor Tyrosine Kinase Trk in Activated CD4-Positive T-Cell Clones," *Proceedings of the National Academy of Sciences (USA)* 90, no. 23 (December 1, 1993): 10984–10988.

Eisenhofer, Graeme, et al., "Substantial Production of Dopamine in the Human Gastrointestinal Tract," *Journal of Clinical Endocrinology and Metabolism* 82, no. 11 (1997): 3864–3871.

Fankhauser, C., et al., "Light Control of Plant Development," *Ann Rev Cell Dev Biol* 13 (1997): 203–229.

Fisher, R. F., et al., "Rhizobium—Plant Signal Exchange," *Nature* 357, no. 6380 (June 25, 1992): 655–660.

Flier, Jeffrey S., M.D., et al., "The Neurologic Basis of Fever," *New England Journal of Medicine* 330, no. 26 (June 30, 1994): 1880–1885.

Freiberg, C., et al., "Molecular Basis of Symbiosis between Rhizobium and Legumes," *Nature* 387, no. 6631 (May 22, 1997): 394–401.

Garcia-Maurino, Sofia, et al., "Melatonin Enhances IL-2, IL-6, and IFN-y Production by Human Circulating CD4+ Cells," *Journal of Immunology* 159 (1997): 574–581.

Gilad, Eli, et al., "Interplay between Sex Steroids and Melatonin in Regulation of Human Benign Prostate Epithelial Cell Growth," *Journal of Clinical Endocrinology and Metabolism* 82, no. 8 (August 1997): 2535–2541.

Glanz, James, "Can 'Resetting' Hormonal Rhythms Treat Illness?" *Science* 269 (September 1, 1995): 1220–1221.

Graf, J., et al., "Host-Derived Amino Acids Support the Proliferation of Symbiotic Bacteria," *Proceedings of the National Academy of Sciences (USA)* 95, no. 4 (February 17, 1998): 1818–1822.

Gura, Trisha, "Obesity Sheds Its Secrets," *Science* 275 (February 7, 1997): 751–753.

Heiss, Cindy J., et al., "Associations of Body Fat Distribution, Circulating Sex Hormones, and Bone Density in Postmenopausal Women," *Journal of Clinical Endocrinology and Metabolism* 80, no. 5 (1995): 1591–1596.

Henry, J. P., "Biological Basis of the Stress Response," *Integrated Physiological Behavioral Sciences* 27, no. 1 (January 1992): 66–83.

Hetts, Steven W., "To Die or Not to Die: An Overview of Apoptosis and Its Role in Disease," *Journal of the American Medical Association* 279, no. 4 (January 28, 1998): 300–307.

Holzapfel, Wilhelm H., et al., "Overview of Gut Flora and Probiotics," *International Journal of Food Microbiology* 41 (1998): 85–101.

Hsu, D. S., et al., "Putative Human Blue-Light Photoreceptors hCRY1 and hCRY2 are Flavoproteins," *Biochemistry* 35, no. 44 (November 5, 1996): 13871–13877.

Illnerova, Helena, et al., "The Circadian Rhythm in Plasma Melatonin Concentration of the Urbanized Man: The Effect of Summer and Winter Time," *Brain Research* 328 (1985): 186–189.

Jibrin, Janis, "Gene Defying Diets," *American Health*, April 1998, 70–74.

Johnson, R. W., et al., "Hormones, Lymphohemopoietic Cytokines and the Neuroimmune Axis," *Comparative Biochemistry and Physiology* 116A, no. 3 (1997): 183–201.

Jones, Peter J. H., et al., "Dietary Cholesterol Feeding Suppresses Human Cholesterol Synthesis Measured by Deuterium Incorporation and Urinary Mevalonic Acid Levels," *Arteriosclerosis, Thrombosis, and Vascular Biology* 16, no. 10 (October 1996): 1222–1228.

Kauppila, Antti, et al., "Inverse Seasonal Relationship between Melatonin and Ovarian Activity in Humans in a Region with a Strong Seasonal Contrast in Luminosity," *Journal of Clinical Endocrinology and Metabolism* 65, no. 5 (1987): 823–828.

Klein, George, "Malign Evolution," *Discover*, August 1997, 46–51.

Kornhauser, J. M., et al., "Light, Immediate-Early Genes, and Circadian Rhythms," *Behavioral Genetics* 26, no. 3 (May 1996): 221–240.

Korth, C., "A Co-Evolutionary Theory of Sleep," *Medical Hypotheses* 45, no. 3 (September 1995): 304–310.

Krieg, Arthur M., "Human Endogenous Retroviruses," *Science and Medicine*, March/April 1997, 34–43.

Lauder, George V., "Evolutionary Transformations," *Science* 276 (April 4, 1997): 46.

Lazazzera, Beth A., et al., "The Ins and Outs of Peptide Signaling," *Trends in Microbiology* 6, no. 7 (1988): 288–294.

Lin, C., et al., "Enhancement of Blue-Light Sensitivity of Arabidopsis Seedlings by a Blue Light Receptor Cryptochrome 2," *Proceedings of the National Academy of Sciences (USA)* 95, no. 5 (March 3, 1998): 2686–2690.

Lisy, V., et al., "On a Simple Model of Low-Frequency Vibrations in DNA Macromolecules," *J Biomol Struc Dyn* 13, no. 4 (February 1996): 707–716.

Liu, Yi, et al., "How Temperature Changes Reset a Circadian Oscillator," *Science* 281 (August 7, 1998): 825–829.

Losick, Richard, et al., "Why and How Bacteria Communicate," *Scientific American*, February 1997, 68–73.

Malhotra, Khushbeer, et al., "Putative Blue-Light Photoreceptors from Arabidopsis thaliana and Sinapsis alba with a High Degree of Sequence Homology to DNA Photolyase Contain the Two Photolyase Cofactors but Lack DNA Repair Activity," *Biochemistry* 34, no. 20 (1995): 6892–6899.

Markos, Anton, "The Ontogeny of Gaia: The Role of Microorganisms in Planetary Information Network," *J Theor Biol* 176 (1995): 175–180.

Marston, Wendy, "Gut Reactions," *Newsweek*, November 17, 1997, 95–99.

McFall-Ngai, M. J., et al., "Symbiont Recognition and Subsequent Morphogenesis As Early Events in an Animal-Bacterial Mutualism," *Science* 254, no. 5037 (December 6, 1991): 1491–1494.

McMillen, I. C., et al., "Melatonin and the Development of Circadian and Seasonal Rhythmicity," *J Reprod Fertil Suppl* 49 (1995): 137–146.

Melnyk, R. B., et al., "Insulin-Induced Feeding in Hibernators," *Behavioral and Neural Biology* 32, no. 1 (May 1981): 70–78.

Miyamoto, Y., et al., "Vitamin B_2-Based Blue-Light Photoreceptors in the Retinohypothalamic Tract As the Photoactive Pigments for Setting the Circadian Clock in Mammals," *Proceedings of the National Academy of Sciences (USA)* 95, no. 11 (May 26, 1998): 6097–6102.

Moldofsky, H., "Sleep and the Immune System," *International Journal of Immunopharmacology* 17, no. 8 (August 1995): 649–654.

Moreau-Hamsany, C., et al., "Hormonal Control of Lipolysis from the White Adipose Tissue of Hibernating Jerboa (Jaculus orientalis)," *Comparative Biochemistry and Physiology* 91, no. 4 (1988): 665–669.

Moss, Robert, "The Problem with Evolution: Where Have We Gone Wrong?" *The Scientist*, October 13, 1997, 7.

Muller-Enoch, D., "Blue Light Mediated Photoreduction of the Flavoprotein NADPH-Cytochrome P450 Reductase: A Forster-Type Energy Transfer," *Z Naturforsch* 52, nos. 9–10 (September 1997): 605–614.

Munoz-Hoyos, A., et al., "Absence of Plasma Melatonin Circadian Rhythm during the First 72 Hours of Life in Human Infants," *Journal of Clinical Endocrinology and Metabolism* 77, no. 3 (1993): 699–703.

Nestler, John E., et al., "Insulin Inhibits Adrenal 17,20-Lyase Activity in Man," *Journal of Clinical Endocrinology and Metabolism* 74, no. 2 (1992): 362–367.

Olsson, Lennart, et al., "Regulation of Receptor Internalization by the Major Histocompatibility Complex Class I Molecule," *Proceedings of the National Academy of Sciences (USA)* 91 (September 1994): 9086–9090.

O'Rahilly, Stephen, "Life without Leptin," *Nature* 392 (March 26, 1998): 330–331.

Overbye, Dennis, "The Cosmos According to Darwin," *The New York Times,* July 13, 1997, 24–33.

Petridou, S., et al., "Light Induces Accumulation of Isocitrate Lyase mRNA in a Carotenoid-Deficient Mutant of Chlamydomonas reinhardtii," *Plant Mol Biol* 33, no. 3 (February 1997): 381–392.

Petrovsky, Nikolai, et al., "Diurnal Rhythmicity of Human Cytokine Production: A Dynamic Disequilibrium in T Helper Cell Type 1/T Helper Cell Type 2 Balance," *Journal of Immunology* 158 (1997): 5163–5168.

Pool, Robert, "Beams of Stuff," *Discover,* December 1997, 103–107.

Reiser, Sheldon, et al., "Isocaloric Exchange of Dietary Starch and Sucrose in Humans: II. Effect on Fasting Blood Insulin, Glucose, and Glucagon and on Insulin and Glucose Response to a Sucrose Load," *American Journal of Clinical Nutrition* 32 (November 1979): 2206–2216.

Rejto, P. A., et al., "Visualization of Fast Energy Flow and Solvent Caging in Unimolecular Dynamics," *Nature* 375, no. 6527 (May 1995): 129–131.

Reppert, S. M., et al., "Forward Genetic Approach Strikes Gold: Cloning of a Mammalian Clock Gene," *Cell* 89, no. 4 (May 16, 1997): 487–490.

Robinson, Gene E., "From Society to Genes with the Honey Bee," *American Scientist* 86 (September/October 1998): 456–461.

Ruoslahti, Erkki, "Stretching Is Good for a Cell," *Science* 276 (May 30, 1997): 1345–1346.

Sainz, R. M., et al., "The Pineal Neurohormone Melatonin Prevents In Vivo and In Vitro Apoptosis in Thymocytes," *Journal of Pineal Research* 19, no. 4 (November 1995): 178–188.

Sassone-Corsi, Paolo, "Molecular Clocks: Mastering Time by Gene Regulation," *Nature* 392 (April 30, 1998): 871–874.

Scislowski, Piotr W. D., et al., "Short Term Dopamine Agonist Treatment Produces Long Lasting Improvement in Diabetes of ob/ob Mice," *Ergo Science* 196 (June 1998): 1–4.

Sinha, M. K., et al., "Nocturnal Rise of Leptin in Lean, Obese, and Non-Insulin-Dependent Diabetes Mellitus Subjects," *Journal of Clinical Investigation* 97, no. 5 (March 1, 1996): 1344–1347.

Slawinski, J., et al., "Stress-Induced Photon Emission from Perturbed Organisms," *Experientia* 48, nos. 11–12 (December 1992): 1041–1058.

Spector, Novera Herbert, Ph.D., "Neuroimmunomodulation: A Brief Review," *Regulatory Toxicology and Pharmacology* 24 (1996): S32-S38.

Spiegel, Karine., et al., "Impact of Sleep Debt on Metabolic and Endocrine Function," *The Lancet* 354 (October 23, 1999): 1435–1439.

Stagsted, Jan, et al., "Regulation of Insulin Receptor Functions by a Peptide Derived from a Major Histocompatibility Complex Class I Antigen," *Cell* 62 (July 27, 1990): 297–307.

Van Cauter, Eve, et al., "Modulation of Glucose Regulation and Insulin Secretion by Circadian Rhythmicity and Sleep," *Journal of Clinical Investigation* 88 (September 1991): 934–942.

Vines, Gail, "There Is More to Heredity than DNA," *New Scientist,* April 19, 1997, 16.

Wehr, Thomas A., et al., "Suppression of Men's Responses to Seasonal Changes in Day Length by Modern Artificial Lighting," *American Journal of Physiology* 269, no. 38 (1995): R173-R178.

Wong, Joyce Y., et al., "Direct Measurement of a Tethered Ligand-Receptor Interaction Potential," *Science* 275 (February 7, 1997): 820–822.

Yeh, I., "Changes in Various Plasma Lipid Components, Glucose, and Insulin in Spermophilus lateralis during Hibernation," *Comparative Biochemistry and Physiology* 111, no. 4 (August 1995): 651–663.

Yuan, Li, et al., "Molecular Actions of Prolactin in the Immune System," *PSEBM* 215 (1997): 35–52.

Zhao, Shaying, et al., "Human Blue-Light Photoreceptor hCRY2 Specifically Interacts with Protein Serine/Threonine Phosphatase 5 and Modulates Its Activity," *Photochemistry and Photobiology* 66, no. 5 (November 1997): 727–731.

Chapter Four: On Ice

Alberts, Arthur S., et al., "Protein Phosphatase 2A Potentiates Activity of Promoters Containing AP-1-Binding Elements," *Molecular and Cellular Biology* 13, no. 4 (April 1993): 2104–2112.

Aujard, F., et al. "Thermoregulatory Responses to Variations of Photoperiod and Ambient Temperature in the Male Lesser Mouse Lemur: a Primitive or an Advanced Adaptive Character?" *Journal of Comparative Physiology.* Volume 168, no. 7 (October 1998): 540–548.

Buresova, Milena, et al., "Human Circadian Rhythm in Serum Melatonin in Short Winter Days and in Simulated Artificial Long Days," *Neuroscience Letters* 136 (1992): 173–176.

Coghlan, Andy, "Shared Roots: Hormones Took Control Long Before Plants and Animals Went Their Separate Ways," *New Scientist,* February 28, 1998, 6.

Essen, Lars-Oliver, et al., "A Cold Break for Photoreceptors," *Nature* 392 (March 12, 1998): 131–133.

Honma, Ken-Ichi, et al., "Seasonal Variation in the Human Circadian Rhythm: Dissociation between Sleep and Temperature Rhythm," *American Journal of Physiology* 262 (1992): R885-R891.

Hopkin, Karen, "Clock Setting," *Scientific American,* April 1998, 20–22.

Hsu, D. S., et al., "Putative Human Blue-Light Photoreceptors hCRY1 and hCRY2 Are Flavoproteins," *Biochemistry* 35, no. 44 (November 5, 1996): 13871–13877.

Kimura, Koutarou D., et al., "Daf-2, an Insulin Receptor-Like Gene That Regulates Longevity and Diapause in Caenorhabditis elegans," *Science* 277 (August 1997): 942–946.

Krauchi, Kurt, et al., "Early Evening Melatonin and S-20098 Advance Circadian Phase and Nocturnal Regulation of Core Body Temperature," *American Journal of Physiology* 272 (April 1997): R1178-R1188.

————, "The Hypothermic Effect of Late Evening Melatonin Does Not Block the Phase Delay Induced by Concurrent Bright Light in Human Subjects," *Neuroscience Letters* 232 (1997): 57–61.

Oren, Dan A., et al., "Restoration of Detectable Melatonin After Entrainment to a 24-Hour Schedule in a 'Free-Running' Man," *Psychoneuroendocrinology* 22, no. 1 (1997): 39–52.

Perret, M., et al., "Influence of Daylength on Metabolic Rate and Daily Water Loss in the Male Prosimian Primate Microcebus Murinus," *Comparative Biochemistry & Physiology & Molecular Integral Physiology* 119, no. 4 (April 1998): 981–989.

Roush, Wade, "Worm Longevity Gene Cloned," *Science* 277 (August 15, 1997): 897–898.

Tattersall, Ian, "Out of Africa Again . . . and Again?" *Scientific American,* April 1997, 60–67.

Vondrasova, Dana, et al., "Exposure to Long Summer Days Affects the Human Melatonin and Cortisol Rhythms," *Brain Research* 759 (1997): 166–170.

Wehr, Thomas A., "Melatonin and Seasonal Rhythms," *Journal of Biological Rhythms* 12, no. 6 (December 1997): 518–527.

Yoon, Carol K., "Antarctica's Frigid Waters Form Evolutionary Caldron," *The New York Times,* March 9, 1999, D2.

Zhao, Shaying, et al., "Human Blue-Light Photoreceptor hCRY2 Specifically Interacts with Protein Serine/Threonine Phosphatase 5 and Modulates Its Activity," *Photochemistry and Photobiology* 66, no. 5 (November 1997): 727–731.

PART III THE TRUTH IS IN HERE
Chapter Five: Deny Everything
Abate, N., et al., "Physico-Chemical Properties of Low Density Lipoproteins in Normolipi-demic Asian Indian Men," *Horm Metab Res* 85, no. 7 (July 1995): 326–331.

Abbassy, A. A., et al., "Hyperprolactinaemia and Male Infertility," *Br J Urol* 54, no. 3 (June 1982): 305–307.

Acheson, Kevin J., et al., "Glycogen Storage Capacity and De Novo Lipogenesis during Massive Carbohydrate Overfeeding in Man," *American Journal of Clinical Nutrition* 48 (1988): 240–247.

"Adult Diabetes Type on Rise in Young," *The New York Times*, July 8, 1997, C7.

Ahima, Rexford S., et al., "Role of Leptin in the Neuroendocrine Response to Fasting," *Nature* 382 (July 18, 1996): 295–297.

Aikens, James E., et al., "Elevated Glycosylated Albumin in NIDDM Is a Function of Recent Everyday Environmental Stress," *Diabetes Care* 20, no. 7 (July 1997): 1111–1113.

AinMelk, Y., et al., "Bromocriptine Therapy in Oligozoospermic Infertile Men," *Arch Androl* 8, no. 2 (March 1982): 135–141.

Akabayashi, A., et al., "Hypothalamic Neuropeptide Y and Its Gene Expression: Relation to Light-Dark Cycle and Circulating Corticosterone," *Molecular and Cellular Neurosciences* 5, no. 3 (June 1994): 210–218.

Alberts, Arthur S., et al., "Protein Phosphatase 2A Potentiates Activity of Promoters Containing AP-1-Binding Elements," *Molecular and Cellular Biology* 13, no. 4 (April 1993): 2104–2112.

Aloia, R. C., et al., "Membrane Function in Mammalian Hibernation," *Biochem Biophys Acta* 988, no. 1 (January 1989): 123–146.

Aloia, R. C., "The Role of Membrane Fatty Acids in Mammalian Hibernation," *Fed Proc* 39, no. 12 (October 1980): 2974–2979.

Ambrosi, B., et al., "Study of the Effects of Bromocriptine on Sexual Impotence," *Clin Endocrinol* 7, no. 5 (November 1977): 417–421.

———, "Effect of Bromocriptine and Metergoline in the Treatment of Hyperprolacti-naemic States," *Acta Endocrinol (Copenh)* 100, no. 1 (May 1982): 10–17.

Ammala, Carina, et al., "Promiscuous Coupling between the Sulphonylurea Receptor and Inwardly Rectifying Potassium Channels," *Nature* 379 (February 8, 1996): 545–548.

Anderson, Erling A., et al., "Hyperinsulinemia Produces Both Sympathetic Neural Activation and Vasodilation in Normal Humans," *Journal of Clinical Investigation* 87 (June 1991): 2246–2252.

Andrews, M. T., et al., "Low-Temperature Carbon Utilization Is Regulated by Novel Gene Activity in the Heart of a Hibernating Mammal," *Proceedings of the National Academy of Sciences (USA)* 95, no. 14 (July 7, 1998): 8392–8397.

Antonetti, D. A., et al., "Insulin Receptor Substrate 1 Binds Two Novel Splice Variants of the Regulatory Subunit of Phosphatidylinositol 3-Kinase in Muscle and Brain," *Molecular and Cellular Biology* 16, no. 5 (May 1996): 2195–2203.

Araki, E., et al., "Characterization and Regulation of the Mouse Insulin Receptor Substrate Gene Promoter," *Mol Endocrinol* 9, no. 10 (October 1995): 1367–1379.

Ault, Alicia, "FDA Warns of Potential Protease-Inhibitor Link to Hyperglycaemia," *The Lancet* 349 (June 21, 1997): 1819.

Auwerx, Johan, et al., "Leptin," *The Lancet* 351 (March 7, 1998): 737–742.

Bancroft, J., et al., "The Effects of Bromocriptine on the Sexual Behaviour of Hyperprolactinaemic Man: A Controlled Case Study," *Clin Endocrinol (Oxf)* 21, no. 2 (August 1984): 131–137.

Bao, Weihang, Ph.D., et al., "Persistent Elevation of Plasma Insulin Levels Is Associated with Increased Cardiovascular Risk in Children and Young Adults," *Circulation* 93, no. 1 (January 1, 1996): 54–59.

Barnes, Brian M., "Freeze Avoidance in a Mammal: Body Temperatures Below 0°C. in an Arctic Hibernator," *Science* 244 (June 30, 1989): 1593–1595.

Bauman, W. A., et al., "Pancreatic Hormones in the Nonhibernating and Hibernating Golden Mantled Ground Squirrel," *Comparative Biochemistry and Physiology* 86, no. 2 (1987): 241–244.

Berent, H., et al., "Hemorrheological Indices, Catecholamines, Neuropeptide Y and Serotonin in Patients with Essential Hypertension," *Blood Pressure* 6, no. 4 (July 1997): 203–208.

Bernard, Marianne, et al., "Chick Pineal Clock Regulates Serotonin N-acetyltransferase mRNA Rhythm in Culture," *Proceedings of the National Academy of Sciences (USA)* 94 (January 1997): 304–309.

Berry, Elliot M., et al., "Effects of Diets Rich in Monounsaturated Fatty Acids on Plasma Lipoproteins—the Jerusalem Nutrition Study: II. Monounsaturated Fatty Acids vs. Carbohydrates 1–3," *American Journal of Clinical Nutrition* 56 (1992): 394–403.

Betteridge, D. J., "Diabetic Dyslipidaemia—What Does It Mean?" *Diabetes News* 18, no. 2 (1997): 1–3.

Blakeslee, Sandra, "Surprising Theory on the Body Clock: Illuminate the Knee," *The New York Times,* January 16, 1998, A1.

Boden, Guenther, et al., "Evidence for a Circadian Rhythm of Insulin Secretion," *American Journal of Physiology* 271 (1996): E246-E252.

Boivin, Diane B., et al., "Dose-Response Relationships for Resetting of Human Circadian Clock by Light," *Nature* 379 (February 8, 1996): 540–544.

Bonora, E., et al., "Relationship between Blood Pressure and Plasma Insulin in Non-Obese and Obese Non-Diabetic Subjects," *Diabetologia* 30 (1987): 719–723.

Born, Jan, et al., "Effects of Sleep and Circadian Rhythm on Human Circulating Immune Cells," *Journal of Immunology* 158 (1997): 4454–4464.

Bornstein, Stefan R., et al., "Plasma Leptin Levels Are Increased in Survivors of Acute Sepsis: Associated Loss of Diurnal Rhythm in Cortisol and Leptin Secretion," *Journal of Clinical Endocrinology and Metabolism* 83, no. 1 (1998): 280–283.

———, "Evidence for a Novel Peripheral Action of Leptin As a Metabolic Signal to the Adrenal Gland," *Diabetes* 16 (July 1997): 1225–1238.

Boswell, T., et al., "NPY and Galanin in a Hibernator: Hypothalamic Gene Expression and Effects on Feeding," *Brain Research Bulletin* 32, no. 4 (1993): 379–384.

Boulware, S. D., et al., "Comparison of the Metabolic Effects of Recombinant Human Insulin-Like Growth Factor-1 and Insulin," *J Clin Invest* 93 (March 1994): 1131–1139.

Bray, George A., et al., "Leptin and Clinical Medicine: A New Piece in the Puzzle of Obesity," *Journal of Clinical Endocrinology and Metabolism* 82, no. 9 (1997): 2271–2276.

Brody, Jane E., "Eating Fish Cited Anew As Good for the Heart," *The New York Times,* April 11, 1997, A12.

Butte, N. F., et al., "Leptin in Human Reproduction: Serum Leptin Levels in Pregnant and Lactating Women," *Journal of Clinical Endocrinology and Metabolism* 82, no. 2 (1997): 585–589.

Buvat, J., "Influence of Primary Hyperprolactinemia on Human Sexual Behavior," *Nouv Presse Med* 11, no. 48 (November 27, 1982): 3561–3563.

Buxton, Orfeu M., et al., "Roles of Intensity and Duration of Nocturnal Exercise in Causing Phase Delays of Human Circadian Rhythms," *American Journal of Physiology* 273 (1997): E536-E542.

Camirand, A., et al., "Thiazolidinediones Stimulate Uncoupling Protein-2 Expression in Cell Lines Representing White and Brown Adipose Tissues and Skeletal Muscle," *Endocrinology* 139, no. 1 (January 1998): 428–431.

Campbell, Scott S., et al., "Extraocular Circadian Phototransduction in Humans," *Science* 279, no. 5349 (January 16, 1998): 396–399.

Cannon, B., et al., "The Biochemistry of an Inefficient Tissue: Brown Adipose Tissue," *Essays in Biochemistry* 20 (1985): 110–164.

Carlson, Lars A., et al., "Ischaemic Heart Disease in Relation to Fasting Values of Plasma Triglycerides and Cholesterol," *The Lancet,* April 22, 1972: 865–868.

Caro, Jose F., et al., "Leptin: The Tale of an Obesity Gene," *Diabetes* 45 (November 1996): 1455–1462.

Castex, C., et al., "Glucose Oxidation by Adipose Tissue of the Edible Dormouse (Glis glis) during Hibernation and Arousal: Effect of Insulin," *Comparative Biochemistry and Physiology* 88, no. 1 (1987): 33–36.

———, "Regulation of Endocrine Pancreas Secretions (Insulin and Glucagon) during the Periodic Lethargy-Waking Cycle of the Hibernating Mammal," *Diabete et Metabolisme* 13, no. 3 (June 1987): 176–181.

———, "Insulin Secretion in the Hibernating Edible Dormouse (Glis glis): In Vivo and In Vitro Studies," *Comparative Biochemistry and Physiology* 79, no. 1 (1984): 179–183.

Chai, Z., et al., "Interleukin (IL)-6 Gene Expression in the Central Nervous System Is Necessary for Fever Response to Lipopolysaccharide or IL-1 Beta: A Study on IL-6-Deficient Mice," *Journal of Experimental Medicine* 183 (January 1996): 311–316.

Chengappa, K. N., et al., "Differences in Serum Interleukin-6 between Healthy Dextral and Non-Dextral Subjects," *Neuroscience Research* 20, no. 2 (August 1994): 185–188.

Cincotta, Anthony H., et al., "Bromocriptine Redirects Metabolism and Prevents Seasonal Onset of Obese Hyperinsulinemic State in Syrian Hamsters," *American Physiological Society* 264 (1993): E285-E292.

———, "Bromocriptine/SKF38393 Treatment Ameliorates Obesity and Associated Metabolic Dysfunctions in Obese (ob/ob) Mice," *Life Sci* 61, no. 10 (1997): 951–956.

————, et al., "Bromocriptine (Ergoset) Reduces Body Weight and Improves Glucose Tolerance in Obese Subjects," *Diabetes Care* 19, no. 6 (June 1996): 667–670.

Cohen, A. M., et al., "Change of Diet of Yemenite Jews in Relation to Diabetes and Ischaemic Heart Disease," *The Lancet* 2 (December 23, 1961): 1399–1401.

————, "Genetics and Diet As Factors in Development of Diabetes Mellitus," *Metabolism* 21, no. 3 (March 1972): 235–240.

Cohen, Batya, et al., "Modulation of Insulin Activities by Leptin," *Science* 274 (November 15, 1996): 1185–1188.

Cole, R. J., et al., "Seasonal Variation in Human Illumination Exposure at Two Different Latitudes," *Journal of Biological Rhythms* 10 (1995): 324–334.

Considine, Robert V., Ph.D., et al., "Serum Immunoreactive Leptin Concentrations in Normal Weight and Obese Humans," *New England Journal of Medicine* 334, no. 5 (February 1, 1996): 292–295.

Cui, Y., et al., "The Modulatory Effects of Mu and Kappa Opioid Agonists on 5-HT Release from Hippocampal Slices of Euthermic and Hibernating Ground Squirrels," *Life Sciences* 53, no. 26 (1993): 1957–1965.

————, "State-Dependent Changes of Brain Endogenous Opioids in Mammalian Hibernation," *Brain Research Bulletin* 40, no. 2 (1996): 129–133.

Daan, S., et al., "An Effect of Castration and Testosterone Replacement on a Circadian Pacemaker in Mice (Mus musculus)," *Proceedings of the National Academy of Sciences (USA)* 72 (1975): 3744–3747.

Dallman, M. F., et al., "The Neural Network That Regulates Energy Balance Is Responsive to Glucocorticoids and Insulin and Regulates HPA Axis Responsivity at a Site Proximal to CRF Neurons," *Annals of the New York Academy of Sciences* 271 (December 29, 1995): 730–742.

Daly, Mark E., et al., "Dietary Carbohydrates and Insulin Sensitivity: A Review of the Evidence and Clinical Implications," *American Journal of Clinical Nutrition* 66 (1997): 1072–1085.

Danilenko, K. V., et al., "Diurnal and Seasonal Variations of Melatonin and Serotonin in Women with Seasonal Affective Disorder," *Arctic Medical Research* 53, no. 3 (July 1994): 137–145.

Davis, Maris R., et al., "Physiologic Hyperinsulinemia Enhances Counterregulatory Hormone Responses to Hypoglycemia in IDDM," *Journal of Clinical Endocrinology and Metabolism* 76, no. 5 (1993): 1383–1385.

Davis, S. N., et al., "Effects of Physiological Hyperinsulinemia on Counterregulatory Response to Prolonged Hypoglycemia in Normal Humans," *American Journal of Physiology* 267, no. 3 (September 1994): E402-E410.

Debreceni, L., et al., "Persistent Hypoglycemia Due to Hyperinsulinemia, Hypoglucagonemia and Mild Adrenal Insufficiency," *Exp Clin Endocrinol* 90, no. 2 (1987): 221–226.

DeFronzo, Ralph A., et al., "Glucose Clamp Technique: A Method for Quantifying Insulin Secretion and Resistance," *American Journal of Physiology* 237, no. 3 (1979): E214-E223.

Demaison, L., et al., "Myocardial Ischemia and In Vitro Mitochondrial Metabolic Efficiency," *Molecular and Cellular Biochemistry* 158, no. 2 (May 24, 1996): 161–169.

De Saint Hilaire, Zara, et al., "Active Immunization of Rats against Insulin Subunits: Effects on Sleep and Feeding," *Physiology & Behavior* 61, no. 5 (1997): 649–651.

Despres, Jean-Pierre, Ph.D., et al., "Hyperinsulinemia As an Independent Risk Factor for Ischemic Heart Disease," *New England Journal of Medicine* 334 (1996): 952–957.

De Zegher, F., et al., "Dopamine Inhibits Growth Hormone and Prolactin Secretion in the Human Newborn," *Pediatric Research* 34, no. 5 (November 1993): 642–645.

Dhurandhar, N. V., et al., "Effect of Adenovirus Infection on Adiposity in Chicken," *Vet Microbiol* 31, nos. 2–3 (June 1, 1992): 101–107.

Diamond, Michael, et al., "Suppression of Counterregulatory Hormone Response to Hypoglycemia by Insulin," *Journal of Clinical Endocrinology and Metabolism* 72, no. 6 (1991): 1388–1390.

Dickinson, C. J., "Cerebral Oxidative Metabolism in Hypertension" (editorial), *Clinical Science* 91, no. 5 (November 1996): 539–550.

Dineen, Sean, "Metabolic Effects of the Nocturnal Rise in Cortisol on Carbohydrate Metabolism in Normal Humans," *Journal of Clinical Investigation* 92, no. 5 (November 1993): 2283–2290.

Doheny, Kathleen, "Zeroing in on Diabetes," *Los Angeles Times,* May 28, 1997, E2.

Donahue, Richard P., et al., "Diabetes Mellitus and Macrovascular Complications," *Diabetes Care* 15, no. 9 (September 1992): 1141–1155.

Duanmu, Zhengbo, et al., "Insulin-Like Growth Factor-1 Decreases Sympathetic Nerve Activity: The Effect Is Modulated by Glycemic Status," *Proceedings of the Society for Experimental Biology and Medicine* 216, no. 1 (October 1997): 93–97.

Dufau, M. L., et al., "Mode of Secretion of Bioactive Luteinizing Hormone in Man," *Journal of Clinical Endocrinology and Metabolism* 57, no. 5 (1983): 993–1000.

Duncan, Wallace C., Jr., "Circadian Rhythms and the Pharmacology of Affective Illness," *Pharmacology* 71, no. 3 (1996): 253–312.

Eastman, C. A., et al., "Can Bright Light Entrain a Free-Runner?" *Sleep Res* 17 (1988): 372.

Eastone, John A., et al., "New-Onset Diabetes Mellitus Associated with Use of Protease Inhibitor," *Annals of Internal Medicine* 127, no. 11 (November 15, 1997): 948.

Edelman, S. V., "Impaired Glucose Tolerance: A Precursor of NIDDM or a Disease Entity in Itself?" *Diabetes News* 16, no. 2 (1995): 1–8.

Emilsson, Valur, et al., "Expression of the Functional Leptin Receptor mRNA in Pancreatic Islets and Direct Inhibitory Action of Leptin on Insulin Secretion," *Diabetes* 46 (February 1997): 313–316.

Endres, Stefan, et al., "The Effect of Dietary Supplementation with n-3 Polyunsaturated Fatty Acids on the Synthesis of Interleukin-1 and Tumor Necrosis Factor by Mononuclear Cells," *New England Journal of Medicine* 320, no. 5 (February 2, 1989): 265–271.

"Epidemiology and Treatment of Hypercholesterolemia: Where We Are Today," *American Journal of Medicine* 102, no. 2A (February 17, 1997): (Editorial)

Ericsson, M., et al., "Common Biological Pathways in Eating Disorders and Obesity," *Addictive Behaviors* 21, no. 6 (November/December 1996): 733–743.

Esler, Murray, et al., "Leptin in Human Plasma Is Derived in Part from the Brain, and Cleared by the Kidneys," *The Lancet* 351 (March 21, 1998): 879.

Essen, Lars-Oliver, et al., "A Cold Break for Photoreceptors," *Nature* 392 (March 12, 1998): 131–133.

Ewald, Paul W., et al., "Catching on to What's Catching," *Natural History,* February 1999: 34–37.

Fankhauser, C., et al., "Light Control of Plant Development," *Ann Rev Cell Dev Biol* 13 (1997): 203–229.

Farquhar, J. W., et al., "Glucose, Insulin, and Triglyceride Responses to High and Low Carbohydrate diets in Man," *Journal of Clinical Investigation* 45, no. 10 (October 1966): 1648–1656.

Fenster, J. M., "The Conquest of Diabetes," *Invention & Technology,* 1999 Winter 1999: 48–55.

Ferrannini, Eleuterio, M.D., et al., "Insulin Resistance in Essential Hypertension," *New England Journal of Medicine* 317, no. 6 (August 6, 1987): 350–357.

Fishman, Alfred P., M.D., "Hibernation in Animals," *Circulation,* August 1961: 433.

Fishman, B., et al., "Daily Rhythms in Hepatic Polysome Profiles and Tyrosine Transaminase Activity: Role of Dietary Protein," *Proceedings of the National Academy of Sciences (USA)* 64 (1969): 677–682.

Florant, Gregory L., et al., "Seasonal Changes in Pancreatic B-cell Function in Euthermic Yellow-Bellied Marmots," *American Journal of Physiology* 249 (1985): R159-R165.

Frankish, H. M., et al., "Neuropeptide Y, the Hypothalamus, and Diabetes: Insights into the Central Control of Metabolism," *Peptides* 16, no. 4 (1995): 757–771.

Freemark, M., et al., "Ontogenesis of Prolactin Receptors in the Human Fetus in Early Gestation: Implications for Tissue Differentiation and Development," *Journal of Clinical Investigation* 99, no. 5 (March 1, 1997): 1107–1117.

Frieboes, Ralf-Michael, et al., "Enhanced Slow Wave Sleep in Patients with Prolactinoma," *Journal of Clinical Endocrinology and Metabolism* 83, no. 8 (1998): 2706–2710.

Gagnon, Anne Marie, et al., "Protease Inhibitors and Adipocyte Differentiation in Cell Culture," *The Lancet* 352 (September 26, 1998): 1032.

Garnacho, Montero J., et al., "Lipids and Immune Function," *Nutricion Hospitalaria* 11, no. 4 (July/August 1996): 230–237.

Genick, Ulrich K., et al., "Structure at 0.85: A Resolution of an Early Protein Photocycle Intermediate," *Nature* 392 (March 12, 1998): 206–209.

Georges, Christopher J., "Studies Link Aggressiveness to Cholesterol," *The New York Times,* September 11, 1990, B5.

Gewolb, I. H., et al., "High Glucose and Insulin Decrease Fetal Lung Insulin Receptor mRNA and Tyrosine Kinase Activity In Vitro," *Biochemical and Biophysical Research Communications* 202, no. 2 (July 29, 1994): 694–700.

"Girls' Body Fat Isn't Related to Cholesterol Levels, Study Finds," *The New York Times,* June 17, 1997, B13.

Giudice, Linda C., "Insulin-Like Growth Factors and Ovarian Follicular Development," *Endocrine Reviews* 13, no. 4 (1992): 641–669.

Glanz, James, "Can 'Resetting' Hormonal Rhythms Treat Illness?" *Science* 269 (September 1, 1995): 1220–1221.

Glass, M. J., et al., "Role of Carbohydrate Type on Diet Selection in Neuropeptide Y-Stimulated Rats," *American Journal of Physiology* 273 (December 1997): R2040-R2045.

Goalstone, Marc L., et al., "Insulin Potentiates Platelet-Derived Growth Factor Action in Vascular Smooth Muscle Cells," *Endocrinology* 139, no. 10 (1998): 4067–4072.

Godo, G., "Hyperprolactinaemia and Female Infertility," *Acta Med Hung* 41, no. 4 (1984): 185–193.

Goldzieher, Joseph W., et al., "Selected Aspects of Polycystic Ovarian Disease," *Reproductive Endocrinology* 21, no. 1 (March 1992): 141–171.

Gong, D. W., et al., "Uncoupling Protein-3 Is a Mediator of Thermogenesis Regulated by Thyroid Hormone, Beta3-Adregergic Agonists, and Leptin," *Journal of Biological Chemistry* 272, no. 39 (September 26, 1997): 24129–24132.

Gorman, Christine, "Doctors' Dilemma," *Time*, August 25, 1997, 64.

Grady, Denise, "Newer Guidelines Redefine Diabetes in Broader Terms: Lowering Level of Blood Sugar Considered Normal Could Mean Tests for Millions," *The New York Times*, June 24, 1997, A1.

Grodum, E., et al., "Dopaminergic Inhibition of Pulsatile Luteinizing Hormone Secretion Is Abnormal in Regularly Menstruating Women with Insulin-Dependent Diabetes Mellitus," *Fertility and Sterility* 64, no. 2 (August 1995): 279–284.

Grunfeld, Carl, et al., "Endotoxin and Cytokines Induce Expression of Leptin, the ob Gene Product, in Hamsters," *Journal of Clinical Investigation* 97, no. 9 (May 1996): 2152–2157.

Gura, Trisha, "Obesity Sheds Its Secrets," *Science* 275 (February 7, 1997): 751–753.

Gurney, M., et al., "The Global Prevalence of Obesity—An Initial Overview of Available Data," *World Health Stat Q* 41, nos. 3–4 (1988): 251–254.

Hademenos, George J., "The Biophysics of Stroke," *American Scientist* 85 (May/June 1997): 226–235.

Hearse, D. J., "Myocardial Hibernation: A Form of Endogenous Protection?" *Eur Heart J* 18, suppl. A (January 1997): A2-A7.

Himms-Hagen, Jean, et al., "Thermogenesis in Brown Adipose Tissue As an Energy Buffer: Implications for Obesity," *New England Journal of Medicine* 311, no. 24 (Dec 13, 1984): 1549–1558.

Hiramatsu, Kazuko, et al., "A Case of Pheochromocytoma with Transient Hyperinsulinemia and Reactive Hypoglycemia," *Jpn J Med* 26, no. 1 (February 1987): 88–90.

Hirsch, Jules, "Some Heat but Not Enough Light," *Nature* 387 (May 1, 1997): 27–28.

Hopfner, Rob L., et al., "Insulin Increases Endothelin-1-Evoked Intracellular Free Calcium Responses by Increased Eta Receptor Expression in Rat Aortic Smooth Muscle Cells," *Diabetes* 47 (June 1998): 937–944.

Hoo-Paris, R., et al., "Role of Glucose and Catecholamines in the Regulation of Insulin Secretion in the Hibernating Hedgehog during Arousal," *General and Comparative Endocrinology* 41, no. 1 (May 1980): 62–65.

———, "In Vitro B Cell Response to Glucose in the Hibernating Hedgehog: Comparison with the Homeothermic Hedgehog and the Rat," *Comparative Biochemistry and Physiology* 78, no. 3 (1984): 559–563.

————, "Glucose Turnover Control by Insulin in the Hibernating Hedgehog," *Hormone and Metabolic Research* 15, no. 1 (January 1983): 47–48.

Hopkin, Karen, "Clock Setting," *Scientific American*, April 1998: 20–22.

Howell, Wanda H., et al., "Plasma Lipid and Lipoprotein Responses to Dietary Fat and Cholesterol: A Meta-Analysis," *American Journal of Clinical Nutrition* 65 (1997): 1747–1764.

Hotamisligil, Gokhan S., et al., "Increased Adipose Tissue Expression of Tumor Necrosis Factor in Human Obesity and Insulin Resistance," *Journal of Clinical Investigation* 95 (May 1995): 2409–2415.

Husten, Larry, "Receptor Offers Clues to How 'Good' Cholesterol Works," *Science* 278 (November 14, 1997): 1228.

Hsu, D. S., et al., "Putative Human Blue-Light Photoreceptors hCRY1 and hCRY2 are Flavoproteins," *Biochemistry* 35, no. 44 (November 5, 1996): 13871–13877.

Illnerova, Helena, et al., "The Circadian Rhythm in Plasma Melatonin Concentration of the Urbanized Man: The Effect of Summer and Winter Time," *Brain Research* 328 (1985): 186–189.

————, "Melatonin Rhythm in Human Milk," *Journal of Clinical Endocrinology and Metabolism* 77, no. 3 (1993): 838–841.

Jarrett, R. J., "Is Insulin Atherogenic?" *Diabetologia* 31 (1988): 71–75.

Johnson, R. W., et al., "Hormones, Lymphohemopoietic Cytokines and the Neuroimmune Axis," *Comparative Biochemistry and Physiology* 116A, no. 3 (1997): 183–201.

Johnston, Colin I., "Renin-Angiotensin System: A Dual Tissue and Hormonal System for Cardiovascular Control," *Journal of Hypertension* 10, suppl. 7 (December 1992): S13-S26.

Jones, Peter J. H., et al., "Dietary Cholesterol Feeding Suppresses Human Cholesterol Synthesis Measured by Deuterium Incorporation and Urinary Mevalonic Acid Levels," *Arteriosclerosis, Thrombosis, and Vascular Biology* 16, no. 10 (October 1996): 1222–1228.

Jun, T., et al., "Increased Superoxide Anion Production in Humans: A Possible Mechanism for the Pathogenesis of Hypertension," *J Hum Hypertens* 10, no. 5 (May 1996): 305–309.

Kahn, Ronald C., "Insulin Action, Diabetogenes, and the Cause of Type II Diabetes," *Diabetes* 43 (August 1994): 1066–1084.

Kamath, Vinaya, M.D., et al., "Effects of a Quick-Release Form of Bromocriptine (Ergoset) on Fasting and Postprandial Plasma Glucose, Insulin, Lipid, and Lipoprotein Concentrations in Obese Nondiabetic Hyperinsulinemic Women," *Diabetes Care* 20, no. 11 (November 1997): 1697–1701.

Kant, G. J., et al., "Effects of Chronic Stress and Time of Day on Preference for Sucrose," *Physiology and Behavior* 54, no. 3 (September 1993): 499–502.

Kilduff, T. S., et al., "Sleep and Mammalian Hibernation: Homologous Adaptations and Homologous Processes? *Sleep* 16, no. 4 (June 16, 1993): 372–386.

King, George L., et al., "Biochemical and Molecular Mechanisms in the Development of Diabetic Vascular Complications," *Diabetes* 45, suppl. 3 (July 1996): S105-S108.

Knott, Cheryl, "Orangutans in the Wild," *National Geographic*, August 1998: 28–56.

Kokkoris, C. P., et al., "Long-Term Ambulatory Temperature Monitoring in a Subject with a Hypernychthemeral Sleep-Wake Cycle Disturbance," *Sleep* 1 (1978): 177–190.

Kolaczynski, Jerzy W., et al., "Acute and Chronic Effect of Insulin on Leptin Production in Humans: Studies In Vivo and In Vitro," *Diabetes* 45, no. 5 (May 1996): 699–701.

————, "Response of Leptin to Short-Term Fasting and Refeeding in Humans: A Link with Ketogenesis but Not Ketones Themselves," *Diabetes* 11 (November 1996): 1511–1515.

————, "Response of Leptin to Short-Term and Prolonged Overfeeding in Humans," *Journal of Clinical Endocrinology and Metabolism* 81, no. 11 (1996): 4162–4165.

Knutson, V. P., et al., "Insulin Resistance is Mediated by a Proteolytic Fragment of the Insulin Receptor," *Journal of Biological Chemistry* 270, no. 42 (October 20, 1995): 24972–24981.

Lakhdar-Ghazal, N., et al., "Vasopressin in the Brain of a Desert Hibernator, the Jerboa (Jaculus orientalis): Presence of Sexual Dimorphism and Seasonal Variation," *Journal of Comparative Neurology* 358, no. 4 (August 7, 1995): 499–517.

LaMarco, Kelly, "Obesity Research: Digesting the Glut of Information," *Exploring Fitness* 21, no. 3 (Fall 1997): 24–25.

Lanni, A., et al., "Induction of UCP2 mRNA by Thyroid Hormones in Rat Heart," *FEBS Letters* 418, nos. 1–2 (November 24, 1997): 171–174.

Lauerman, John F., "A Persistent Plague," *Harvard Magazine* (September/October 1998): 22–25.

Lelkes, P. I., et al., "Microgravity Decreases Tyrosine Hydroxylase Expression in Rat Adrenals," *FASEB J* 8, no. 14 (November 1994): 1177–1182.

Licinio, Julio, et al., "Human Leptin Levels Are Pulsatile and Inversely Related to Pituitary-Adrenal Function," *Nature Medicine* 3, no. 5 (May 1997): 575–579.

Lin, C., et al., "Enhancement of Blue-Light Sensitivity of Arabidopsis Seedlings by a Blue Light Receptor Cryptochrome 2," *Proceedings of the National Academy of Sciences (USA)* 95, no. 5 (March 3, 1998): 2686–2690.

Lin, Yuzhong J., et al., "Direct Stimulation of Immediate-Early Genes by Intranuclear Insulin in Trypsin-Treated H35 Hepatoma Cells," *Proceedings of the National Academy of Sciences (USA)* 89 (October 1992): 9691–9694.

Lincoln, G. A., et al., "Does Melatonin Act on Dopaminergic Pathways in the Mediobasal Hypothalamus to Mediate Effects of Photoperiod on Prolactin Secretion in the Ram?" *Neuroendocrinology* 62, no. 5 (November 1995): 425–433.

————, "Evidence That Melatonin Acts in the Pituitary Gland through a Dopamine-Independent Mechanism to Mediate Effects of Day Length on the Secretion of Prolactin in the Ram," *Journal Neuroendocrinol* 7, no. 8 (August 1995): 637–643.

Liu, Li Sen, et al., "Tumor Necrosis Factor Alpha Acutely Inhibits Insulin Signaling in Human Adipocytes: Implication of the p80 Tumor Necrosis Factor Receptor," *Diabetes* 47 (April 1998): 515–522.

Liu, Zhenqi, et al., "Insulin and Glucose Suppress Hepatic Glycogenolysis by Distinct Enzymatic Mechanisms," *Metabolism* 42, no. 12 (December 1993): 1536–1551.

Lonnqvist, Fredrik, "Leptin Secretion from Adipose Tissue in Women," *Journal of Clinical Investigation* 99, no. 10 (May 10, 1997): 2398–2404.

Lunt, H., "Diabetes Mellitus in Older Patients: Is Tight Blood Glucose Control Warranted?" *Drugs Aging* 8, no. 6 (June 1996): 401–407.

Lyman, Charles P., "Hibernation in Mammals," *Circulation* (August 1961): 434–445.

Malhotra, Khushbeer, et al., "Putative Blue-Light Photoreceptors from Arabidopsis thaliana and Sinapsis alba with a High Degree of Sequence Homology to DNA Photolyase Contain the Two Photolyase Cofactors but Lack DNA Repair Activity," *Biochemistry* 34, no. 20 (1995): 6892–6899.

Mantzoros, Christos S., et al., "Leptin Concentrations in Relation to Body Mass Index and the Tumor Necrosis Factor-alpha System in Humans," *Journal of Clinical Endocrinology and Metabolism* 82, no. 10 (1997): 3408–3413.

———, "Short-Term Hyperthyroidism Has No Effect on Leptin Levels in Man," *Journal of Clinical Endocrinology and Metabolism* 82, no. 2 (1997): 497–499.

Marin, Per, et al., "Assimilation and Mobilization of Triglycerides in Subcutaneous Abdominal and Femoral Adipose Tissue In Vivo in Men: Effects of Androgens," *Journal of Clinical Endocrinology and Metabolism* 80, no. 1 (1995): 239–243.

Marsden, P. J., "Severe Impairment of Insulin Action in Adipocytes from Amenorrheic Subjects with Polycystic Ovary Syndrome," *Metabolism* 43, no,. 12 (December 1994): 1536–1542.

Masaki, T., et al., "Enhanced Expression of Uncoupling Protein 2 Gene in Rat White Adipose Tissue and Skeletal Muscle Following Chronic Treatment with Thyroid Hormone," *FEBS Letters* 418, no. 3 (December 1, 1997): 323–326.

Masson-Pevet, M., et al., "An Attempt to Correlate Brain Areas Containing Melatonin-Binding Sites with Rhythmic Functions: A Study in Five Hibernator Species," *Cell and Tissue Research* 278, no. 1 (October 1994): 97–106.

Masucci-Magoulas, Lori, et al., "A Mouse with Features of Familiar Combined Hyperlipidemia," *Science* 275 (January 17, 1997): 391–394.

Masuzaki, Hiroaki, et al., "Nonadipose Tissue Production of Leptin: Leptin As a Novel Placenta-Derived Hormone in Humans," *Nature Medicine* 3, no. 9 (September 1997): 1029–1033.

Matkovic, Velimir, et al., "Leptin Is Inversely Related to Age at Menarche in Human Females," *Journal of Clinical Endocrinology* 82, no. 10 (1997): 3239–3245.

Matsumoto, Kazunari, et al., "Increase of Lipoprotein (a) with Trogolitazone," *The Lancet* 350 (December 13, 1997): 1748–1749.

McCarty, M. F., "Insulin Resistance in Mexican Americans—A Precursor to Obesity and Diabetes?" *Medical Hypotheses* 41, no. 4 (October 1993): 308–315.

McMillen, I. C., et al., "Melatonin and the Development of Circadian and Seasonal Rhythmicity," *J Reprod Fertil Suppl* 49 (1995): 137–146.

Melnyk, Roman B., et al., "Insulin and Central Regulation of Spontaneous Fattening and Weight Loss," *American Journal of Physiology* 249 (1985): R203-R208.

Metherall, James E., et al., "Progesterone Inhibits Cholesterol Biosynthesis in Cultured Cells," *American Society for Biochemistry and Molecular Biology* 271, no. 5 (1996): 2627–2633.

Millet, L., et al., "Increased Uncoupling Protein-2 and -3 mRNA Expression during Fasting in Obese and Lean Humans," *Journal of Clinical Investigation* 100, no. 11 (December 1, 1997): 2665–2670.

Mitchell, Peter, "Cancelled IGF-1 Trials Bode Ill for Diabetic Patients," *The Lancet* 350 (November 29, 1997): 1606.

Miyamoto, Y., et al., "Vitamin B$_2$-Based Blue-Light Photoreceptors in the Retinohypothalamic Tract As the Photoactive Pigments for Setting the Circadian Clock in Mammals," *Proceedings of the National Academy of Sciences (USA)* 95, no. 11 (May 26, 1998): 6097–6102.

Monamaney, Terence, "TV Viewing, Childhood Obesity Linked," *Los Angeles Times*, March 25, 1998, A1.

Monteleone, P., et al., "The Human Pineal Gland Responds to Stress-Induced Sympathetic Activation in the Second Half of the Dark Phase: Preliminary Evidence," *Journal of Neural Transmission* 92, no. 1 (1993): 25–32.

Montelongo, Adela, et al., "Longitudinal Study of Plasma Lipoproteins and Hormones during Pregnancy in Normal and Diabetic Women," *Diabetes* 41 (December 1992): 1651–1659.

Mooney, Michael, et al., "Protease Inhibitors and Potbelly," *Metabolism* 2, no. 2 (March 17, 1998): 1–6.

Moreau-Hamsany, C., et al., "Hormonal Control of Lipolysis from the White Adipose Tissue of Hibernating Jerboa (Jaculus orientalis)," *Comparative Biochemistry and Physiology* 91, no. 4 (1988): 665–669.

Morell, Virginia, "A 24-Hour Circadian Clock Is Found in the Mammalian Retina," *Science* 272 (April 19, 1995): 349.

Morimoto, Y., et al., "Complements in Diabetes Mellitus: Activation of Complement System Evidenced by C3d Elevation in IDDM," *Diabetes Research Clinical Practice* 5, no. 4 (October 14, 1988): 309–312.

Morkawa, K., et al., "Immunosuppressive Property of Bromocriptine on Human B Lymphocyte Function In Vitro," *Clinical and Experimental Immunology* 93, no. 2 (August 1993): 200–205.

Morris, Jason Z., et al., "A Phosphatidylinositol-3-OH Kinase Family Member Regulating Longevity and Diapause in Caenorhabditis elegans," *Nature* 382 (August 8, 1996): 536–538.

Morrow, Linda A., et al., "Effects of Epinephrine on Insulin Secretion and Action in Humans," *Diabetes* 42 (February 1993): 307–315.

Muller-Enoch, D., "Blue Light Mediated Photoreduction of the Flavoprotein NADPH-Cytochrome P450 Reductase: A Forster-Type Energy Transfer," *Z Naturforsch* 52, nos. 9–10 (September 1997): 605–614.

Munoz-Hoyos, A., et al., "Absence of Plasma Melatonin Circadian Rhythm during the First 72 Hours of Life in Human Infants," *Journal of Clinical Endocrinology and Metabolism* 77, no. 3 (1993): 699–703.

Nagulesparen, M., et al., "Bromocriptine Treatment of Males with Pituitary Tumours, Hyperprolactinaemia, and Hypogonadism," *Clin Endocrinolo (Oxf)* 9, no. 1 (July 1978): 73–79.

Nakata, Masanori, et al., "Leptin Promotes Aggregation of Human Platelets via the Long Form of Its Receptor," *Diabetes* 48 (1999): 426–429.

Nevretdinova, Zelya, et al., "Some Aspects of Lipid Metabolism and Thyroid Function in Arctic Ground Squirrel, Citellus parryi, during Hibernation," *Arctic Medical Research* 51 (1992): 196–204.

Nilsson, P. M., "Premature Ageing: The Link between Psychosocial Risk Factors and Disease," *Medical Hypotheses* 47, no. 1 (July 1996): 39–42.

Niskanen, L., "Insulin Treatment in Elderly Patients with Non-Insulin-Dependent Diabetes Mellitus: A Double-Edged Sword?" *Drugs Aging* 8, no. 3 (March 1996): 183–192.

Nurnberger, F., et al., "The Somatostatin System of the Brain and Hibernation on the European Hamster (Cricetus cricetus)," *Cell and Tissue Research* 288, no. 3 (June 1997): 441–447.

O'Connell, Y., et al., "The Effect of Prolactin, Human Chorionic Gonadotropin, Insulin and Insulin-Like Growth Factor 1 on Adrenal Steroidogenesis in Isolated Guinea-Pig Adrenal Cells," *Journal of Steroid Biochemistry and Molecular Biology* 48, nos. 2–3 (February 1994): 235–240.

Odawara, M., "Involvement of Mitochondrial Gene Abnormalities in the pathogenesis of Diabetes Mellitus," *Annals of the New York Academy of Sciences* 786 (June 15, 1996): 72–81.

Okutani, M., et al., "What Time Is the 'Biologic Zero Hour' of Circadian Variability?" *American Journal of Hypertension* 10, no. 7 (July 1997): 756–762.

Olefsky, Jerrold M., et al., "Reappraisal of the Role of Insulin in Hypertriglyceridemia," *American Journal of Medicine* 57 (October 1974): 551–560.

Omura, Y., et al., "Non-Invasive Evaluation of the Effects of Opening and Closing of Eyes, and of Exposure to a Minute Light Beam, As Well As to Electrical or Magnetic Field, on the Melatonin, Serotonin, and Other Neuro-Transmitters of Human Pineal Gland Representation Areas and the Heart," *Acupuncture and Electro-Therapeutics Research* 18, no. 2 (April-June 1993): 125–151.

O'Rahilly, Stephen, "Life without Leptin," *Nature* 392 (March 26, 1998): 330–331.

Oren, Dan A., et al., "Restoration of Detectable Melatonin After Entrainment to a 24-Hour Schedule in a 'Free-Running' Man," *Psychoneuroendocrinology* 22, no. 1 (1997): 39–52.

———, "Tweaking the Human Circadian Clock with Light," *Science* 279 (January 16, 1998): 333–334.

Ormseth, O. A., et al., "Leptin Inhibits Prehibernation Hyperphagia and Reduces Body Weight in Arctic Ground Squirrels," *American Journal of Physiology* 271, no. 6 (December 1996): R1775-R1779.

Ornish, Dean, M.D., et al., "Dietary Treatment of Hyperlipidemia," *Journal of Cardiovascular Risk* 1, no. 4 (December 1994): 283–286.

Ornish, Dean, M.D., "Treatment of and Screening for Hyperlipidemia," *New England Journal of Medicine* 329, no. 15 (October 7, 1993): 1124–1125; 1127–1128.

Orosco, M., et al., "Hypothalamic Monoamines and Insulin in Relation to Feeding in the Genetically Obese Zucker Rat As Revealed by Microdialysis," *Obesity Research*, suppl. 5 (December 3, 1995): 655S-665S.

Jackson, F. R., et al., "Oscillating Molecules and Circadian Clock Output Mechanisms," *Molecular Psychiatry* 3 (1998): 381–385.

Ouchi, Yasuyoshi, et al., "Augmented contractile Function and Abnormal Ca2+ Handling in the Aorta of Zucker Obese Rats with Insulin Resistance," *Diabetes* 45, suppl. 3 (July 1996): S55-S57.

Pagliassotti, Michael J., et al., "Increased Net Hepatic Glucose Output from Gluconeogenic Precursors After High-Sucrose Diet Feeding in Male Rats," *American Journal of Physiology* 272 (1997): R526-R531.

Pal, B., et al., "Limitation of Joint Mobility and Shoulder Capsulitis in Insulin- and Non-Insulin-Dependent Diabetes Mellitus," *Br J Rheumatol* 25, no. 2 (May 1986): 147–151.

Parke-Davis (a division of Warner-Lambert Company), *"How Rezulin* [troglitazone] *Fits into Your Diabetes Control Plan: A New Therapy for Type II Diabetes,"* (1997): 2–19.

Pasolini, G., et al., "Effects of Aging on Dehydroepiandrosterone Sulfate in Relation to fasting Insulin Levels and Body Composition Assessed by Bioimpedance Analysis," *Metabolism* 46, no. 7 (July 1997): 826–832.

Pastor, J. Feliz-De Vargas, et al., "Hipoglucemia por Hiperinsulinismo: Estudio de Cuatro Casos," *Ann Esp Pediatr* 39, no. 6 (1993): 507–511.

Peeke, P. M., et al., "Hypercortisolism and Obesity," *Annals of the New York Academy of Sciences* 771 (December 29, 1995): 665–676.

Pendergast, D. R., et al., "The Role of Dietary Fat on Performance, Metabolism, and Health," *American Journal of Sports Medicine* 24, no. 6 (1996): S53-S58.

Peschke, E., et al., "Evidence for a Circadian Rhythm of Insulin Release from Perifused Rat Pancreatic Islets," *Diabetologia* 41 (1998): 1085–1092.

Petrovsky, Nikolai, et al., "Diurnal Rhythmicity of Human Cytokine Production: A Dynamic Disequilibrium in T Helper Cell Type 1/T Helper Cell Type 2 Balance," *Journal of Immunology* 158 (1997): 5163–5168.

Phillips, D. I. W., et al., "Elevated Plasma Cortisol Concentrations: A Link between Low Birth Weight and the Insulin Resistance Syndrome?" *Journal of Clinical Endocrinology and Metabolism* 83, no. 3 (1998): 757–760.

Pierini, A. A., et al., "Male Diabetic Sexual Impotence: Effects of Dopaminergic Agents," *Arch Androl* 6, no. 4 (June 1981): 347–350.

Pombo, M., et al., "Nocturnal Rise of Leptin in Normal Prepubertal and Pubertal Children and in Patients with Perinatal Stalk-Transection Syndrome," *Journal of Clinical Endocrinology and Metabolism* 82, no. 8 (1997): 2751–2754.

Poretsky, L., et al., "Insulin Receptor Mediates Inhibitory Effect of Insulin, but Not of Insulin-Like Growth Factor 1 (IGF-1), on IGF Binding Protein 1 (IGFBP-1) Production in Human Granulosa Cells," *Journal of Clinical Endocrinology and Metabolism* 81, no. 2 (February 1996): 493–496.

Porte, Daniel, Jr., et al., "Diabetes Complications: Why Is Glucose Potentially Toxic?" *Science* 272 (May 3, 1996): 699–700.

Porter, T. E., et al., "Evidence That Stimulatory Dopamine Receptors May Be Involved in the Regulation of Prolactin Secretion," *Endocrinology* 134, no. 3 (March 1994): 1263–1268.

Prentki, Marc, et al., "Glucolipoxia and the Etiology of Obesity-Associated Type II Diabetes," *Exp Clin Endocrinol Diabetes* 105 (1997): 89–96.

Preuss, Harry G., M.D., et al., "Sugar-Induced Blood Pressure Elevations over the Life Span of Three Substrains of Wistar Rats," *Journal of the American College of Nutrition* 17, no. 1 (1998): 36–47.

Prins, Johannes B., et al., "Tumor Necrosis Factor Induces Apoptosis of Human Adipose Cells, *Diabetes* 46 (December 1997): 1939–1944.

Ramakrishnan, R., et al., "Brain Dopamine in Experimental Diabetes," *Indian Journal of Physiology and Pharmacology* 40, no. 2 (April 1996): 193–195.

Rasmussen, Ole W., M.D., et al., "Effects on Blood Pressure, Glucose, and Lipid Levels of a High-Monounsaturated-Fat Diet Compared with a High-Carbohydrate Diet in NIDDM Subjects," *Diabetes Care* 16, no. 12 (December 1993): 1565–1571.

Ravussin, Eric, et al., "Relatively Low Plasma Leptin Concentrations Precede Weight Gain in Pima Indians," *Nature Medicine* 3, no. 2 (February 1997): 238–240.

Reaven, Gerald M., et al., "Effect of a High Carbohydrate Diet on Insulin Binding to Adipocytes and on Insulin Action In Vivo in Man," *Diabetes* 28 (August 1979): 731–736.

———, "Studies of the Mechanism of Fructose-Induced Hypertriglyceridemia in the Rat," *Metabolism* 31, no. 11 (November 1982): 1077–1083.

———, "Increased Plasma and Insulin Responses to High Carbohydrate Feedings in Normal Subjects," *Journal of Clinical Endocrinology and Metabolism* 38, no. 1 (1974): 151–154.

———, "Induction of Hypertriglyceridemia by a Low-Fat Diet," *Journal of Clinical Endocrinology and Metabolism* 42, no. 4 (1976): 729–735.

———, "Kinetics of Triglyceride Turnover of Very Low Density Lipoproteins of Human Plasma," *Journal of Clinical Investigation* 44, no. 11 (November 1965): 1826–1833.

———, "Reappraisal of the Role of Insulin in Hypertriglyceridemia," *American Journal of Medicine* 57 (October 1974): 551–560.

———, "Role of Insulin in Endogenous Hypertriglyceridemia," *Journal of Clinical Investigation* 46, no. 11 (November 1967): 1756–1767.

———, "Steady State Plasma Insulin Response to Continuous Glucose Infusion in Normal and Diabetic Subjects," *Diabetes* 18, no. 5 (May 1969): 273–279.

———, "Study of the Relationship between Plasma Insulin Concentration and Efficiency of Glucose Uptake in Normal and Mildly Diabetic Subjects," *Diabetes* 19, no. 8 (August 1970): 571–578.

———, "Hypertension and Associated Metabolic Abnormalities: The Role of Insulin Resistance and the Sympathoadrenal System," *New England Journal of Medicine* 334, no. 6 (February 8, 1996): 374–381.

Reber, Paul M., "Prolactin and Immunomodulation," *American Journal of Medicine* 95 (December 1993): 637–644.

Regland, B., et al., "Homocysteinemia and Schizophrenia As a Case of Methylation Deficiency," *Journal of Neural Transmission* 98, no. 2 (1994): 143–152.

Reiser, Sheldon, et al., "Isocaloric Exchange of Dietary Starch and Sucrose in Humans," *American Journal of Clinical Nutrition* 32 (August 1979): 1659–1669.

———, "Isocaloric Exchange of Dietary Starch and Sucrose in Humans: II. Effect on Fasting Blood Insulin, Glucose, and Glucagon and on Insulin and Glucose Response to a Sucrose Load," *American Journal of Clinical Nutrition* 32 (November 1979): 2206–2216.

Remme, W. J., "Effect of ACE Inhibition on Neurohormones," *European Heart Journal* 19, suppl. J (1998): J16-J23.

Reppert, S. M., et al., "Forward Genetic Approach Strikes Gold: Cloning of a Mammalian Clock Gene," *Cell* 89, no. 4 (May 16, 1997): 487–490.

Rivkees, Scott A., et al., "Newborn Primate Infants Are Entrained by Low Intensity Lighting," *Proceedings of the National Academy of Sciences (USA)* 94 (February 1997): 292–297.

Robillon, J. F., et al., "Type I Diabetes Mellitus and Homocysteine," *Diabete et Metabolisme* 20, no. 5 (September 1994): 494–496.

Russom, J. M., et al., "Plasma Lipoprotein Cholesterol Concentrations in the Golden-Mantled Ground Squirrel (Spermophilus lateralis): A Comparison between Pre-Hibernators and Hibernators," *Comp Biochem Physiol* B, 102, no. 3 (1992): 573–578.

———, "Circulating Lipoprotein Cholesterol Concentrations in the Summer-Active Ground Squirrel (Spermophilus lateralis): A Comparison with Those in Humans and Rabbits," *Comp Biochem Physiol* A, 99, nos. 1–2 (1991): 21–25.

Rybkin, I. I., et al., "Effect of Restraint Stress on Food Intake and Body Weight Is Determined by Time of Day," *American Journal of Physiology* 273, no. 5 (November 1997): R1612-R1622.

Saad, Mohammed F., et al., "Physiological Insulinemia Acutely Modulates Plasma Leptin," *Diabetes* 47 (1998): 544–549.

Saarela, S., et al., "Function of Melatonin in Thermoregulatory Processes," *Life Sciences* 54, no. 5 (1994): 295–311.

Saladin, Regis, et al., "Transient Increase in Obese Gene Expression After Food Intake or Insulin Administration," *Nature* 377 (October 12, 1995): 527–529.

Salimuddin, et al., "Effects of Vanadate and Insulin on the Activities of Selected Enzymes of Amino Acid Metabolism in Alloxan Diabetic Rat Kidney," *Biochem Mol Biol Int* 40, no. 4 (November 1996): 853–860.

Sassone-Corsi, Paolo, "Molecular Clocks: Mastering Time by Gene Regulation," *Nature* 392 (April 30, 1998): 871–874.

Schorah, C. J., et al., "Blood Vitamin C Concentrations in Patients with Diabetes Mellitus," *Int J Vitam Nutr Res* 58, no. 3 (1988): 312–318.

Schwartz, William J., "Internal Timekeeping," *Science & Medicine* (May/June 1996), 44–53.

Scislowski, P. W., et al., "Biochemical Mechanisms Responsible for the Attenuation of Diabetic and Obese Conditions in ob/ob Mice Treated with Dopaminergic Agonists." *The International Journal of Obesity and Related Metabolic Disorders*, 23 no. 4 (April 1999): 425–431.

Seeley, R. J., et al., "Melanocortin Receptors in Leptin Effects," *Nature* 390 (November 27, 1997): 349.

Seidell, Jacob C., et al., "Assessing Obesity: Classification and Epidemiology," *British Medical Bulletin* 53, no. 2 (1997): 238–252.

Semenkovich, Clay F., et al., "The Mystery of Diabetics and Atherosclerosis," *Diabetes* 46 (March 1997): 327–334.

Sensi, S., et al., "Chronobiology in Endocrinology," *Annali dell Instituto Superiore di Sanita* 29, no. 4 (1993): 613–631.

Sigal, Ronald J., et al., "Codon 972 Polymorphism in the Insulin Receptor Substrate-1 Gene, Obesity, and Risk of Noninsulin-Dependent Diabetes Mellitus," *Journal of Clinical Endocrinology and Metabolism* 81, no. 4 (1996): 1657–1659.

Sinha, M. K., et al., "Nocturnal Rise of Leptin in Lean, Obese, and Non-Insulin-Dependent Diabetes Mellitus Subjects," *Journal of Clinical Investigation* 97, no. 5 (March 1, 1996): 1344–1347.

Solanes, G., et al., "The Human Uncoupling Protein-3 Gene: Genomic Structure, Chromosomal Localization, and Genetic Basis for Short and Long Form Transcripts," *Journal of Biological Chemistry* 272, no. 41 (October 10, 1997): 25433–25436.

Sotowska-Brochocka, J., et al., "Dopaminergic Inhibition of Gonadotropic Release in Hibernating Frogs, Rana temporaria," *General and Comparative Endocrinology* 93, no. 2 (February 1994): 192–196.

Sowers, James R., "Effects of Insulin and IGF-1 on Vascular Smooth Muscle Glucose and Cation Metabolism," *Diabetes* 45, suppl. 3 (July 1996): S47-S58.

Spiegel, Karine, et al., "Effect of a Sleep Debt on Glucose Regulation and Counterregulatory Hormones," *Diabetes* 47, Abstract, suppl. (1998): A301.

————, "Prolactin Secretion and Sleep," *Sleep* 17, no. 1 (February 1994): 20–27.

Srere, Hilary K., et al., "Central Role for Differential Gene Expression in Mammalian Hibernation," *Proceedings of the National Academy of Sciences (USA)* 89 (August 1992): 7119–7123.

Stegmayr, B., et al., "Hyperprolactinaemia and Testosterone Production: Observations in Two Men on Long-Term Dialysis," *Horm Res* 21, no. 4 (1985): 224–228.

Stokkan, K. A., et al., "Food Restriction Retards Aging of the Pineal Gland," *Brain Res* 545, nos. 1–2 (April 5, 1991): 66–72.

Storey, K. B., "Metabolic Regulation in Mammalian Hibernation: Enzyme and Protein Adaptations," *Comp Biochem Physiol A Physiol* 118, no. 4 (December 1997): 1115–1124.

————, "Organic Solutes in Freezing Tolerance," *Comp Biochem Physiol A Physiol* 117, no. 3 (July 1997): 319–326.

Stout, Robert W., M.D., "Insulin and Atheroma," *Diabetes Care* 13, no. 6 (June 1990): 631–654.

Suzuki, Masaaki, et al., "Mechanism and Clinical Implication of Insulin Resistance Syndrome," *Diabetes* 45, suppl. 3 (July 1996): S52-S54.

Suzuki, Y., et al., "Diabetes Mellitus Associated with the 3243 Mitochondrial tRNA (Leu)(UUR) Mutation: Insulin Secretion and Sensitivity," *Metabolism* 46, no. 9 (September 1997): 1019–1023.

Svensson, A. M., et al., "Diet-Induced Obesity and Pancreatic Islet Blood Flow in the Rat: A Preferential Increase in Islet Blood Perfusion Persists After Withdrawal of the Diet and Normalization of Body Weight," *Journal of Endocrinology* 151 (1996): 507–511.

Takahashi, Joseph S., "Circadian Clocks a la CREM," *Nature* 365 (September 23, 1993): 299–300.

Takahashi, S., et al., "Inhibition of Tumor Necrosis Factor Attenuates Physiological Sleep in Rabbits," *Neuroreport* 7, no. 2 (January 31, 1996): 642–646.

Taylor, Simeon I., "Does Leptin Contribute to Diabetes Caused by Obesity?" *Science* 274 (November 15, 1996): 1151–1152.

Thibault, L., "Dietary Carbohydrates: Effects on Self-Selection, Plasma Glucose and Insulin, and Brain Indoleaminergic Systems in Rat," *Appetite* 3 (December 23, 1994): 275–286.

Thompson, D. B., et al., "Structure and Sequence Variation at the Human Leptin Receptor Gene in Lean and Obese Pima Indians," *Human Molecular Genetics* 6, no. 5 (May 1997): 675–679.

Toyoda, Hiroo, et al., "Effect of 5-a Dihydrotestosterone on T-Cell Proliferation of the Female Nonobese Diabetic Mouse," *PSEBM* 213 (1996): 287–293.

Tsaur, M. L., et al., "Isolation of a cDNA Clone Encoding a KATP Channel-Like Protein Expressed in Insulin-Secreting Cells, Localization of the Human Gene to Chromosome Band 21q22.1, and Linkage Studies with NIDDM," *Diabetes* 44, no. 5 (May 1995): 592–596.

Tsigos, C., et al., "Dose Effects of Recombinant Human Interleukin-6 on Pituitary Hormone Secretion and Energy Expenditure," *Neuroendocrinology* 66, no. 1 (July 1997): 54–62.

Tung, P., et al., "Nephropathy in Non-Insulin-Dependent Diabetes Mellitus," *American Journal of Medicine* 85, no. 5A (November 28, 1988): 131–136.

Uysal, Teoman K., et al., "Protection from Obesity-Induced Insulin Resistance in Mice Lacking TNF Function," *Nature* 389 (October 1997): 610–614.

Van Cauter, Eve, et al., "Modulation of Glucose Regulation and Insulin Secretion by Circadian Rhythmicity and Sleep," *Journal of Clinical Investigation* 88 (September 1991): 934–942.

Van Eck, M., et al., "The Effects of Perceived Stress, Traits, Mood States, and Stressful Daily Events on Salivary Cortisol," *Psychosomatic Medicine* 58, no. 5 (September 1996): 447–458.

Van Itallie, Theodore B., M.D., "Prevalence of Obesity," *Endocrinology and Metabolism Clinics of North America* 25, no. 4 (December 1996): 887–905.

Vasquez, Robles M., et al., "The Prevalence of Non-Insulin-Dependent Diabetes Mellitus and the Associated Risk Factors in a Population of Mexico, D.F.," *Gaceta Medica de Mexico* 129, no. 3 (May/June 1993): 191–199.

Verma, M., et al., "Biophysical Profile of Blood Pressure in School Children," *Indian Pediatr* 85, no. 7 (July 1995): 749–754.

Vidal-Puig, A., et al., "UCP3: An Uncoupling Protein Homologue Expressed Preferentially and Abundantly in Skeletal Muscle and Brown Adipose Tissue," *Biochemical and Biophysical Research Communications* 235, no. 1 (June 9, 1997): 79–82.

Visnegarwala, Fehmida, et al., "Severe Diabetes Associated with Protease Inhibitor Therapy," *Annals of Internal Medicine* 127, no. 11 (November 15, 1997): 947.

Von Brackel-Bobdenhausen, A., et al., "Effects of Photoperiod and Slow-Release Preparations of Bromocriptine and Melatonin on Reproductive Activity and Prolactin Secretion in Female Goats," *J Anim Sci* 72, no. 4 (April 1994): 955–962.

Vondrasova, Dana, et al., "Exposure to Long Summer Days Affects the Human Melatonin and Cortisol Rhythms," *Brain Research* 759 (1997): 166–170.

Von Treuer, K., et al., "Overnight Human Plasma Melatonin, Cortisol, Prolactin, TSH, under Conditions of Normal Sleep, Sleep Deprivation, and Sleep Recovery," *Journal of Pineal Research* 20, no. 1 (January 1996): 7–14.

———, "Can Social Behavior of Man Be Glimpsed in a Lowly Worm?" *The New York Times,* September 8, 1998, B9.

Wang, L. C., et al., "The 'Hibernation Induction Trigger': Specificity and Validity of Bioassay Using the 13-Lined Ground Squirrel," *Cryobiology* 25, no. 4 (August 1998): 355–362.

Wehr, Thomas A., et al., "Conservation of Photoperiod-Responsive Mechanisms in Humans," *American Journal of Physiology* 265 (October 1993): R846-R857.

———, "The Duration of Human Melatonin Secretion and Sleep Respond to Changes in Day Length (Photoperiod)," *Journal of Clinical Endocrinology and Metabolism* 73, no. 6 (1991): 1276–1280.

———, "Suppression of Men's Responses to Seasonal Changes in Day Length by Modern Artificial Lighting," *American Journal of Physiology* 269, no. 38 (1995): R173-R178.

———, "Melatonin and Seasonal Rhythms," *Journal of Biological Rhythms* 12, no. 6 (December 1997): 518–527.

Wei, Y., et al., "Tissue-Specific Expression of the Human Receptor for Glucagon-Like Peptide-I: Brain, Heart, and Pancreatic Forms Have the Same Deduced Amino Acid Sequences," *FEBS Letters* 358, no. 3 (January 30, 1995): 219–224.

"Weight Control: What Works and Why," *Mayo Clinic Health Letter* supplement (1994), 1–8.

Weigle, David S., et al., "Effect of Fasting, Refeeding, and Dietary Fat Restrictions on Plasma Leptin Levels," *Journal of Clinical Endocrinology and Metabolism* 82, no. 2 (1997): 561–565.

Whitworth, Judith A., et al., "Mechanisms of Cortisol-Induced Hypertension in Humans," *Steroids* 60 no. 1 (January 1995): 76–80.

Williams, Stephen, "A Six Pack of Stout and a Coffin to Go," *Newsweek,* October 20, 1997, 76.

Willis, D., et al., "Insulin Action in Human Granulosa Cells from Normal and Polycystic Ovaries Is Mediated by the Insulin Receptor and Not the Type-I Insulin-Like Growth Factor Receptor," *Journal of Clinical Endocrinology and Metabolism* 80, no. 12 (December 1995): 3788–3790.

Wolf, G., "High-Fat, High-Cholesterol Diet Raises Plasma HDL Cholesterol: Studies on the Mechanism of This Effect," *Nutrition Reviews* 54 (January 1996): 34–35.

Wolk, Alocja, Ph.D., et al., "A Prospective Study of Association of Monounsaturated Fat and Other Types of Fat with Risk of Breast Cancer," *Arch Intern Med* 158 (January 12, 1998): 41–45.

Wong, Joyce Y., et al., "Direct Measurement of a Tethered Ligand-Receptor Interaction Potential," *Science* 275 (February 7, 1997): 820–822.

Wood, Diana, "Sugarland Express: Beware! Your Favorite Foods Could Be Raising Your Insulin Level to Dizzying Heights," *W,* October 1997, 159–160.

Wurtman, Richard J., et al., "Daily Rhythms in the Concentrations of Various Amino Acids in Human Plasma," *New England Journal of Medicine* 279 (1968): 171–175.

Wurtman, Richard J., "Daily Rhythms in Mammalian Protein Metabolism," *Mammalian Protein Metabolism* 4 (1970): 445–479.

Yeh, I., "Changes in Various Plasma Lipid Components, Glucose, and Insulin in Spermophilus lateralis during Hibernation," *Comparative Biochemistry and Physiology* 111, no. 4 (August 1995): 651–663.

Yehuda, Rachel, "Stress and Glucocorticoid," *Science* 275 (March 14, 1997): 1662.

Yerboeket-van de Venne, W. P., et al., "Effects of Dietary Fat and Carbohydrate Exchange on Human Energy Metabolism," *Appetite* 26, no. 3 (June 1996): 287–300.

Yoshida, H., et al., "Transient Suppression of Pancreatic Endocrine Function in Patients Following Brain Death," *Clinical Transplantation* 10 (February 1996): 28–33.

Yoshimura, Ryohei, et al., "Impact of Natural IRS-1 Mutations on Insulin Signals," *Diabetes* 46 (June 1997): 929–936.

Yu, W. H., et al., "Role of Leptin in Hypothalamic-Pituitary Function," *Proceedings of the National Academy of Sciences (USA)* 94 (February 1997): 1023–1028.

Yuan, Li, et al., "Molecular Actions of Prolactin in the Immune System," *PSEBM* 215 (1997): 35–52.

Yudkin, John, M.D., "Sucrose, Coronary Heart Disease, Diabetes, and Obesity: Do Hormones Provide a Link?" *American Heart Journal* 115, no. 2 (February 1988): 493–498.

Zavaroni, Ivana, et al., "Studies of the Mechanism of Fructose-Induced Hypertriglyceridemia in the Rat," *Metabolism* 31, no. 11 (November 1982): 1077–1083.

Zawilska, J. B., et al., "Serotonin N-Acetyltransferase Activity in Chicken Retina: In Vivo Effects of Phosphodiesterase Inhibitors, Forskolin, and Drugs Affecting Dopamine Receptors," *Journal of Pineal Research* 11, nos. 3–4 (October 1991): 116–122.

Zgliczynski, S., et al., "Effect of Testosterone Replacement Therapy on Lipids and Lipoproteins in Hypogonadal and Elderly Men," *Atherosclerosis* 121, no. 1 (March 1996): 35–43.

Zhang, S. Q., et al., "Bromocriptine-Induced Blockade of Pregnancy Affects Sleep Patterns in Rats," *Neuroimmunomodulation* 3, no. 4 (July 1996): 219–226.

Zhao, Shaying, et al., "Human Blue-Light Photoreceptor hCRY2 Specifically Interacts with Protein Serine/Threonine Phosphatase 5 and Modulates Its Activity," *Photochemistry and Photobiology* 66, no. 5 (November 1997): 727–731.

Zheng, Lixin, et al., "Induction of Apoptosis in Mature T Cells by Tumor Necrosis Factor," *Nature* 377 (September 28, 1995): 348–351.

Zhong, H. H., et al., "Effects of Synergistic Signaling by Phytochrome A and Cryptochrome 1 on Circadian Clock-Regulated Catalase Expression," *Plant Cell* 9, no. 6 (June 1997): 947–955.

Zhou, Jian, et al., "Anatomy of the Human Ovarian Insulin-Like Growth Factor System," *Biology of Reproduction* 48 (1993): 467–482.

Zimmet, P. Z., et al., "The Global Epidemiology of Non-Insulin-Dependent Diabetes Mellitus and the Metabolic Syndrome," *Journal of Diabetes and Its Complications* 11, no. 2 (March/April 1997): 60–68.

Chapter Six: It *Is* All in Your Head

Accili, Domenico, et al., "A Targeted Mutation of the D₃ Dopamine Receptor Gene Is Associated with Hyperactivity in Mice," *Proceedings of the National Academy of Sciences (USA)* 93 (March 1996): 1945–1949.

Ahima, Rexford S., et al., "Role of Leptin in the Neuroendocrine Response to Fasting," *Nature* 382 (July 18, 1996): 295–297.

Ahren, B., et al., "Plasma Neuropeptide Y in Impaired Glucose Tolerance," *Acta Diabetologia* 33, no. 4 (December 1996): 295–297.

Al'Absi, M., et al., "Cortisol Concentrations in Serum of Borderline Hypertensive Men Exposed to a Novel Experimental Setting," *Psychoneuroendocrinology* 18, nos. 5–6 (1993): 355–363.

Aldhous, Peter, "What's Serotonin Got to Do with It?" *New Scientist,* February 13, 1997, 13.

Al-Mudallal, A. S., et al., "Diet-Induced Ketosis Does Not Cause Cerebral Acidosis," *Epilepsia* 37, no. 2 (March 1996): 258–261.

Altun-Gultekin, Z. F., et al., "Activation of Rho-Dependent Cell Spreading and Focal Adhesion Biogenesis by the v-Crk Adaptor Protein," *Mol Cell Biol* 18, no. 8 (May 1998): 3044–3058.

Ambrosi, B., et al., "Effect of Bromocriptine and Metergoline in the Treatment of Hyperprolactinaemic States," *Acta Endocrinol (Copenh)* 100, no. 1 (May 1982): 10–17.

Avraham, Y., et al., "Behavioral and Neurochemical Alterations Caused by Diet Restriction—The Effect of Tyrosine Administration in Mice," *Brain Research* 732, nos. 1–2 (September 2, 1996): 133–144.

Ayers, N. A., et al., "Circadian Variation of Nitric Oxide Synthase Activity and Cytosolic Protein Levels in Rat Brain," *Brain Research* 707, no. 1 (January 22, 1996): 127–130.

Bamberger, Christoph M., et al., "Human Lymphocytes Produce Urocortin, but Not Corticotropin-Releasing Hormone," *Journal of Clinical Endocrinology and Metabolism* 83, no. 2 (1998): 708–711.

Bancroft, J., et al., "The Effects of Bromocriptine on the Sexual Behaviour of Hyperprolactinaemic Man: A Controlled Case Study," *Clin Endocrinol (Oxf)* 21, no. 2 (August 1984): 131–137.

Barinaga, Marcia, "No-New-Neurons Dogma Loses Ground," *Science* 279 (March 27, 1998): 2041–2042.

Bechter, K., et al., "Pathofenicity of Borna Disease Virus in Psychiatric and Neurologic Disorders of Humans: Current Status of Research and Critical Comments," *Nervenarzt* 68, no. 5 (May 1997): 425–430.

Beck, K. D., "Functions of Brain-Derived Neurotrophic Factor, Insulin-Like Growth Factor-I, and Basic Fibroblast Growth Factor in the Development and Maintenance of Dopaminergic Neurons," *Progress in Neurobiology* 44, no. 5 (December 1994): 497–516.

Begley, Sharon, "Psychiatrists Are Ridiculed for Calling Every Quirk a Mental Illness, but New Research on Genes and the Brain Suggests They Might Be Right," *Newsweek,* January 26, 1998, 51–55.

Beijani, Boulos-Paul, M.D., et al., "Transient Acute Depression Induced by High-Frequency Deep-Brain Stimulation," *New England Journal of Medicine* 340, no. 19 (May 13, 1999): 1476–1480.

Bennet, W. M., et al., "Presence of Neuropeptide Y and Its Messenger Ribonucleic Acid in Human Islets: Evidence for a Possible Paracrine Role," *Journal of Clinical Endocrinology and Metabolism* 81, no. 6 (June 1996): 2117–2120.

Bettahi, I., et al., "Melatonin Reduces Nitric Oxide Synthase Activity in Rat Hypothalamus," *Journal of Pineal Research* 20, no. 4 (May 1996): 205–210.

Blakeslee, Sandra, "Old Brains Can Learn New Language Tricks," *The New York Times,* April 20, 1999, D3.

———, "Running Late? Researchers Blame Aging Brain," *The New York Times,* March 24, 1998, B13.

Blundell, J. E., et al., "Control of Human Appetite: Implications for the Intake of Dietary Fat," *Annual Review of Nutrition* 16 (1996): 285–319.

Boatright, J. H., et al., "Regulation of Endogenous Dopamine Release in Amphibian Retina by Melatonin: The Role of GABA," *Visual Neuroscience* 11, no. 5 (September/October 1994): 1013–1018.

Boden, G., et al., "Effect of Fasting on Serum Leptin in Normal Human Subjects," *Journal of Clinical Endocrinology and Metabolism* 81, no. 9 (1996): 3419–3423.

Bornstein, Stefan R., et al., "Evidence for a Novel Peripheral Action of Leptin As a Metabolic Signal to the Adrenal Gland: Leptin Inhibits Cortisol Release Directly," *Diabetes* 46, no. 7 (July 1997): 1235–1238.

Botchkarev, V. A., et al., "A New Role for Neurotrophins: Involvement of Brain-Derived Neurotrophic Factor and Neurotrophin-4 in Hair Cycle Control," *FASEB J* 13, no. 2 (February 1999): 395–410.

Brandenberger, G., et al., "Disruption of Endocrine Rhythms in Sleeping Sickness with Preserved Relationship between Hormonal Pulsatility and the REM-NREM Sleep Cycles," *Journal of Biological Rhythms* 11, no. 3 (September 1996): 258–267.

Brenner, I. K., et al., "The Impact of Heat Exposure and Repeated Exercise on Circulating Stress Hormones," *European Journal of Applied Physiology and Occupational Physiology* 76, no. 5 (1997): 445–454.

Brody, Jane E., "Many Smokers Who Can't Quit Are Mentally Ill, A Study Finds," *The New York Times,* August 27, 1997, C8.

———, "Obesity Drugs: Weighing the Risks to Health against the Small Victories," *The New York Times,* September 3, 1997, B9.

———, "New Tack Promising on Winter Depression," *The New York Times,* March 31, 1998, B13.

Brown, Richard, et al., "Are Antibiotic Effects on Sleep Behavior in the Rat Due to Modulation of Gut Bacteria?" *Physiology and Behavior* 48 (1990): 561–565.

Brown, R., et al., "Differences in Nocturnal Melatonin Secretion between Melancholic Depressed Patients and Control Subjects," *American Journal of Psychiatry* 142, no. 7 (July 1985): 811–816.

Burnham, John, "Methods and Madness," *Nature* 389 (October 30, 1997): 927–928.

Buvat, J., "Influence of Primary Hyperprolactinemia on Human Sexual Behavior," *Nouv Presse Med* 11, no. 48 (November 27, 1982): 3561–3563.

Buxton, Orfeu M., et al., "Roles of Intensity and Duration of Nocturnal Exercise in Causing Phase Delays of Human Circadian Rhythms," *American Journal of Physiology* 273 (1997): E536–E542.

Cacioppo, J. T. et al., "Heterogeneity in Neuroendocrine and Immune Responses to Brief Psychological Stressors As a Function of Autonomic Cardiac Activation," *Psychosomatic Medicine* 57, no. 2 (March/April 1995): 154–164.

Cajochen, Christian, et al., "Melatonin and S-20098 Increase REM Sleep and Wake-Up Propensity without Modifying NREM Sleep Homeostasis," *American Journal of Physiology* 272 (1997): R1189–R1196.

Carney, R. M., et al., "Major Depression, Heart Rate, and Plasma Norepinephrine in Patients with Coronary Heart Disease," *Biol Psychiatry* 45, no. 4 (February 15, 1999): 458–463.

Casper, R. C., "Carbohydrate Metabolism and Its Regulatory Hormones in Anorexia Nervosa," *Psychiatry Research* 62, no. 1 (April 16, 1996): 85–96.

Castel, M., et al., "Light-Induced c-Fos Expression in the Mouse Suprachiasmatic Nucleus: Immunoelectron Microscopy Reveals Co-Localization in Multiple Cell Types," *Eur J Neurosci* 9, no. 9 (September 1997): 1950–1960.

Cheng, J. G., et al., "Cardiotrophin-1 Induces the Same Neuropeptides in Sympathetic Neurons As Do Neuropoietic Cytokines," *Journal of Neurochemistry* 69, no. 6 (December 1997): 2278–2284.

Clark, W. L., et al., "Metabolic and Cutaneous Events Associated with Hypoglycemia Detected by Sleep Sentry," *Diabetes Care* 11, no. 8 (September 1988): 630–635.

Cleophas, T. J., "Depression and Myocardial Infarction: Implications for Medical Prognosis and Options for Treatment," *Neth J Med* 52, no. 2 (February 1998): 82–89.

Cohen, Batya, et al., "Modulation of Insulin Activities by Leptin," *Science* 274 (November 15, 1996): 1185–1188.

Cohen, Philip, "Death Wish Gene," *New Scientist*, January 24, 1998, 21.

———, "Disarming Gene Is a Lucky Strike for Smokers," *New Scientist*, November 29, 1997, 19.

———, "Nicotine May Block Formation of Alzheimer's Plaques," *New Scientist*, November 2, 1996, 8.

———, "Can Gene Drugs Help You Dry Out?" *New Scientist*, June 7, 1997, 18.

Coleman, Richard M., et al., "Sleep-Wake Disorders Based on a Polysomnographic Diagnosis," *Journal of the American Medical Association* 247 (1982): 997–1003.

Condic, M. L., et al., "Ligand-Induced Changes in Itergin Expression Regulate Neuronal Adhesion and Neurite Outgrowth," *Nature* 389 (October 23, 1997): 852–853.

"Coping with Insomnia," *Health News*, March 4, 1997, 1–8.

Corpas, Emiliano, et al., "Human Growth Hormone and Human Aging," *Endocrine Reviews* 14, no. 1 (1993): 20–38.

Cowen, P. J., et al., "Why Is Dieting So Difficult?" *Nature* 376 (August 17, 1995): 557.

Cui, Y., et al., "The Modulatory Effects of Mu and Kappa Opioid Agonists on 5-HT Release from Hippocampal Slices of Euthermic and Hibernating Ground Squirrels," *Life Sciences* 53, no. 26 (1993): 1957–1965.

————, "State-Dependent Changes of Brain Endogenous Opioids in Mammalian Hibernation," *Brain Research Bulletin* 40, no. 2 (1996): 129–133.

Ogilvie, Alan D., et al., "Polymorphism in Serotonin Transporter Gene Associated with Susceptibility to Major Depression," *The Lancet* 347 (March 16, 1996): 731–733.

Dallman, M. F., et al., "The Neural Network That Regulates Energy Balance Is Responsive to Glucocorticoids and Insulin and Regulates HPA Axis Responsivity at a Site Proximal to CRF Neurons," *Annals of the New York Academy of Sciences* 771 (December 29, 1995): 730–742.

Danilenko, K. V., et al., "Diurnal and Seasonal Variations of Melatonin and Serotonin in Women with Seasonal Affective Disorder," *Arctic Medical Research* 53, no. 3 (July 1994): 137–145.

Davis, S. N., et al., "Brain of the Conscious Dog Is Sensitive to Physiological Changes in Circulating Insulin," *American Journal of Physiology* 272 (1997): E567–E575.

Delagrange, P., et al., "Melatonin, Its Receptors, and Relationships with Biological Rhythm Disorders," *Clin Neuropharmacol* 20, no. 6 (December 1997): 482–510.

De Zegher, F., et al, "Dopamine Inhibits Growth Hormone and Prolactin Secretion in the Human Newborn," *Pediatric Research* 34, no. 5 (November 1993): 642–645.

Dhurandhar, N. V., et al., "Association of Adenovirus Infection with Human Obesity," *Obes Res* 5, no. 5 (September 1997): 464–469.

Ding, J. M., et al., "Resetting the Biological Clock: Mediation of Nocturnal CREB Phosphorylation via Light, Glutamate, and Nitric Oxide," *J Neurosci* 17, no. 2 (January 1997): 667–675.

Dinges, David F., et al., "Leukocytosis and Natural Killer Cell Function Parallel Neurobehavioral Fatigue Induced by 64 Hours of Sleep Deprivation," *Journal of Clinical Investigation* 93 (1994): 1930–1939.

Dooley, Audrey E., et al., "Serotonin Promotes the Survival of Cortical Glutamatergic Neurons In Vitro," *Experimental Neurology* 148 (1997): 205–214.

Duman, R. S., et al., "Novel Therapeutic Approaches beyond the Serotonin Receptor," *Biol Psychiatry* 44, no. 5 (September 1, 1998): 324–335.

Duncan, Wallace C., Jr., "Circadian Rhythms and the Pharmacology of Affective Illness," *Pharmacology* 71, no. 3 (1996): 253–312.

During, Matthew J., et al., "Glucose Modulates Rat Substantia Nigra GABA Release In Vivo via ATP-Sensitive Potassium Channels," *Journal of Clinical Investigation* 95 (May 1995): 2403–2408.

Easton, John, "Probable Site of Alcohol and Anesthetic Actions Discovered," *University of Chicago Chronicle* 17, no. 1 (September 25, 1997): 3; 12.

Ericsson, M., et al., "Common Biological Pathways in Eating Disorders and Obesity," *Addictive Behaviors* 21, no. 6 (November/December 1996): 733–743.

Erecinska, M., et al., "Regulation of GABA Level in Rat Brain Synaptosomes: Fluxes through Enzymes of GABA Shunt and Effects of Glutamate, Calcium, and Ketone Bodies," *Journal of Neurochemistry* 67, no. 6 (December 1996): 2325–2334.

Falcini, F., et al., "Nerve Growth Factor Circulating Levels Are Increased in Kawasaki Disease: Correlation with Disease Activity and Reduced Angiotensin Converting Enzyme Levels," *J Rheumatol* 23, no. 10 (October 1996): 1798–1802.

Feleder, C., et al., "Bacterial Endotoxin Inhibits LHRH Secretion Following the Increased Release of Hypothalamic GABA Levels: Different Effects on Amino Acid Neurotransmitter Release," *Neuroimmunomodulation* 3, no. 6 (November/December 1996): 342–351.

Fernstrom, John D., et al., "Brain Serotonin Content: Physiological Regulation by Plasma Neutral Amino Acids," *Science* 178 (June 6, 1972): 414–416.

———, "Nutrition and the Brain," *Scientific American* 230 (February 1974): 84–91.

———, "Control of Brain Serotonin Levels by the Diet," *Advances in Biochemical Psychopharmacology* 11 (1974): 133–138.

Figlewicz, D. P., et al., "Diabetes Causes Differential Changes in CNS Noradrenergic and Dopaminergic Neurons in the Rat: A Molecular Study," *Brain Research* 736, nos. 1–2 (October 14, 1996): 54–60.

Formby, Bent, "The In Vivo and In Vitro Effect of Diphenylhydantoin and Phenobarbitone on K+-Activated Phosphohydrolase and (Na+, K+)-Activated ATPase in Particulate Membrane Fractions from Rat Brain," *Journal of Pharmacy and Pharmacology* 22, no. 2 (February 1970): 81–85.

Foulkes, N. S., et al., "Rhythmic Transcription: The Molecular Basis of Circadian Melatonin Synthesis," *Trends Neurosci* 20, no. 10 (October 1997): 487–492.

Fuller, Ray W., "Neural Functions of Serotonin," *Scientific American Science and Medicine*, July/August 1995, 48–57.

Ganguli, R., et al., "Serum Interleukin-6 Concentration in Schizophrenia: Elevation Associated with Duration of Illness," *Psychiatry Research* 51, no. 1 (January 1994): 1–10.

———, "Autoimmunity in Schizophrenia: A Review of Recent Findings," *Annals of Medicine* 25, no. 5 (October 1993): 489–496.

Gastel, J. A., et al., "Melatonin Production: Proteasomal Proteolysis in Serotonin N-acetyltransferase Regulation," *Science* 279, no. 5355 (February 27, 1998): 1358–1360.

Gauer, F., et al., "Differential Seasonal Regulation of Melatonin Receptor Density in the Pars Tuberalis and the Suprachiasmatic Nuclei: A Study in the Hedgehog," *Journal of Neuroendocrinology* 5, no. 6 (December 1993): 685–690.

"Gene Believed to Make Some Susceptible to Bipolar Illness," *Santa Barbara News Press,* October 27, 1997, A4.

Gershon, Elliot S., et al., "Closing in on Genes for Manic-Depressive Illness and Schizophrenia," *Neuropsychopharmacology* 18, no. 4 (April 1998) 233–242.

Geusz, M. E., et al., "Long-Term Monitoring of Circadian Rhythms in C-fos Gene Expression from Suprachiasmatic Nucleus Cultures," *Curr Biol* 7, no. 10 (October 1997): 758–766.

Gillard, E. R., et al., "Evidence That Neuropeptide Y and Dopamine in the Perifornical Hypothalamus Interact Antagonistically in the Control of Food Intake," *Brain Research* 628, nos. 1–2 (November 19, 1993): 128–136.

Glanz, James, "Can 'Resetting' Hormonal Rhythms Treat Illness?" *Science* 269 (September 1, 1995): 1220–1221.

Glass, Michael J., et al., "Potency of Naloxone's Anorectic Effect in Rats Is Dependent on Diet Preference," *American Journal of Physiology* 271 (1996): R217-R221.

Glassman, Alexander H., M.D., et al., "Depression and the Course of Coronary Artery Disease," *American Journal of Psychiatry* 155 (1998): 4–11.

Glausiusz, Josie, "Brain, Heal Thyself," *Discover,* August 1996, 28.

Glund, C., et al., "No Effect of Oral Testosterone Treatment on Sexual Dysfunction in Alcoholic Cirrhotic Men," *Gastroenterology* 95, no. 6 (December 1988): 1582–1587.

Goldberg, A. David, M.D., et al., "Ischemic, Hemodynamic, and Neurohormonal Responses to Mental and Exercise Stress: Experience from the Psychophysiological Investigations of Myocardial Ischemia Study (PIMI)," *Circulation* 94, no. 10 (November 15, 1996): 2402–2409.

Goode, Erica, "Study Shows Role of Time and Place of Birth in Schizophrenia," *The New York Times,* February 25, 1999, A20.

Gooren, L. J., "Androgen Levels and Sex Functions in Testosterone-Treated Hypogonadal Men," *Arch Sex Behav* 16, no. 6 (December 1987): 463–473.

Gorman, Christine, "Anatomy of Melancholy," *Time,* May 5, 1997, 78.

Grady, Denise, "Brain-Tied Gene Defect May Explain Why Schizophrenics Hear Voices," *The New York Times,* January 21, 1997, B14.

Granata, A. R., et al., "Relationship between Sleep-Related Erections and Testosterone Levels in Men," *J Androl* 18, no. 5 (September 1997): 522–527.

Green, C. B., et al., "Tryptophan Hydroxylase mRNA Levels Are Regulated by the Circadian Clock, Temperature, and cAMP in Chick Pineal Cells," *Brain Research* 738, no. 1 (October 28, 1996): 1–7.

Grey, Neil, M.D., et al., "Effect of Diet Composition on the Hyperinsulinemia of Obesity," *New England Journal of Medicine* 285, no. 15 (October 7, 1971): 827–831.

Guerrero, J. M., et al., "Nocturnal Decreases in Nitric Oxide and Cyclic GMP Contents in the Chick Brain and Their Prevention by Light," *Neurochem Int* 29, no. 4 (October 1996): 417–421.

Gura, Trisha, "Obesity Sheds Its Secrets," *Science* 275 (February 7, 1997): 751–753.

Hansen, M. K., et al., "Subdiaphragmatic Vagotomy Blocks the Sleep and Fever-Promoting Effects of Interleukin-1 Beta," *American Journal of Physiology* 273, no. 4 (October 1997): 1246–1253.

Harley, C. W., "A Role for Norepinephrine in Arousal, Emotion, and Learning? Limbic Modulation by Norepinephrine and the Kety Hypothesis," *Progress in Neuropsychopharmacology and Biological Psychiatry* 11, no. 4 (1987): 419–458.

Hamilton, Josh, et al., " 'Quick-Fix' Pills and Internet Peddling Condemned in World Narcotics Report," *The Lancet* 349 (March 15, 1997): 784.

Hasselbalch, S. G., et al., "Blood-Brain Barrier Permeability of Glucose and Ketone Bodies during Short-Term Starvation in Humans," *American Journal of Physiology* 268, no. 6 (June 1995): 1161–1166.

————, "Changes in Cerebral Blood Flow and Carbohydrate Metabolism during Acute Hyperketonemia," *American Journal of Physiology* 270, no. 5 (May 1996): E746-E751.

————, "Brain Metabolism during Short-Term Starvation in Humans," *Journal of Cerebral Blood Flow and Metabolism* 14, no. 1 (January 1994): 125–131.

Heath, B. M., et al., "Overexpression of Nerve Growth Factor in the Heart Alters Ion Channel Activity and Beta-Adrenergic Signalling in an Adult Transgenic Mouse," *J Physiol (Lond)* 512, no. 3 (November 1, 1998): 779–791.

Henry, J. P., "Psychological and Physiological Responses to Stress: The Right Hemisphere and the Hypothalamo-Pituitary-Adrenal Axis—An Inquiry into Problems of Human Bonding," *Acta Physiologica Scandinavia* 640 (suppl.) (1997): 10–25.

Hicks, B. H., et al., "Metergoline As an Alternative to Bromocriptine in Amenorrhea," *Acta Endocrinol (Copenh)* 107, no. 4 (December 1994): 439–444.

Hilts, Philip J., "Diet Drug Tests on Children Reviewed," *Santa Barbara News Press*, April 15, 1998, A1.

Holden, J. P., et al., "Regulation of Insulin-Like Growth Factor Binding Protein-1 during the 24-Hour Metabolic Clock and in Response to Hypoinsulinemia Induced by Fasting and Somatostatin in Normal Women," *J Soc Gynecol Investig* 2, no. 1 (January 1995): 38–44.

Holden, R. J., et al., "Schizophrenia Is a Diabetic Brain State: An Elucidation of Impaired Neurometabolism," *Medical Hypotheses* 43, no. 6 (December 1994): 420–435.

Hsu, D. S., et al., "Putative Human Blue-Light Photoreceptors hCRY1 and hCRY2 are Flavoproteins," *Biochemistry* 35, no. 44 (November 5, 1996): 13871–13877.

Huang, X. C., et al., "Modulation of Angiotensin II Type 2 Receptor mRNA in Rat Hypothalamus and Brain Stem Neuronal Cultures by Growth Factors," *Brain Res Mol Brain Res* 47, nos. 1–2 (July 1997): 229–236.

Hulihan-Giblin, B. A., et al., "Regional Analysis of 5-HT1A Receptors in Two Species of Peromyscus," *Pharmacology, Biochemistry and Behavior* 45, no. 1 (May 1993): 143–145.

Inder, W. J., et al., "Elevated Basal Adrenocorticotropin and Evidence for Increased Central Opioid Tone in Highly Trained Male Athletes," *Journal of Clinical Endocrinology and Metabolism* 80, no. 1 (1995): 244–248.

Iuvone, P. M., et al., "Functional Interaction of Melatonin Receptors and D1 Dopamine Receptors in Cultured Chick Retinal Neurons," *Journal of Neuroscience* 15, no. 3 (March 1995): 2179–2185.

Jarry, H., et al., "In Vitro Prolactin but Not LH and FSH Release Is Inhibited by Compounds in Extracts of Agnus Castus: Direct Evidence for a Dopaminergic Principle by the Dopamine Receptor Assay," *Experimental and Clinical Endocrinology* 102, no. 6 (1994): 448–454.

Johnson, R. W., et al., "Hormones, Lymphohemopoietic Cytokines and the Neuroimmune Axis," *Comparative Biochemistry and Physiology* 116A, no. 3 (1997): 183–201.

Kahn, R. S., et al., "Effects of Ipsapirone in Healthy Subjects: A Dose-Response Study," *Psychopharmacology* 114, no. 1 (February 1994): 155–160.

Kaas, Jon H., "Phantoms of the Brain," *Nature* 391 (January 22, 1998): 331–333.

Kawai, K., et al., "Severe Depression Associated with ACTH, PRL, and GH Deficiency: a Case Report," *Endocrine Journal* 41, no. 2 (June 1994): 275–279.

Kennedy, Sidney H., et al., "Changes in Melatonin Levels but Not Cortisol Levels Are Associated with Depression in Patients with Eating Disorders," *Arch Gen Psychiatry* 46 (1989): 73–78.

Kerschensteiner, M., et al., "Activated Human T Cells, B Cells, and Monocytes Produce Brain-Derived Neurotrophic Factor In Vitro and in Inflammatory Brain Lesions: A Neuroprotective Role in Inflammation?" *Journal of Experimental Medicine* 189, no. 5 (March 1, 1999): 865–870.

Klatt, P., et al., "Characterization of Heme-Deficient Neuronal Nitric-Oxide Synthase Reveals a Role for Heme in Subunit Dimerization and Binding of the Amino Acid Substrate and Tetrahydrobiopterin," *Journal of Biological Chemistry* 271, no. 13 (March 29, 1996): 7336–7342.

Klein, D. C., et al., "The Melatonin Rhythm-Generating Enzyme: Molecular Regulation of Serotonin N-Acetyltransferase in the Pineal Gland," *Recent Progress in Hormone Research* 52 (1997): 307–357.

Korth, C., "A Co-Evolutionary Theory of Sleep," *Medical Hypotheses* 45, no. 3 (September 1995): 304–310.

Kunugi, H., et al., "Low Serum Cholesterol in Suicide Attempters," *Biological Psychiatry* 41, no. 2 (January 15, 1997): 196–200.

Landry, Donald W., "Immunotherapy for Cocaine Addiction," *Scientific American,* February 1997, 42–45.

Lange, K. W., et al., "Subjective Time Estimation in Parkinson's Disease," *J Neural Transm Suppl* 46 (1995): 433–438.

Lebouille, J. L., et al., "Properties of a Leu-Phe-Cleaving Endopeptidase Activity Putatively Involved in Beta-Endorphin Metabolism in Rat Brain," *J Neurochem* 52, no. 6 (June 1989): 1714–1721.

Lephart, E. D., et al., "Inhibition of Brain 5 Alpha-Reductase in Pregnant Rats: Effects on Enzymatic and Behavioral Activity," *Brain Research* 739, nos. 1–2 (November 11, 1996): 356–360.

Levin, Barry E., "Obesity-Prone and Resistant Rats Differ in Their Brain (3H) Paraminoclonidine Binding," *Brain Research* 512 (1990): 54–59.

Lieberman, Harris R., Ph.D., et al., "Changes in Mood After Carbohydrate Consumption among Obese Individuals," *American Journal of Clinical Nutrition* 44 (1986): 772–778.

Lingenfelser, Thomas, et al., "Insulin-Associated Modulation of Neuroendocrine Counterregulation, Hypoglycemia Perception, and Cerebral Function in Insulin-Dependent Diabetes Mellitus: Evidence for an Intrinsic Effect of Insulin on the Central Nervous System," *Journal of Clinical Endocrinology and Metabolism* 81, no. 3 (1996): 1197–1205.

Lockhart, Sybil T., et al., "Nerve Growth Factor Modulates Synaptic Transmission between Sympathetic Neurons and Cardiac Myocytes," *Journal of Neuroscience* 17, no. 24 (December 15, 1997): 9573–9582.

Lonnqvist, Fredrik, "Leptin Secretion from Adipose Tissue in Women," *Journal of Clinical Investigation* 99, no. 10 (May 10, 1997): 2398–2404.

Lord, Graham M., et al., "Leptin Modulates the T-Cell Immune Responses and Reverses Starvation-Induced Immunosuppression," *Nature* 394 (August 1998): 897–901.

Lowenstein, Charles J., et al., "Nitric Oxide: A Novel Biologic Messenger," *Cell* 70 (September 4, 1992): 705–707.

Lyons, Philippa M., et al., "Serotonin Precursor Influenced by Type of Carbohydrate Meal in Healthy Adults," *American Journal of Clinical Nutrition* 47 (1988): 433–439.

Mainen, Zachary F., et al., "Reliability of Spike Timing in Neocortical Neurons," *Science* 268 (June 9, 1995): 1503–1506.

Maldonado, Rafael, et al., "Absence of Opiate Rewarding Effects in Mice Lacking Dopamine D2 Receptors," *Nature* 388 (August 7, 1997): 586–589.

Malhotra, Khushbeer, et al., "Putative Blue-Light Photoreceptors from Arabidopsis thaliana and Sinapsis alba with a High Degree of Sequence Homology to DNA Photolyase Contain the Two Photolyase Cofactors but Lack DNA Repair Activity," *Biochemistry* 34, no. 20 (1995): 6892–6899.

Marano, Hara Estroff, "Depression: Beyond Serotonin," *Psychology Today*, March/April 1999, 30–76.

Marshall, John C., "Everyday Tales of Ordinary Madness," *Nature* 389 (September 4, 1997): 29.

Martins, J. Martin, et al., "Transport of CRH from Mouse Brain Directly Affects Peripheral Production of B-Endorphin by the Spleen," *American Journal of Physiology* 273 (1997): E1083–1089.

Masuzaki, Hiroaki, et al., "Glucocorticoid Regulation of Leptin Synthesis and Secretion in Humans: Elevated Plasma Leptin Levels in Cushing's Syndrome," *Journal of Clinical Endocrinology and Metabolism* 82, no. 8 (1997): 2542–2547.

McCann, U. D., et al., "Brain Serotonin Neurotoxicity and Primary Pulmonary Hypertension from Fenfluramine and Dexfenfluramine: A Systematic Review of the Evidence," *Journal of the American Medical Association* 278, no. 8 (August 27, 1997): 666–672.

McCrone, John, "Wild Minds," *New Scientist* 156, no. 2112 (December 13, 1997): 26–30.

McCullers, D. L., et al., "Mineralocorticoid Receptors Regulate Bcl–2 and P53 mRNA Expression in Hippocampus," *Neuroreport* 9, no. 13 (September 14, 1998): 3085–3089.

McIntyre, I. M., et al., "Plasma Melatonin Concentrations in Depression," *Aust N Z J Psychiatry* 20, no. 3 (September 1986): 381–383.

Mellman, Michael J., et al., "Effect of Physiological Hyperinsulinemia on Counterregulatory Hormone Response during Hypoglycemia in Humans," *Journal of Clinical Endocrinology and Metabolism* 75, no. 5 (1992): 1293–1297.

Mellon, Synthia H., "Neurosteroids: Biochemistry, Modes of Action, and Clinical Relevance," *Journal of Clinical Endocrinology and Metabolism* 78, no. 5 (1994): 1003–1008.

Melo, L., et al., "Regulation of Circadian Photic Responses by Nitric Oxide," *Journal of Biological Rhythms* 12, no. 4 (August 1997): 319–326.

Mihailovic, L. J., et al., "Effects of Hibernation on Learning and Retention," *Nature* 218 (April 13, 1998): 191–192.

Mikhail, Adel A., et al., "Leptin Stimulates Fetal and Adult Erythroid and Myeloid Development," *Blood* 89, no. 5 (March 1, 1997): 1507–1512.

Mitchell, G. A., et al., "Medical Aspects of Ketone Body Metabolism," *Clinical and Investigative Medicine* 18, no. 3 (June 1995): 193–216.

Miwa, S., et al., "A Novel Function of Tetrahydrobiopterin," *Nippon Yakurigaku Zasshi* 100, no. 5 (November 1992): 367–381.

Modai, I., et al., "Blood Levels of Melatonin, Serotonin, Cortisol, and Prolactin in Relation to the Circadian Rhythm of Platelet Serotonin Uptake," *Psychiatry Res* 43, no. 2 (August 1992): 161–166.

Moguid, M. M., et al., "The Gut-Brain Brain-Gut Axis in Anorexia: Toward an Understanding of Food Intake Regulation," *Nutrition,* suppl. 1 (January 12, 1996): S57–S62.

MohanKumar, Puliyur S., et al., "Effects of Chronic Hyperprolactinemia on Tuberoinfundibular Dopaminergic Neurons," *PSEBM* 217 (1998): 461–465.

Moldofsky, H., "Sleep and the Immune System," *International Journal of Immunopharmacology* 17, no. 8 (August 1995): 649–654.

Mondaini, F., et al., "Sexuality Changes in a Hemodialysis Patient with Hyperprolactinemia: Therapeutic Possibilities," *Riv Ital Ginecol* 59 (1980): 93–96.

Monmaney, Terrence, "Seeking a Biological Link to Violence," *Los Angeles Times,* February 26, 1998, A1.

Morris, Lois B., "Mood News," *Allure,* April 1998, 104.

Morrow, Linda A., et al., "Effects of Epinephrine on Insulin Secretion and Action in Humans," *Diabetes* 42 (February 1993): 307–315.

Motluck, Alison, "Calm Before the Storm," *New Scientist* 158, no. 2130 (April 18, 1998): 46–47.

Muller, N., "Role of the Cytokine Network in the CNS and Psychiatric Disorders," *Nervenarzt* 68, no. 1 (January 1997): 11–20.

Murphy, D. L., et al., "Neuroendocrine Responses to Serotonergic Agonists As Indices of the Functional Status of Central Serotonin Neurotransmission in Humans: A Preliminary Comparative Analysis of Neuroendocrine Endpoints versus Other Endpoint Measures," *Behav Brain Res* 73, nos. 1–2 (1996): 209–214.

Myrsen-Axcrona, U., et al., "Dexamethasone Induces Neuropeptide Y (NPY) Expression and Impairs Insulin Release in the Insulin-Producing Cell Line RINm5F: Release of NPY and Insulin through Different Pathways," *Journal of Biological Chemistry* 272, no. 16 (April 18, 1997): 10790–10796.

Nakamura, Y., "Isolation of Borna Disease Virus from the Autopsy Brain of a Schizophrenia Patient," *Hokkaido Igaku Zasshi* 73, no. 3 (May 1998): 287–297.

Nair, N. P., et al., "Circadian Rhythm of Plasma Melatonin in Endogenous Depression," *Progress in Neuropsychopharmacology and Biological Psychiatry* 8, nos. 4–6 (1984): 715–718.

Nehlig, A., et al., "Caffeine-Diazepam Interaction and Local Cerebral Glucose Utilization in the Conscious Rat," *Brain Research* 419, nos. 1–2 (September 1, 1987): 272–278.

Nibert, Max L., et al., "Mechanisms of Viral Pathogenesis," *Journal of Clinical Investigation* 88 (September 1991): 727–734.

Nierenberg, Andrew, M.D., "Should You Take St. John's Wort?" *Healthnews,* April 20, 1998, 5; 6.

"The Nightmare World of Sleep Deprivation: It Costs You Money . . . and Animals Their Lives," *PETA's Animal Times* (Spring 1998): 18–19.

Nimgaonkar, V. L., et al., "Association Study of Schizophrenia and the IL-2 Receptor Beta Chain Gene," *American Journal of Medical Genetics* 60, no. 5 (October 9, 1995): 448–451.

Noach, E. L., "Appetite Regulation by Serotoninergic Mechanisms and Effects of D-Fenfluramine," *Netherlands Journal of Medicine* 45, no. 3 (September 1994): 123–133.

Norrgren, Gunilla, et al., "Nerve Growth Factor in Medium Conditioned by Embryonic Chicken Heart Cells," *In J Devl Neuroscience* 4, no. 1 (1986): 41–49.

Odawara, Masato, et al., "Diabetes, Hypertension, and Manic Episodes," *The Lancet* 348 (1996): 518.

Okutani, M., et al., "What Time Is the 'Biologic Zero Hour' of Circadian Variability?" *American Journal of Hypertension* 10, no. 7 (July 1997): 756–762.

Opp, M. R., et al., "Human Immunodeficiency Virus Envelope Glycoprotein 120 Alters Sleep and Induces Cytokine mRNA Expression in Rats," *American Journal of Physiology* 270, no. 5 (May 1996): 963–970.

Oren, Dan A., et al., "Adaptation to Dim Light in Depressed Patients with Seasonal Affective Disorder," *Psychiatry Res* 36 (1991): 187–193.

————, "Restoration of Detectable Melatonin After Entrainment to a 24-Hour Schedule in a 'Free-Running' Man," *Psychoneuroendocrinology* 22, no. 1 (1997): 39–52.

Orosco, M., et al., "Hypothalamic Monoamines and Insulin in Relation to Feeding in the Genetically Obese Zucker Rat As Revealed by Microdialysis," *Obesity Research,* suppl. 5 (December 3, 1995): 655S–665S.

Papanicolaou, Dimitris A., M.D., et al., "The Pathophysiologic Roles of Interleukin-6 in Human Disease," *Annals of Internal Medicine* 128, no. 2 (January 15, 1998): 127–137.

Pare, C. M. B., et al., "5-Hydroxytryptamine, Noradrenaline, and Dopamine in Brain Stem, Hypothalamus, and Caudate Nucleus of Controls and of Patients Committing Suicide by Coal-Gas Poisoning," *The Lancet* 2 (July 19, 1969): 133–135.

Penttinen, Jyrki, "Hypothesis: Low Serum Cholesterol, Suicide, and Interleukin-2," *American Journal of Epidemiology* 141 (1995): 716–718.

Pereira, de Vasconcelos A., et al., "Consequences of Chronic Phenobarbital Treatment on Local Cerebral Glucose Utilization in the Developing Rat," *Brain Research and Developmental Brain Research* 53, no. 2 (May 1, 1990): 168–178.

Picciotto, Marina R., et al., "Acetylcholine Receptors Containing the B2 Subunit Are Involved in the Reinforcing Properties of Nicotine," *Nature* 391 (January 8, 1998): 173–176.

Pidoplichko, Volodymyr I., et al., "Nicotine Activates and Desensitizes Midbrain Dopamine Neurons," *Nature* 390 (November 27, 1997): 401–404.

Pierini, A. A., et al., "Male Diabetic Sexual Impotence: Effects of Dopaminergic Agents," *Arch Androl* 6, no. 4 (June 1981): 347–350.

Pierotti, A. R., et al., "Endopeptidase-24.15 in Rat Hypothalamic/Pituitary/Gonadal Axis," *Mol Cell Endocrinol* 76, nos. 1–3 (April 1991): 95–103.

Pijl, H., et al., "Evidence for Brain Serotonin-Mediated Control of Carbohydrate Consumption in Normal Weight and Obese Humans," *International Journal of Obesity and Related Metabolic Disorders* 17, no. 9 (September 1993): 513–520.

————, "Plasma Amino Acid Ratios Related to Brain Serotonin Synthesis in Response to Food Intake in Bulimia Nervosa," *Biological Psychiatry* 38, no. 10 (November 15, 1995): 659–668.

Power, Ronan F., et al., "Dopaminergic and Ligand-Independent Activation of Steroid Hormone Receptors," *Science* 254 (December 13, 1991): 1636–1639.

Pratley, R. E., et al., "Plasma Leptin Responses to Fasting in Pima Indians," *American Journal of Physiology* 273, no. 3 (September 1997): E644-E649.

————, "Effects of Acute Hyperinsulinemia on Plasma Leptin Concentrations in Insulin-Sensitive and Insulin-Resistant Pima Indians," *Journal of Clinical Endocrinology and Metabolism* 81, no. 12 (December 1996): 4418–4421.

Purvis, C. C., et al., "Discrete Thalamic Lesions Attenuate Winter Adaptations and Increase Body Weight," *American Journal of Physiology* 273 (July 1997): R226-R235.

Ramakrishnan, R., et al., "Brain Dopamine in Experimental Diabetes," *Indian Journal of Physiology and Pharmacology* 40, no. 2 (April 1996): 193–195.

Rao, K., et al., "Serum Prolactin Levels in Male Patients with Erectile Dysfunction," *Indian J Med Res* 74 (September 1981): 412–414.

Rasika, S., et al., "BDNF Mediates the Effects of Testosterone on the Survival of New Neurons in an Adult Brain," *Neuron* 22, no. 1 (January 1999): 53–62.

Ravussin, Eric, et al., "Effects of a Traditional Lifestyle on Obesity in Pima Indians," *Diabetes Care* 17, no. 9 (September 1994): 1067–1074.

————, "Relatively Low Plasma Leptin Concentrations Precede Weight Gain in Pima Indians," *Nature Medicine* 3, no. 2 (February 1997): 238–240.

Regland, B., et al., "Homocysteinemia and Schizophrenia As a Case of Methylation Deficiency," *Journal of Neural Transmission* 98, no. 2 (1994): 143–152.

————, "Homocysteinemia Is a Common Feature of Schizophrenia," *Journal of Neural Transmission* 100, no. 2 (1995): 165–169.

Reichlin, Seymour, M.D., "Neuroendocrine-Immune Interactions," *New England Journal of Medicine* 329, no. 17 (October 21, 1993): 1246–1253.

Remme, W. J., "The Sympathetic Nervous System and Ischaemic Heart Disease," *European Heart Journal* 19, suppl. F (1998): F62-F71.

Rizza, Robert A., et al., "Cortisol-Induced Insulin Resistance in Man: Impaired Suppression of Glucose Production and Stimulation of Glucose Utilization Due to a Postreceptor Defect of Insulin Action," *Journal of Clinical Endocrinology and Metabolism* 54, no. 1 (1982): 131–138.

Rohner-Jeanrenaud, Francoise, Ph.D., et al., "Obesity, Leptin, and the Brain," *New England Journal of Medicine* 334, no. 5 (February 1, 1996): 324–325.

Roncari, Daniel A. K., "Relationships between the Hypothalamus and Adipose Tissue Mass," *Advanced Experimental Medicine and Biology* 291 (1991): 99–104.

Roose, S. P., et al., "Depression: Treating the Patient with Comorbid Cardiac Disease," *Geriatrics* 54, no. 2 (February 1999): 20–21; 25–26; 29–31.

Ruiz, Maria Luisa, et al., "Single Cyclic Nucleotide-Gated Channels Locked in Different Ligand-Bound States," *Nature* 389 (September 25, 1997): 389–390.

Salkovic, M., et al., "Striatal Dopaminergic D1 and D2 Receptors After Intracerebroventricular Application of Alloxan and Streptozocin in Rat," *Journal of Neural Transmission* 100, no. 2 (1995): 137–145.

Sarada, B., et al., "Increased Expression of an Endopeptidase (gamma-EGE/IDE) Hydrolyzing Beta-Endorphin during Differentiation and Maturation of Bone Marrow Macrophages," *J Leukoc Biol* 62, no. 6 (December 1997): 753–760.

Sejnowski, Terrence J., "The Year of the Dendrite," *Science* 275 (January 1997): 178–179.

Schaaf, M. J., et al., "Downregulation of BDNF mRNA and Protein in the Rat Hippocampus by Corticosterone," *Brain Research* 813, no. 1 (November 30, 1998): 112–120.

Schlingensiepen, K. H., et al., "The Role of Jun Transcription Factor Expression and Phosphorylation in Neuronal Differentiation, Neuronal Cell Death, and Plastic Adaptations In Vivo," *Cell Mol Neurobiol* 14, no. 5 (October 1994): 487–505.

Schoeller, D. A., et al., "Entrainment of the Diurnal Rhythm of Plasma Leptin to Meal Timing," *Journal of Clinical Investigation* 100, no. 7 (October 1997): 1882–1887.

Schroeder, H., et al., "Long-Term Consequences of Neonatal Exposure to Diazepam on Cerebral Glucose Utilization, Learning, Memory and Anxiety," *Brain Research* 766, nos. 1–2 (August 22, 1997): 142–152.

Schroeder, H., et al., "Short- and Long-Term Effects of Neonatal Diazepam Exposure on Local Cerebral Glucose Utilization in the Rat," *Brain Research* 660, no. 1 (October 10, 1994): 144–153.

Schulte, H. M., et al., "Systemic Interleukin-1 Alpha and Interleukin-2 Secretion in Response to Acute Stress to Corticotrophin-Releasing Hormone in Humans," *European Journal of Clinical Investigation* 24, no. 11 (November 1994): 773–777.

Schuman, Erin, "Growth Factors Sculpt the Synapse," *Science* 275 (February 28, 1997): 1277–1278.

Schuman, E. M., "Neurotrophin Regulation of Synaptic Transmission," *Curr Opin Neurobiol* 9, no. 1 (February 1999): 105–109.

Schwartz, Jeffrey M., "Obsessive-Compulsive Disorder," *Science and Medicine,* March/April 1997, 14–23.

Schwartz, Michael W., et al., "Insulin in the Brain: A Hormonal Regulator of Energy Balance," *Endocrine Reviews* 13, no. 3 (1992): 387–413.

Sheline, Yvette I., et al., "How Safe Are Serotonin Reuptake Inhibitors for Depression in Patients with Coronary Heart Disease?" *American Journal of Medicine* 102, no. 1 (January 1997): 54–59.

Sheps, D. S., et al., "Does Depression Predict More Symptoms or More Disease?" *American Heart Journal* 137, no. 3 (March 1999): 386–387.

Shimizu, K., et al., "Sympathetic Dysfunction in Heart Failure," *Bailieres Clinical Endocrinology and Metabolism* 7, no. 2 (April 1993): 439–463.

Shinohara, M. L., et al., "Glyceraldehyde-3-Phosphate Dehydrogenase Is Regulated on a Daily Basis by the Circadian Clock," *Journal of Biological Chemistry* 273, no. 1 (January 2, 1998): 446–452.

Shono, N., et al., "The Relationships of Testosterone, Estradiol, Dehydroepiandrosterone-Sulfate and Sex Hormone-Binding Globulin to Lipid and Glucose Metabolism in Healthy Men," *J Atheroscler Thromb* 3, no. 1 (1996): 45–51.

Silverstein, J. T., et al., "Neuropeptide Y-Like Gene Expression in the Salmon Brain Increases with Fasting," *Gen Comp Endocrinol* 110, no. 2 (May 1998): 157–165.

Simko, M., et al., "Effects of 50 EMF Exposure on Micronucleus Formation and Apoptosis in Transformed and Nontransformed Human Cell Lines." *Bioelectromagnetics*, 19, no. 2 (1998): 85–91.

Smith, K. A., et al., "Relapse of Depression After Rapid Depletion of Tryptophan," *The Lancet* 349 (March 29, 1997): 915–919.

Smith, Sheryl S., et al., "GABAa Receptor a4 Subunit Suppression Prevents Withdrawal Properties of an Endogenous Steroid," *Nature* 392 (April 30, 1998): 926–930.

Solomon, Andrew, "Anatomy of Melancholy," *The New Yorker*, January 12, 1998, 46–61.

Spector, Novera Herbert, Ph.D., "Neuroimmunomodulation: A Brief Review," *Regulatory Toxicology and Pharmacology* 24 (1996): S32-S38.

Spessert, R., et al., "In the Rat Pineal Gland, but Not in the Suprachiasmatic Nucleus, the Amount of Constitutive Neuronal Nitric Oxide Synthase Is Regulated by Environmental Lighting Conditions," *Biochemical and Biophysical Research Communications* 212, no. 1 (July 6, 1995): 70–76.

Spiegel, K., et al., "Temporal Relationship between Prolactin Secretion and Slow-Wave Electroencephalic Activity during Sleep," *Sleep* 18, no. 7 (September 1995): 543–548.

———, "Prolactin Secretion and Sleep," *Sleep* 17, no. 1 (February 1994): 20–27.

Squadrito, F., et al., "Food Deprivation Increases Brain Nitric Oxide Synthase and Depresses Brain Serotonin Levels in Rats," *Neuropharmacology* 33, no. 1 (January 1994): 83–86.

Stegmayr, B., et al., "Hyperprolactinaemia and Testosterone Production: Observations in Two Men on Long-Term Dialysis," *Horm Res* 21, no. 4 (1985): 224–228.

Stephens, Thomas W., et al., "The Role of Neuropeptide Y in the Antiobesity Action of the Obese Gene Product," *Nature* 377 (October 12, 1995): 530–532.

Sudo, A., et al., "Dissociation of Catecholamine and Corticosterone Responses to Different Types of Stress in Rats," *Industrial Health* 31, no. 3 (1993): 101–111.

Sutin, E. L., et al., "Light-Induced Gene Expression in the Suprachiasmatic Nucleus of Young and Aging Rats," *Neurobiol Aging* 14, no. 5 (September 1993): 441–446.

Takahashi, S., et al., "Inhibition of Tumor Necrosis Factor Attenuates Physiological Sleep in Rabbits," *Neuroreport* 7, no. 2 (January 31, 1996): 642–646.

Taubes, Gary, "Double Helix Does Chemistry at a Distance—But How?" *Science* 275 (March 7, 1997): 1420–1421.

Thibault, L., "Dietary Carbohydrates: Effects on Self-Selection, Plasma Glucose and Insulin, and Brain Indoleaminergic Systems in Rat," *Appetite* 3 (December 23, 1994): 275–286.

Thompson, D. B., et al., "Structure and Sequence Variation at the Human Leptin Receptor Gene in Lean and Obese Pima Indians," *Human Molecular Genetics* 6, no. 5 (May 1997): 675–679.

———, "A Physical Map at 1p31 Encompassing the Acute Insulin Response Locus and the Leptin Receptor," *Genomics* 39, no. 2 (January 15, 1997): 227–230.

Thorner, M. O., et al., "Bromocriptine Treatment of Hyperprolactinaemic Hypogonadism," *Acta Endocrinol Suppl (Copenh)* 216 (1978): 131–146.

Thun, Michael J., et al., "Alcohol Consumption and Mortality among Middle-Aged and Elderly U.S. Adults," *New England Journal of Medicine* 337, no. 24 (December 11, 1997): 1705–1764.

Tosini, Gianluca, et al., "Circadian Rhythms in Cultured Mammalian Retina," *Science* 272 (April 19, 1996): 419–421.

"Tracing the Background of Phen-Fen: Rise and Fall of a Diet 'Miracle'," *The New York Times,* September 23, 1997, B1; B12.

Tsigos, C., et al., "Dose Effects of Recombinant Human Interleukin-6 on Pituitary Hormone Secretion and Energy Expenditure," *Neuroendocrinology* 66, no. 1 (July 1997): 54–62.

Tuomisto, Jouko, et al., "Decreased Uptake of 5-Hydroxytryptamine in Blood Platelets from Depressed Patients," *Nature* 262, no. 5569 (August 12, 1976): 596–598.

Van Cauter, Eve, et al., "Modulation of Glucose Regulation and Insulin Secretion by Circadian Rhythmicity and Sleep," *Journal of Clinical Investigation* 88 (September 1991): 934–942.

Veneman, Thiemo, et al., "Effect of Hyperketonemia and Hyperlacticacidemia on Symptoms, Cognitive Dysfunction, and Counterregulatory Hormone Responses during Hypoglycemia in Normal Humans," *Diabetes* 43 (November 1994): 1311–1317.

Venkatraman, Jaya T., et al., "Influence of the Level of Dietary Lipid Intake and Maximal Exercise on the Immune Status in Runners," *Medicine and Science in Sports and Exercise* 29 (1997): 333–344.

Vermeulen, A., "Biological Manifestations of the Andropause," *Fiziol Zh* 36, no. 5 (September 1990): 90–93.

Vogel, Gretchen, "Neuroscience's Meeting of the Minds in Washington," *Science* 274 (November 29, 1996): 1466–1467.

Voultsios, A., et al., "Salivary Melatonin As a Circadian Phase Marker: Validation and Comparison to Plasma Melatonin," *Journal of Biological Rhythms* 12, no. 5 (October 1997): 457–466.

Wan, Q., et al., "Recruitment of Functional GABAa Receptors to Postsynaptic Domains by Insulin," *Nature* 388 (August 14, 1997): 686–690.

Wand, Gary S., et al., "Relationship between Plasma Adrenocorticotropin, Hypothalamic Opioid Tone, and Plasma Leptin," *Journal of Clinical Endocrinology and Metabolism* 83, no. 6 (1988): 2138–2142.

Wang, J., et al., "Central Insulin Inhibits Hypothalamic Galanin and Neuropeptide Y Gene Expression and Peptide Release in Intact Rats," *Brain Research* 777, nos. 1–2 (November 28, 1997): 231–236.

Want, Qiong, et al., "Interactions between Leptin and Hypothalamic Neuropeptide Y Neurons in the Control of Food Intake and Energy Homeostasis in the Rat," *Diabetes* 46 (March 1997): 335–341.

Watkins, L. R., et al., "Mechanisms of Tumor Necrosis Factor-Alpha (TNF-Alpha) Hyperalgesia," *Brain Research* 692, nos. 1–2 (September 18, 1995): 244–250.

Weaver, David R., "The Suprachiasmatic Nucleus: A 25-Year Retrospective," *Journal of Biological Rhythms* 13, no. 2 (April 1998): 100–112.

Weber, E. Todd, et al., "Neuropeptide Y Blocks Light-Induced Phase Advances but Not Delays of the Circadian Activity Rhythm in Hamsters," *Neuroscience Letters* 231 (1997): 159–162.

Wehr, Thomas A., "Melatonin and Seasonal Rhythms," *Journal of Biological Rhythms* 12, no. 6 (December 1997): 518–527.

————, "Effect of Seasonal Changes in Day Length on Human Neuroendocrine Function," *Hormone Research* 49 (1998): 118–124.

————, "Suppression of Men's Responses to Seasonal Changes in Day Length by Modern Artificial Lighting," *American Journal of Physiology* 269, no. 38 (1995): R173-R178.

Welch, Catherine C., et al., "Palatability-Induced Hyperphagia Increases Hypothalamic Dynorphin Peptide and mRNA Levels," *Brain Research* 721 (1996): 126–131.

Weibel, L., et al., "Comparative Effect of Night and Daytime Sleep on the 24-Hour Cortisol Secretory Profile," *Sleep* 18, no. 7 (September 1995): 549–556.

Weyerbrock, A., et al., "Effects of Light and Chronotherapy on Human Circadian Rhythms in Delayed Sleep Phase Syndrome: Cytokines, Cortisol, Growth Hormone, and the Sleep-Wake Cycle," *Biological Psychiatry* 40, no. 8 (October 15, 1996): 794–797.

Whitworth, J. A., et al., "Mechanisms of Cortisol-Induced Hypertension in Humans," *Steroids* 60, no. 1 (January 1995): 76–80.

Wickelgren, Ingrid, "Tracking Insulin to the Mind," *Science* 280 (April 24, 1998): 517–519.

Wikholm, Gary, M.D., "Dangerous Anti-Depressant Drugs," *Doctor's Prescription for Healthy Living* 2, no. 2 (1998): 1; 14.

Williams, Carol J., "Something Is Rotund in Denmark," *Los Angeles Times*, February 9, 1999, A1.

Wilson, C. A., et al., "Relationship of the White Blood Cell Count to Body Fat: Role of Leptin," *British Journal of Haematology* 99, no. 2 (November 1997): 447–451.

Winerip, Michael, "Schizophrenia's Most Zealous Foe," *The New York Times Magazine*, February 22, 1998: 26–29.

Winters, S. J., et al., "Altered Pulsatile Secretion of Luteinizing Hormone in Hypogonadal Men with Hyperprolactinaemia," *Clin Endocrinol (Oxf)* 21, no. 3 (September 1984): 257–263.

Wise, Phyllis M., et al., "Aging Alters the Circadian Rhythm of Glucose Utilization in the Suprachiasmatic Nucleus," *Proceedings of the National Academy of Sciences (USA)* 85 (July 1988): 5305–5309.

Wolfe, Barbara E., et al., "The Effects of Dieting on Plasma Tryptophan Concentration and Food Intake in Healthy Women," *Physiology and Behavior* 61, no. 4 (1997): 537–541.

Wolfovitz, E., et al., "Effects of Hypercortisolemia or Hyperinsulinemia on Neurochemical Indices of Catecholamine Release and Synthesis in Conscious Rats," *Journal of the Autonomic Nervous System* 54, no. 2 (August 4, 1995): 104–112.

Wozniak, Magdalena, et al., "The Cellular and Physiological Actions of Insulin in the Central Nervous System," *Neurochemistry International* 22, no. 1 (1993): 1–10.

Wurtman, Richard J., et al., "Brain Catechol Synthesis: Control by Brain Tyrosine Concentration," *Science* 18 (February 26, 1974): 183–184.

———, "Brain Serotonin, Carbohydrate Craving, Obesity and Depression," *Obesity Research* 4 (November 3, 1995): 477S-480S.

Yanagimoto, M., et al., "Afferents Originating from the Dorsal Penile Nerve Excite Oxytocin Cells in the Hypothalamic Paraventricular Nucleus of the Rat," *Brain Research* 733, no. 2 (September 16, 1996): 292–296.

Yang, Z. W., et al., "An Association between Anti-Hippocampal Antibody Concentration and Lymphocyte Production of IL-2 in Patients with Schizophrenia," *Psychological Medicine* 24, no. 2 (May 24, 1994): 449–455.

Yehuda, Rachel, "Stress and Glucocorticoid," *Science* 275 (March 14, 1997): 1662.

Yie, Shang-Mian, et al., "Melatonin Receptors on Human Granulosa Cell Membranes," *Journal of Clinical Endocrinology and Metabolism* 80, no. 5 (1995): 1747–1749.

Yoshida, H., et al., "Transient Suppression of Pancreatic Endocrine Function in Patients Following Brain Death," *Clinical Transplantation* 10 (February 1996): 28–33.

Youdim, Moussa B. H., et al., "Understanding Parkinson's Disease," *Scientific American,* January 1997, 52–59.

Young, L. J., et al., "Gene Targeting Approaches to Neuroendocrinology: Oxytocin, Maternal Behavior, and Affiliation," *Hormones and Behavior* 31, no. 3 (June 1997): 221–231.

Zarrindast, M. R., et al., "Effects of Monoamine Receptor Antagonists on Nicotine-Induced Hypophagia in the Rat," *European Journal of Pharmacology* 321, no. 2 (February 26, 1997): 157–162.

Zawilska, J. B., et al., "Serotonin N-Acetyltransferase Activity in Chicken Retina: In Vivo Effects of Phosphodiesterase Inhibitors, Forskolin, and Drugs Affecting Dopamine Receptors," *Journal of Pineal Research* 11, nos. 3–4 (October 1991): 116–122.

Zelissen, P. M., "Drug Treatment of Sex Disorders in Men," *Ned Tijdschr Geneeskd* 140, no. 50 (December 14, 1996): 2528.

Zhong, H. H., et al., "Effects of Synergistic Signaling by Phytochrome A and Cryptochrome 1 on Circadian Clock-Regulated Catalase Expression," *Plant Cell* 9, no. 6 (June 1997): 947–955.

Zureik, Mahmoud, et al., "Serum Cholesterol Concentration and Death from Suicide in Men: Paris Prospective Study I," *BMJ* 313 (September 14, 1996): 648–651.

Chapter Seven: The Best Place to Hide a Lie Is Between Two Truths

Agardh, C. D., et al., "Lack of Association between Plasma Homocysteine Levels and Microangiopathy in Type I Diabetes Mellitus," *Scandinavian Journal of Clinical Lab Investigation* 54, no. 8 (December 1994): 637–641.

Al'Absi, M., et al., "Cortisol Concentrations in Serum of Borderline Hypertensive Men Exposed to a Novel Experimental Setting," *Psychoneuroendocrinology* 18, nos. 5–6 (1993): 355–363.

American Heart Association Steering Committee, "Dietary Guidelines for Healthy American Adults," *Circulation* 74, no. 6 (December 1986): 1465A-1468A.

Araki, A., et al., "Plasma Homocysteine Concentrations in Japanese Patients with Non-Insulin-Dependent Diabetes Mellitus: Effect of Parenteral Methylcobalamin Treatment," *Atherosclerosis* 103, no. 2 (November 1993): 149–157.

Arangino, Serenella, M.D., et al., "Effects of Melatonin on Vascular Reactivity, Catecholamine Levels, and Blood Pressure in Healthy Men," *American Journal of Cardiology* 83 (May 1, 1999): 1417–1419.

Artino, M., et al., "The Effect of Continuous Illumination and an Inverse Rhythm (Light-Darkness) on Fibrinolysis," *Rev Med Chir Soc Nat Iasi* 100, nos. 3–4 (July 1996): 114–117.

Ascherio, Alberto, M.D., et al., "Trans-Fatty Acids Intake and Risk of Myocardial Infarction," *Circulation* 89 (1994): 94–101.

Ash, Caroline, "Like Frogs Disguised As Leaves," *Trends in Microbiology* 7 (1999): 142.

Attali, Bernard, "A New Wave for Heart Rhythms," *Nature* 384 (November 7, 1996): 24–25.

Balkau, Beverly, Ph.D., et al., "High Blood Glucose Concentration Is a Risk Factor for Mortality in Middle-Aged Nondiabetic Men," *Diabetes Care* 21, no. 3 (March 1998): 360–367.

Bang, H. O., et al., "Plasma Lipid and Lipoprotein Pattern in Greenlandic West-Coast Eskimos," *The Lancet* 1 (June 5, 1971) 1143–1146.

Barhanin, Jacques, et al., "KvLQT1 and IsK (Mink) Proteins Associate to Form the I ks Cardiac Potassium Current," *Nature* 384 (November 7, 1996): 78–80.

Barinaga, Marcia, "How Much Pain for Cardiac Gain?" *Science* 276 (May 30, 1997): 1324–1327.

Barker, D. J. P., et al., "Fetal Nutrition and Cardiovascular Disease in Adult Life," *The Lancet* 341 (1993): 938–941.

Bartels, Claus, et al., "Detection of Chlamydia pneumoniae but Not Cytomegalovirus in Occluded Saphenous Vein Coronary Artery Bypass Grafts," *Circulation* 99 (1999): 879–882.

Baumgartner, E. R., et al., "Congenital Defect in Intracellular Cobalamin Metabolism Resulting in Homocysteinuria and Methylmalonic Aciduria: I. Case Report and Histopathology," *Helv Paediatr Acta* 34, no. 5 (1979): 465–482.

Becker, Lewis C., M.D., et al., "Left Ventricular, Peripheral Vascular, and Neurohumoral Responses to Mental Stress in Normal Middle-Aged Men and Women," *Circulation* 94 (1996): 2768–2777.

Bergendahl, Matti, et al., "Fasting As a Metabolic Stress Paradigm Selectively Amplifies Cortisol Secretory Burst Mass and Delays the Time of Maximal Nyctohemeral Cortisol Concentrations in Healthy Men," *Journal of Clinical Endocrinology and Metabolism* 81, no. 2 (1996): 692–699.

Bergers, Gabriele, et al., "Effects of Angiogenesis Inhibitors on Multistage Carcinogenesis in Mice," *Science* 284 (April 30, 1999): 808–812.

Bierhaus, Angelika, et al., "Advanced Glycation End Product-Induced Activation of NF-kB Is Suppressed by a-Lipoic Acid in Cultured Endothelial Cells," *Diabetes* 46 (September 1997): 1481–1490.

Bjorntorp, P., "Visceral Fat Accumulation: The Missing Link between Psychosocial Factors and Cardiovascular Disease?" *Journal of Internal Medicine* 230, no. 3 (September 1991): 195–201.

Blakeslee, Sandra, "What Controls Blood Flow in Tissues? It Could Be Blood Itself," *The New York Times,* July 22, 1997, C1.

Blum, Arnon, M.D., et al., "High Anti-Cytomegalovirus (CMV) lgG Antibody Titer Is Associated with Coronary Artery Disease and May Predict Post-Coronary Balloon Angioplasty Restenosis," *American Journal of Cardiology* 81 (1998): 866–868.

Blumenthal, James A., et al., "Mental Stress-Induced Ischemia in the Laboratory and Ambulatory Ischemia during Daily Life," *Circulation* 92 (1995): 2102–2108.

Boulton, M. I., et al., "Prostaglandin F2alpha-Induced Nest-Building in Pseudopregnant Pigs: Space Restriction Stress Does Not Influence Secretion of Oxytocin, Prolactin, Oestradiol, or Progesterone," *Physiology and Behavior* 62, no. 5 (November 1997): 1079–1085.

Boyce, Nell, ". . . Fear Itself," *New Scientist,* March 6, 1999, 34–37.

Brand, K., et al., "Oxidized LDL Enhances Lipopolysaccharide-Induced Tissue Factor Expression in Human Adherent Monocytes," *Arterioscler Thromb* 14, no. 5 (May 1994): 790–797.

Brestrich, M., et al., "Preventing and Arresting Coronary Atherosclerosis," *American Heart Journal* 85, no. 6 (September 1995): 580–600.

Brewitt, B., "Homeopathic Growth Factors: Understanding Like Cures from the Scientific and Medical Literature," *Alternative Therapies* 3, no. 2 (March 1997): 92–93.

Brody, Jane E., "Eating Fish Cited Anew As Good for the Heart," *The New York Times,* April 11, 1997, A12.

Brugger, P., et al., "Impaired Nocturnal Secretion of Melatonin in Coronary Heart Disease," *The Lancet* 345 (1995): 1408.

Buchanan, Mark, "The Heart That Just Won't Die," *New Scientist,* March 20, 1999, 24–28.

Buttiker, M., "Electron Statistical Effects: Bunches of Photons—Antibunches of Electrons," *Science* 284 (April 9, 1999): 275.

Buxton, Orfeu M., et al., "Roles of Intensity and Duration of Nocturnal Exercise in Causing Phase Delays of Human Circadian Rhythms," *American Journal of Physiology* 273 (1997): E536-E542.

Carlson, Lars A., et al., "Ischaemic Heart Disease in Relation to Fasting Values of Plasma Triglycerides and Cholesterol," *The Lancet* (April 22, 1972) 865–868.

Carney, R. M., et al., "Reproducibility of Mental Stress-Induced Myocardial Ischemia in the Psychophysiological Investigations of Myocardial Ischemia (PIMI)," *Psychosomatic Medicine* 60, no. 1 (January/February 1998): 64–70.

Chan, H., et al., "Expression and Characterization of Human Tissue Kallikrein Variants," *Protein Expr Purif* 12, no. 3 (April 1998): 361–370.

Chan, T. Y., et al., "Effect of Melatonin on the Maintenance of Cholesterol Homeostasis in the Rat," *Endocr Res* 21, no. 3 (August 1995): 681–696.

Chen, Li-Dun, et al., "In Vivo and In Vitro Effects of the Pineal Gland and Melatonin on [Ca(2+)+Mg(2+)]-Dependent ATPase in Cardiac Sarcolemma," *Journal of Pineal Research* 14, no. 4 (May 1993): 178–183.

———, "Melatonin Prevents the Suppression of Cardiac Ca(2+)-Stimulated ATPase Activity Induced by Alloxan," *American Journal of Physiology* 267 (July 1994): E57-E62.

———, "Melatonin Reduces 3H-Nitrendipine Binding in the Heart," *Melatonin and Calcium Channels* 207 (1994): 34–37.

Cheng, J. G., et al., "Cardiotrophin-1 Induces the Same Neuropeptides in Sympathetic Neurons As Do Neuropoietic Cytokines," *Journal of Neurochemistry* 69, no. 6 (December 1997): 2278–2284.

Chuang, J. I., et al., "Pineal Stimulation Produces Both Hypertension and Tachycardia in Rats," *Brain Research Bulletin* 33, no. 5 (1994): 473–476.

Clark, Robert, et al., "Lowering Blood Homocysteine with Folic Acid Based Supplements: Meta-Analysis of Randomised Trials," *British Medical Journal* 316 (March 21, 1998): 894–898.

———, "Hyperhomocysteinemia: An Independent Risk Factor for Vascular Disease," *New England Journal of Medicine* 324, no. 17 (April 25, 1991): 1149–1155.

Colwell, J. A., et al., "Forum Two: Unanswered Research Questions about Metabolic control in Non-Insulin-Dependent Diabetes Mellitus," *Annals of Internal Medicine* 124, no. 1 (January 1, 1996): 178–179.

Coghlan, Andy, "Electric DNA," *New Scientist,* February 13, 1999, 19.

———, "Fix for Fury Arteries," *New Scientist,* November 15, 1997, 6.

Confalonieri, M., et al., "Heterozygosity for Homocysteinuria: A Detectable and Reversible Risk Factor for Pulmonary Thromboembolism," *Monaldi Arch Chest Dis* 50, no. 2 (April 1995): 114–115.

Connor, Sonja, et al., "Are Fish Oils Beneficial in the Prevention and Treatment of Coronary Artery Disease?" *American Journal of Clinical Nutrition* 66 (1997): 1020S–1031S.

Coombes, B. K., et al., "Chlamydia pneumoniae Infection of Human Endothelial Cells Induces Proliferation of Smooth Muscle Cells via an Endothelial Cell-Derived Soluble Factor(s)," *Infect Immun* 67, no. 6 (1999): 2909–2915.

Cowley, Geoffrey, et al., "Healer of Hearts," *Newsweek,* March 16, 1998, 50–56.

———, "Is There a Sixth Sense?" *Newsweek,* October 13, 1997, 67.

Cravatt, Benjamin F., et al., "Molecular Characterization of an Enzyme That Degrades Neuromodulatory Fatty-Acid Amines," *Nature* 384 (November 1996): 83.

Crawford, Michael A., et al. "Are Fish Oils Beneficial in Disease Prevention and Treatment?" *American Journal of Clinical Nutrition* 66 (1997): 1042S–1043S.

Csonka, E., et al., "Influence of the Measles Virus on the Proliferation and Protein Synthesis of Aortic Endothelial and Smooth Muscle Cells," *Acta Microbiol Hung* 37, no. 2 (1990): 193–200.

Da Silva, Wilson, "A Steady Heart," *New Scientist,* August 1, 1997, 12.

Dajer, Tony, "Hearts and Minds," *Discover,* December 1997, 49–53.

Demaison, L., et al., "Myocardial Ischemia and In Vitro Mitochondrial Metabolic Efficiency," *Molecular and Cellular Biochemistry* 158, no. 2 (May 24, 1996): 161–169.

Despres, Jean-Pierre, et al., "Hyperinsulinemia As an Independent Risk Factor for Ischemic Heart Disease," *New England Journal of Medicine* 334 (1996): 952–957.

Dhurandhar, N. V., et al., "Association of Adenovirus Infection with Human Obesity," *Obes Res* 5, no. 5 (September 1997): 464–469.

Dickinson, C. J., "Cerebral Oxidative Metabolism in Hypertension," *Clinical Science* 91, no. 5 (November 1996): 539–550.

Dold, Catherine, "Needles Nerves," *Discover,* September 1998, 59–62.

Doyama, K., et al., "Tumour Necrosis Factor Is Expressed in Cardiac Tissues of Patients with Heart Failure," *International Journal of Cardiology* 54, no. 3 (June 1996): 217–225.

Duanmu, Zhengbo, et al., "Insulin-Like Growth Factor-1 Decreases Sympathetic Nerve Activity: The Effect Is Modulated by Glycemic Status," *Proceedings of the Society for Experimental Biology and Medicine* 216, no. 1 (October 1997): 93–97.

Eggesbo, J. B., et al., "LPS Induced Procoagulant Activity and Plasminogen Activator Activity in Mononuclear Cells from Persons with High or Low Levels of HDL Lipoprotein," *Thromb Res* 77, no. 5 (March 1, 1995): 441–452.

Endres, Stefan, et al., "The Effect of Dietary Supplementation with n-3 Polyunsaturated Fatty Acids on the Synthesis of Interleukin-1 and Tumor Necrosis Factor by Mononuclear Cells," *New England Journal of Medicine* 320, no. 5 (February 2, 1989): 265–271.

"Fake Cells," *Discover*, May 1997, 26.

Favaretto, A. L., et al., "Oxytocin Releases Atrial Natriuretic Peptide from Rat Atria In Vitro That Exerts Negative Inotropic and Chronotropic Action," *Peptides* 18, no. 9 (1997): 1377–1381.

Ferrannini, Eleuterio, M.D., et al., "Insulin Resistance in Essential Hypertension," *New England Journal of Medicine* 317, no. 6 (August 6, 1987): 350–357.

Ferrari, R., "Effect of ACE Inhibition of Myocardial Ischaemia," *European Heart Journal* 19, suppl. J (September 1998): J30–J35.

Fimognari, F. L., et al., "Associated Daily Biosynthesis of Cortisol and Thromboxane A2: A Preliminary Report," *J Lab Clin Med* 128, no. 1 (July 1996): 115–121.

Finstad, Hanne S., et al., "Effect of n-3 and n-6 Fatty Acids on Proliferation and Differentiation of Promyelocytic Leukemic HL-60 Cells," *Blood* 84, no. 11 (December 1, 1994): 3799–3809.

Fisher, W. E., et al., "Insulin Promotes Pancreatic Cancer: Evidence for Endocrine Influence on Exocrine Pancreatic Tumors," *J Surg Res* 63, no. 1 (June 1996): 310–313.

Fontbonne, A., et al., "Hyperinsulinaemia As a Predictor of Coronary Heart Disease Mortality in a Healthy Population: The Paris Prospective Study 15-Year Follow-Up," *Diabetologia* 34 (1991): 356–361.

Fraser, G. E., et al., "Risk Factors for All-Cause and Coronary Heart Disease Mortality in the Oldest-Old: The Adventist Health Study," *Arch Intern Med* 348, no. 9024 (October 27, 1997): 2249–2258.

Garnacho, Montero J., et al., "Lipids and Immune Function," *Nutricion Hospitalaria* 11, no. 4 (July/August 1996): 230–237.

Gillman, Matthew W., M.D., et al., "Inverse Association of Dietary Fat with Development of Ischemic Stroke in Men," *Journal of the American Medical Association* 278, no. 24 (December 24–31, 1997): 2145–2150.

Glaser, J. L., et al., "Elevated Serum Dehydroepiandrosterone Sulfate Levels in Practitioners of the Transcendental Meditation (TM) and TM-Sidhi Programs," *Journal of Behavioral Medicine* 15, no. 4 (August 1992): 327–341.

Glausiusz, Josie, "Infected Hearts," *Discover*, September 1998, 30–33.

Glueck, Charles J., et al., "Evidence That Homocysteine Is an Independent Risk Factor for Atherosclerosis in Hyperlipidemic Patients," *American Journal of Cardiology* 75 (January 15, 1995): 132–136.

Goalstone, J. L., et al., "Insulin Potentiates Platelet-Derived Growth Factor Action in Vascular Smooth Muscle Cells," *Endocrinology* 139, no. 10 (October 1998): 4067–4072.

Goenjian, A. K., et al., "Basal Cortisol, Dexamethasone Suppression of Cortisol, and MHPG in Adolescents After the 1988 Earthquake in Armenia," *American Journal of Psychiatry* 153, no. 7 (July 1996): 929–934.

Goldberg, A. David, M.D., et al., "Ischemic, Hemodynamic, and Neurohormonal Responses to Mental and Exercise Stress: Experience from the Psychophysiological Investigations of Myocardial Ischemia Study (PIMI)," *Circulation* 94, no. 10 (November 15, 1996): 2402–2409.

Golomb, Beatrice A., M.D., "Cholesterol and Violence: Is There a Connection?" *Annals of Internal Medicine* 128 (1998): 478–487.

Goodnight, Scott H., "The Fish Oil Puzzle," *Science & Medicine,* September/October 1996, 42–51.

Goodwin, Liza, "Change of Hearts," *Mirabella,* March 1999, 92.

Gornel, Daniel L., M.D., "Rates of Death from Coronary Heart Disease," *New England Journal of Medicine* 340, no. 9 (March 4, 1999): 730.

Gould, K. L., et al., "Changes in Myocardial Perfusion Abnormalities by Positron Emission Tomography After Long-Term, Intense Risk Factor Modification," *Journal of the American Medical Association* 274, no. 11 (September 20, 1995): 894–901.

Grady, Denise, "Some Antibiotics May Reduce Risk of Heart Attack, Study Finds," *The New York Times,* February 3, 1999, A14.

Graham, Barbara, "A Meditation from the Heart," *Self,* April 1998, 60.

Grayston, J. Thomas, et al., "Chlamydia pneumoniae (TWAR) in Atherosclerosis of the Carotid Artery," *Circulation* 92 (1995): 3397–3400.

Green, Laurence H., et al., "Platelet Activation during Exercise-Induced Myocardial Ischemia," *New England Journal of Medicine* 302 (1980): 193–197.

Gura, Trisha, "Chlamydia Protein Linked to Heart Disease," *Science* 283 (February 26, 1999): 1238–1239.

Guterman, Lila, "Why We're All Charged Up over DNA," *New Scientist,* August 22, 1998, 21.

Gutkowska, Jolanta, et al., "Oxytocin Releases Atrial Natriuretic Peptide by Combining with Oxytocin Receptors in the Heart," *Proceedings of the National Academy of Sciences (USA)* 94 (October 1997): 11704–11709.

Haanwinckel, M. A., et al., "Oxytocin Mediates Atrial Natriuretic Peptide Release and Natriuresis After Volume Expansion in the Rat," *Proceedings of the National Academy of Sciences (USA)* 92, no. 17 (August 15, 1995): 7902–7906.

Hademenos, George J., "The Biophysics of Stroke," *American Scientist* 85 (May/June 1997): 226–235.

Hajjar, David P., et al., "Lipoprotein Trafficking in Vascular Cells," *Journal of Biological Chemistry* 272, no. 37 (September 12, 1997): 22975–22978.

Hansen, J. C., et al., "Fatty Acids and Antioxidants in the Inuit Diet: Their Role in Ischemic Heart Disease (IHD) and Possible Interactions with Other Dietary Factors—A Review," *Arctic Medical Research* 53 (1994): 4–17.

Hata, M., et al., "A Correlation between Atrial Natriuretic Peptide, Brain Natriuretic Peptide, and Perioperative Cardiac and Renal Functions in Open Heart Surgery," *Thoracic Surgery* 45, no. 11 (November 1997): 1797–1802.

Hobbs, C. G., et al., "Lipoproteins in Non-Insulin-Dependent Diabetes Mellitus (NIDDM)," *Biochem Soc Trans* 24, no. 2 (May 1996): 153S.

Holden, Arun V., "A Last Wave from the Dying Heart," *Nature* 392 (March 1998): 20–21.

Holmang, A., et al., "The Effects of Hyperinsulinaemia on Myocardial Mass, Blood Pressure Regulation and Central Haemodynamics in Rats," *European Journal of Clinical Investigation* 26, no. 11 (November 1996): 973–978.

Holmes, Bob, "Jabs Take a Stab at Heart Disease," *New Scientist,* April 12, 1997, 18.

Hooper, L. V., "Host-Microbial Symbiosis in the Mammalian Intestine: Exploring an Internal Ecosystem," *Bioessays* 20, no. 4 (April 1998): 336–343.

Hopfner, Rob L., et al., "Insulin Increases Endothelin-1-Evoked Intracellular Free Calcium Responses by Increased Eta Receptor Expression in Rat Aortic Smooth Muscle Cells," *Diabetes* 47 (June 1998): 937–944.

Hsu, D. S., et al., "Putative Human Blue-Light Photoreceptors hCRY1 and hCRY2 are Flavoproteins," *Biochemistry* 35, no. 44 (November 5, 1996): 13871–13877.

Hu, Frank B., M.D., et al., "Dietary Fat Intake and the Risk of Coronary Heart Disease in Women," *New England Journal of Medicine* 337, no. 21 (November 20, 1997): 1491–1545.

Ida, T., et al., "Heterogeneity of Non-Insulin-Dependent Diabetes Mellitus in HLA Types and Clinical Features: Comparison with Insulin-Dependent Diabetes Mellitus," *Endocrinol Jpn* 39, no. 1 (February 1991): 9–13.

Ikeda, Uichi, M.D., et al., "Homocysteine Increases Nitric Oxide Synthesis in Cytokine-Stimulated Vascular Smooth Muscle Cells," *Circulation* 99 (1999): 1230–1235.

Ivanov, Eugene, "Molecular Mimicry Implicated in Heart Disease," *Molecular Medicine Today* 5, no. 5 (January 1999): 8.

Jarrett, R. J., "Is Insulin Atherogenic?" *Diabetologia* 31 (1988): 71–75.

Jennings, J. R., et al., "Aging or Disease? Cardiovascular Reactivity in Finnish Men over the Middle Years," *Psychology and Aging* 12, no. 2 (June 12, 1997): 225–238.

Jeppesen, Jorgen, et al., "Effects of Low-Fat, High-Carbohydrate Diets on Risk Factors for Ischemic Heart Disease in Postmenopausal Women," *American Journal of Clinical Nutrition* 65 (1997): 1027–1033.

Jevning, R., et al., "The Physiology of Meditation—A Review: A Wakeful Hypometabolic Integrated Response," *Neuroscience and Biobehavioral Reviews* 16, no. 3 (Fall 1992): 415–442.

Jiang, W., et al., "Mental Stress-Induced Myocardial Ischemia and Cardiac Events," *Journal of the American Medical Association* 275, no. 21 (June 5, 1996): 1651–1656.

Johnson, R. W., et al., "Hormones, Lymphohemopoietic Cytokines and the Neuroimmune Axis," *Comparative Biochemistry and Physiology* 116A, no. 3 (1997): 183–201.

Johnston, Colin I., "Renin-Angiotensin System: A Dual Tissue and Hormonal System for Cardiovascular Control," *Journal of Hypertension* 10, suppl. 7 (December 1992): S13–S26.

Jones, Peter J. H., et al., "Dietary Cholesterol Feeding Suppresses Human Cholesterol Synthesis Measured by Deuterium Incorporation and Urinary Mevalonic Acid Levels," *Arteriosclerosis, Thrombosis, and Vascular Biology* 16, no. 10 (October 1996): 1222–1228.

Jourdheuil-Rahmani, D., et al., "Homocysteine Induces Synthesis of a Serine Elastase in Arterial Smooth Muscle Cells from Multi-Organ Donors," *Cardiovascular Research* 34, no. 3 (June 1997): 597–602.

Joven, J., et al., "Concentrations of Lipids and Apolipoproteins in Patients with Clinically Well Controlled Insulin-Dependent and Non-Insulin-Dependent Diabetes," *Clinical Chemistry* 35, no. 5 (May 1989): 813–816.

Kamarck, T. W., et al., "Exaggerated Blood Pressure Responses during Mental Stress Are Associated with Enhanced Carotid Atherosclerosis in Middle-Aged Finnish Men: Findings from the Kuopio Ischemic Heart Disease Study," *Circulation* 96, no. 11 (December 2, 1996): 3842–3848.

Kark, Jeremy D., M.D., et al., "Iraqi Missile Attacks on Israel," *Journal of the American Medical Association* 273, no. 15 (April 19, 1995): 1208–1210.

Katan, Martijn B., "High-Oil Compared with Low-Fat, High-Carbohydrate Diets in the Prevention of Ischemic Heart Disease," *American Journal of Clinical Nutrition* 66 (1997): 974S-979S.

Kelly, Ralph A., et al., "de Modulatione Cordis," *Circulation* 94, no. 10 (1996): 2361–2363.

Kelly, Shana O., et al., "Electron Transfer between Bases in Double Helical DNA," *Science* 283 (January 15, 1999): 375–381.

Kenny, James, "Low-Fat, High-Carbohydrate Diets and Risk Factors for Ischemic Heart Disease," *American Journal of Clinical Nutrition* 66 (1997): 1293–1296.

Kleiner, Kurt, "Hard Hearts Blamed on Misplaced Bone," *New Scientist,* April 4, 1998, 5.

Kloner, R. A., et al. "Population-Based Analysis of the Effect of the Northridge Earthquake on Cardiac Death in Los Angeles County, California," *J Am Coll Cardiol* 30, no. 5 (November 1, 1997): 1174–1180.

Knight, Jonathan, "Cunning Plumbing," *New Scientist,* February 6, 1999, 32–37.

Knuiman, M. W., et al., "Prevalence of Diabetic Complications in Relation to Risk Factors," *Diabetes* 35, no. 12 (December 1986): 1332–1339.

Kok, F. W., et al., "Endocrine and Cardiovascular Responses to a Series of Graded Physical and Psychological Stress Stimuli in Healthy Volunteers," *European Neuropsychopharmacology* 5, no. 4 (December 1995): 515–522.

Komukai, K., et al., "Oscillatory Changes in the Intracellular Ca2+ Concentration in Cardiac Muscles," *Nippon Rinsho* 54, no. 8 (August 1996): 2045–2049.

Koprovicova, J., et al., "Levels of Lp(a) and Apolipoproteins in Vegetarians and Their Informative Value in Hyperlipidemia," *Bratisl Lek Listy* 98, no. 1 (January 1997): 17–21.

Koschinsky, T., et al., "Vascular Growth Factors and the Development of Macrovascular Disease in Diabetes Mellitus," *Horm Metab Res Suppl* 15 (1985): 23–27.

Krauchi, Kurt, et al., "Early Evening Melatonin and S-20098 Advance Circadian Phase and Nocturnal Regulation of Core Body Temperature," *American Journal of Physiology* 272 (April 1997): R1178-R1188.

Krieg, Arthur M., "Human Endogenous Retroviruses," *Science and Medicine,* March/April 1997, 34–43.

Kromhout, Daan, "Fish Consumption and Sudden Cardiac Death," *Journal of the American Medical Association* 279, no. 1 (January 7, 1998): 65–66.

Krucoff, Carol, "Tai Chi As Effective As Aerobics in Study on Hypertension," *Los Angeles Times,* May 11, 1998, S3.

Kunugi, H., et al., "Low Serum Cholesterol in Suicide Attempters," *Biological Psychiatry* 41, no. 2 (January 15, 1997): 196–200.

Kuvin, Jeffrey T., et al., "Infectious Causes of Atherosclerosis," *American Heart Journal* 137, no. 2 (February 1999): 216–226.

Ladwig, K. H., et al., "Extracardiac Contributions to Chest Pain Perception in Patients Six Months After Acute Myocardial Infarction," *American Heart Journal* 137 no. 3 (March 1, 1999): 528–534.

Lakatta, E. G., "Functional Implications of Spontaneous Sarcoplasmic Reticulum Ca2+ Release in the Heart," *Cardiovasc Res* 26, no. 3 (March 1992): 193–214.

Lakatta, E. G., et al., "Spontaneous Myocardial Calcium Oscillations: Are They Linked to Ventricular Fibrillation?" *J Cardiovasc Electrophysiol* 4, no. 4 (August 1993): 473–489.

Leclerc, D., et al., "Cloning and Mapping of a cDNA for Methionine Synthase Reductase, a Flavoprotein Defective in Patients with Homocysteinuria," *Proceedings of the National Academy of Sciences (USA)* 95, no. 6 (March 17, 1998): 3059–3064.

Leddy, John, et al., "Effect of a High or a Low Fat Diet on Cardiovascular Risk Factors in Male and Female Runners," *Medicine and Science in Sports and Exercise* 29 (1997): 17–25.

Leor, Jonathan, M.D., et al., "The Northridge Earthquake As a Trigger for Acute Myocardial Infarction," *Am J Cardiol* 77, no. 14 (June 1, 1996): 1230–1232.

———, "Sudden Cardiac Death Triggered by an Earthquake," *New England Journal of Medicine* 334, no. 7 (February 15, 1996): 413–439.

Levin, Ellis R., M.D., et al., "Natriuretic Peptides," *Mechanisms of Disease* 339, no. 5 (July 30, 1998): 321–328.

Levy, Daniel, M.D., "Rates of Death from Coronary Heart Disease, *New England Journal of Medicine* 339, no. 13 (September 24, 1998): 915–916.

Lewis, Frederick D., et al., "Distance-Dependent Electron Transfer in DNA Hairpins," *Science* 277 (August 1, 1997): 673–676.

Liang, F., et al., "Mechanical Strain Increases Expression of the Brain Natriuretic Peptide Gene in Rat Cardiac Myocytes," *Journal of Biological Chemistry* 272, no. 44 (October 31, 1997): 28050–28056.

Lin, C., et al., "Enhancement of Blue-Light Sensitivity of Arabidopsis Seedlings by a Blue Light Receptor Cryptochrome 2," *Proceedings of the National Academy of Sciences (USA)* 95, no. 5 (March 3, 1998): 2686–2690.

Lissoni, P., et al., "A Study of Heart-Pineal Interactions: Atrial Natriuretic Peptide Response to Melatonin Administration in Healthy Humans," *Journal of Pineal Research* 9, no. 3 (1990): 167–170.

———, "Melatonin Response to Atrial Natriuretic Peptide Administration in Healthy Volunteers," *Journal of Cardiovascular Pharmacology* 16, no. 5 (November 1990): 850–852.

Lockhart, Sybil T., et al., "Nerve Growth Factor Modulates Synaptic Transmission between Sympathetic Neurons and Cardiac Myocytes," *Journal of Neuroscience* 17, no. 24 (December 15, 1997): 9573–9582.

Lopes-Virella, M. F., et al., "Interactions between Bacterial Lipopolysaccharides and Serum Lipoproteins and Their Possible Role in Coronary Heart Disease," *European Heart Journal* 14 (December 1993): 9573–9582.

Lopez-Lopez, Jose Ramon, et al., "Local Calcium Transients Triggered by Single L-Type Calcium Channel Currents in Cardiac Cells," *Science* 268 (May 19, 1995): 1042–1049.

Mackenzie, Dana, "New Clues to Why Size Equals Destiny," *Science* 284 (June 4, 1999): 1607–1609.

MacLean, C. R., et al., "Effects of the Transcendental Meditation Program on Adaptive Mechanisms: Changes in Hormone Levels and Responses to Stress After Four Months of Practice," *Psychoneuroendocrinology* 22, no. 4 (May 1997): 277–295.

Malhotra, Khushbeer, et al., "Putative Blue-Light Photoreceptors from Arabidopsis thaliana and Sinapsis alba with a High Degree of Sequence Homology to DNA Photolyase Contain the Two Photolyase Cofactors but Lack DNA Repair Activity," *Biochemistry* 34, no. 20 (1995): 6892–6899.

Marktl, W., et al., "Melatonin and Coronary Heart Disease," *Wiener Klinische Wochenschrift* 109, no. 18 (October 3, 1997): 747–749.

Marz, Pia, et al., "Sympathetic Neurons Can Produce and Respond to Interleukin-6," *Proceedings of the National Academy of Sciences (USA)* 95, no. 6 (March 17, 1998): 3521–3526.

Mason, Michael, "Could My Blood Pressure Pills Kill Me?" *Health*, November/December 1996, 26.

Mattila, K. J., et al., "Role of Infection As a Risk Factor for Atherosclerosis, Myocardial Infarction, and Stroke," *Clinical Infectious Diseases* 26 (1998): 719–734.

McArthur, John H., et al, "The Two Cultures and the Health Care Revolution," *Journal of the American Medical Association* 277, no. 12 (March 26, 1997): 985–1005.

McCarthy, N. M., et al., "Estrogen Modulation of Oxytocin and Its Relation to Behavior," *Advances in Experimental Medicine and Biology* 395 (1995): 235–245.

———, "An Anxiolytic Action of Oxytocin Is Enhanced by Estrogen in the Mouse," *Physiology and Behavior* 60, no. 5 (November 1996): 1209–1215.

McCully, Kilmer S., "Chemical Pathology of Homocysteine III: Cellular Function and Aging: *Annual of Clinical Lab Scientists* 24, no. 2 (1994): 134–152.

McEvoy, L. M., et al., "Novel Vascular Molecule Involved in Monocyte Adhesion to Aortic Endothelium in Models of Atherogenesis," *J Exp Med* 185, no. 12 (June 16, 1997): 2069–2077.

Miguez, J. M., et al., "Evidence for a Regulatory Role of Melatonin on Serotonin Release and Uptake in the Pineal Gland," *Journal of Neuroendocrinology* 7, no. 12 (December 1995): 949–956.

Minshall, Richard D., et al., "Ovarian Steroid Protection against Coronary Artery Hyperactivity in Rhesus Monkeys," *Journal of Clinical Endocrinology and Metabolism* 83, no. 2 (1998): 649–659.

Miralles, F., et al., "Expression of Nerve Growth Factor and Its High-Affinity Receptor Trk-A in the Rat Pancreas during Embryonic and Fetal Life," *J Endocrinol* 156, no. 3 (March 1998): 431–439.

Miyagawa, Koichi, et al., "Medroxyprogesterone Interferes with Ovarian Steroid Protection against Coronary Vasospasm," *Nature Medicine* 3, no. 3 (March 1997): 324–327.

Modai, I., et al., "Blood Levels of Melatonin, Serotonin, Cortisol, and Prolactin in Relation to the Circadian Rhythm of Platelet Serotonin Uptake," *Psychiatry Res* 43, no. 2 (August 1992): 161–166.

Moller, J. M., et al., "Homocysteine in Greenland Inuits," *Thrombosis Research* 86, no. 4 (May 15, 1997): 333–335.

Much, Marilyn, "The New America: Feeling Fit," *Investors Business Daily,* January 30, 1996, A8.

Munshi, M. N., et al., "Hyperhomocysteinemia Following a Methionine Load in Patients with Non-Insulin-Dependent Diabetes Mellitus and Macrovascular Disease," *Metabolism* 45, no. 1 (January 1996): 133–135.

Murphy, Mark, et al., "Cytokines Which Signal through the LIF Receptor and Their Actions in the Nervous System," *Progress in Neurobiology* 52 (1997): 355–378.

Nagtegaal, E., et al., "Melatonin Secretion and Coronary Heart Disease," *The Lancet* 346, no. 8595 (November 11, 1995): 1299.

Natelson, B. H., et al., "The Pineal Affects Life Span in Hamsters with Heart Disease," *Physiology and Behavior* 62, no. 5 (November 1997): 1059–1064.

Nathan, D. M., "Prevention of Long-Term Complications of Non-Insulin-Dependent Diabetes Mellitus," *Clin Invest Med* 18, no. 4 (August 1995): 332–339.

Nechad, M., et al., "Production of Nerve Growth Factor by Brown Fat in Culture: Relation with the In Vivo Developmental Stage of the Tissue," *Comp Biochem Physiol Comp Physiol* 107, no. 2 (February 1994): 381–388.

Nieminen, M. S., et al., "Infection and Inflammation As Risk Factors for Myocardial Infarction," *European Heart Journal* 14, suppl. K (1993): 12–16.

Nishikimi, T., et al., "Increased Plasma Levels of Adrenomedullin in Patients with Heart Failure," *Journal of the American College of Cardiology* 26, no. 6 (November 15, 1995): 1424–1431.

Nisoli, E., et al., "Expression of Nerve Growth Factor in Brown Adipose Tissue: Implications for Thermogenesis and Obesity," *Endocrinology* 137, no. 2 (February 1996): 495–503.

Nistratova, S. N., et al., "Seasonal Characteristics of the Emergence from Inhibition by and Desensitization to Acetylcholine of the Frog Heart Muscle," *Fiziol Zh SSSR* 74, no. 6 (June 1988): 827–832.

Norrgren, G., et al., "Nerve Growth Factor in Medium Conditioned by Embryonic Chicken Heart Cells," *Int J Dev Neurosci* 4, no. 1 (1986): 41–49.

O'Byrne, S., et al., "Plasma Protein Binding of Lidocaine and Warfarin in Insulin-Dependent and Non-Insulin-Dependent Diabetes Mellitus," *Clin Pharmacokinet* 24, no. 2 (February 1993): 183–186.

Oei, Howard H. H., et al., "Platelet Serotonin Uptake during Myocardial Ischemia," *American Heart Journal* 106 (1983): 1077.

Olcese, J., et al. "Natriuretic Peptides Elevate Cyclic 3, 5-Guanosine Monophosphate Levels in Cultured Rat Pinealocytes: Evidence for Guanylate Cyclase-Linked Membrane Receptors," *Molecular Cellular Endocrinology* 103, nos. 1–2 (July 1994): 95–100.

Olson, Melodie, M.D., et al., "Stress-Induced Immunosuppression and Therapeutic Touch," *Alternative Therapies in Health and Medicine* 3, no. 2 (March 1997): 68–74.

Omenn, Gilbert S., M.D., et al., "Preventing Coronary Heart Disease," *Circulation* 97 (1998): 421–424.

Ornish, Dean, M.D., et al., "Dietary Treatment of Hyperlipidemia," *Journal of Cardiovascular Risk* 1, no. 4 (December 1994): 283–286.

Ornish, Dean, M.D., "Can Lifestyle Changes Reverse Coronary Heart Disease?" *World Review of Nutrition and Dietetics* 72 (1993): 38–48.

Orth-Gomer, K., et al., "Fresh Start After Heart Disease: Changed Life Style Is an Important Part of Rehabilitation," *Lakartidningen* 91, no. 5 (February 2, 1994): 379–384.

Ouchi, Yasuyoshi, et al., "Augmented Contractile Function and Abnormal Ca2+ Handling in the Aorta of Zucker Obese Rats with Insulin Resistance," *Diabetes* 45, suppl. 3 (July 1996): S55–S57.

Pablos, M. I., et al., "Iron Decreases the Nuclear but Not the Cytosolic Content of the Neurohormone Melatonin in Several Tissues in Chicks," *Journal of Cellular Biochemistry* 60, no. 3 (March 1, 1996): 317–321.

Pais, P., et al., "Risk Factors for Acute Myocardial Infarction in Indians: A Case-Control Study," *The Lancet* 348, no. 9024 (August 10, 1996): 358–363.

Palinski, Wulf, et al., "Low-Density Lipoprotein Undergoes Oxidative Modification In Vivo," *Proceedings of the National Academy of Sciences (USA)* 86 (February 1989): 1372–1376.

Pang, C. S., et al., "2-[125I] Iodomelatonin Binding Sites in the Lung and Heart: A Link between the Photoperiodic Signal, Melatonin, and the Cardiopulmonary System," *Biological Signals* 2, no. 4 (July 1993): 228–236.

———, "2-[125I] Iodomelatonin Binding Sites in the Quail Heart: Characteristics, Distribution and Modulation by Guanine Nucleotides and Cations," *Life Sciences* 58, no. 13 (1996): 1047–1057.

Panteghini, M., et al., "Nonensymic Glycation of Apolipoprotein B in Patients with Insulin- and Non-Insulin-Dependent Diabetes Mellitus," *Clin Biochem* 28, no. 6 (December 1995): 587–592.

Pauletto, Paolo, et al., "Blood Pressure and Atherogenic Lipoprotein Profiles of Fish-Diet and Vegetarian Villagers in Tanzania: The Lugalawa Study," *The Lancet* 348 (September 21, 1996): 784–788.

Pauschinger, Matthias, M.D., et al., "Eneroviral RNA Replication in the Myocardium of Patients with Left Ventricular Dysfunction and Clinically Suspected Myocarditis," *Circulation* 99 (1999): 889–895.

Pennica, D., et al., "Cardiotrophin-1, a Cytokine Present in Embryonic Muscle, Supports Long-Term Survival of Spinal Motoneurons," *Neuron* 17, no. 1 (July 1996): 63–74.

————, "Human Cardiotrophin-1: Protein and Gene Structure, Biological and Binding Activities, and Chromosomal Localization," *Cytokine* 8, no. 3 (March 1996): 183–189.

Pilgeram, L., "Perspective: A Mechanism Underlying Homocysteinemia and Increased Risk of Coronary Artery and Cerebrovascular Disease," *Circulation* 94, no. 11 (December 1, 1996): 2990.

Pinkney, Jonathan H., et al., "Endothelial Dysfunction: Cause of the Insulin Resistance Syndrome," *Diabetes* 46, suppl. 2 (September 1997): S9-S13.

Polak, M., et al., "Nerve Growth Factor Induces Neuron-Like Differentiation of an Insulin-Secreting Pancreatic Beta Cell Line," *Proceedings of the National Academy of Sciences (USA)* 90, no. 12 (June 15, 1993): 5781–5785.

Poon, M., et al., "Apolipoprotein(a) Induces Monocyte Chemotactic Activity in Human Vascular Endothelial Cells," *Circulation* 96, no. 8 (October 21, 1997): 2514–2519.

Press, Raymond I., et al., "The Effect of Chromium Picolinate on Serum Cholesterol and Apolipoprotein Fractions in Human Subjects," *Western Journal of Medicine* 152 (January 1990): 41–45.

Proebstle, T., et al., "Recombinant Interleukin-2 Acts Like a Class 1 Antiarrhythmic Drug on Human Cardiac Sodium Channels," *European Journal of Physiology* 429, no. 4 (February 1995): 462–469.

Putsep, K., et al., "Antibacterial Peptide from H. pylori," *Nature* 398 (April 22, 1999): 671–672.

Pyorala, Marja, M.D., et al., "Hyperinsulinemia Predicts Coronary Heart Disease Risk in Healthy Middle-Aged Men," *Circulation* 98 (1998): 398–404.

Raloff, J., "Hormone Therapy: Issues of the Heart," *Science* 151 (March 8, 1997): 140.

Rao, G. M., "Oxytocin Induces Intimate Behaviors," *Indian Journal of Medical Sciences* 49, no. 11 (November 1995): 261–266.

Ray, B. K., et al., "Induction of Serum Amyloid A (SAA) Gene by SAA-Activating Sequence-Binding Factor (SAF) in Monocyte/Macrophage Cells: Evidence for a Functional Synergy between SAF and Sp1," *Journal of Biological Chemistry* 272, no. 46 (November 14, 1997): 28948–28953.

Reaven, Gerald M., M.D., et al., "Effects of Low-Fat, High-Carbohydrate Diets on Risk Factors for Ischemic Heart Disease in Postmenopausal Women," *American Journal of Clinical Nutrition* 65 (1997): 1027–1033.

Reaven, Gerald M., M.D., "Syndrome X: Past, Present, and Future," *Clinical Research in Diabetes and Obesity* 2 (1995): 357–382.

Reaven, Peter, et al., "Effects of Oleate-Rich and Linoleate-Rich Diets on the Susceptibility of Low Density Lipoprotein to Oxidative Modification in Mildly Hypercholesterolemic Subjects," *Journal of Clinical Investigation* 91 (February 1993): 668–676.

Regland, B., et al., "Homocysteinemia and Schizophrenia As a Case of Methylation Deficiency," *Journal of Neural Transmission* 98, no. 2 (1994): 143–152.

————, "Homocysteinemia Is a Common Feature of Schizophrenia," *Journal of Neural Transmission* 100, no. 2 (1995): 165–169.

Reiter, R. J., et al., "Tryptophan Administration Inhibits Nocturnal N-acetyltransferase Activity and Melatonin Content in the Rat Pineal Gland: Evidence That Serotonin Modulates Melatonin Production via a Receptor-Mediated Mechanism," *Neuroendocrinology* 52, no. 3 (September 1990): 291–296.

———, "Attenuated Nocturnal Rise in Pineal and Serum Melatonin in a Genetically Cardiomyopathic Syrian Hamster with a Deficient Calcium Pump," *Journal of Pineal Research* 11, nos. 3–4 (October/November 1991): 156–162.

Remme, W. J., et al., "Neurohumoral Activation during Acute Myocardial Ischaemia: Effects of ACE Inhibition," *European Heart Journal* 11, suppl. B (April 1990): 162–171.

Robbins, Mark, "All Stressed Out," *Nature* 389 (September 25, 1997): 331–332.

Robillon, J. F., et al., "Type I Diabetes Mellitus and Homocysteine," *Diabete et Metabolisme* 20, no. 5 (September 1994): 494–496.

Robinson, Killian, M.D., et al., "Low Circulating Folate and Vitamin B$_6$ Concentrations: Risk Factors for Stroke, Peripheral Vascular Disease, and Coronary Artery Disease," *Circulation* 97 (1998): 437–443.

Robledo, O., et al., "Hepatocyte-Derived Cell Lines Express a Functional Receptor for Cardiotrophin-1," *European Cytokine Network* 8, no. 3 (September 1997): 245–252.

———, "Regulation of Interleukin-6 Expression by Cardiotrophin-1," *Cytokine* 9, no. 9 (September 1997): 666–671.

———, "Signaling of the Cardiotrophin-1 Receptor: Evidence for a Third Receptor Component," *Journal of Biological Chemistry* 272, no. 8 (February 21, 1997): 4855–4863.

Rosenbaum, T., et al., "Pancreatic Beta Cells Synthesize and Secrete Nerve Growth Factor," *Proceedings of the National Academy of Sciences (USA)* 95, no. 13 (June 23, 1998): 7784–7788.

Ross, Russell, "The Pathogenesis of Atherosclerosis: A Perspective for the 1990s," *Nature* 362 (April 29, 1993): 801–809.

———, "Cell Biology of Atherosclerosis," *Annual Review of Physiology* 57 (1995): 791–804.

Rozanski, A., et al., "Mental Stress and the Induction of Silent Myocardial Ischemia in Patients with Coronary Artery Disease," *New England Journal of Medicine* 318, no. 16 (April 21, 1998): 1005–1012.

Rubin, Rita, "Why Low Cholesterol Should Be Lower," *U.S. News and World Report*, (May 29, 1995): 65.

Saikku, Pekka, M.D., et al., "Chronic Chlamydia pneumoniae Infection As a Risk Factor for Coronary Heart Disease in the Helsinki Heart Study," *Annals of Internal Medicine* 116 (1992): 273–278.

Sanguinetti, M. C., et al., "Coassembly of KvLQT1 and minK (IsK) Proteins to Form Cardiac I ks Potassium Channel," *Nature* 384 (November 7, 1996): 80–82.

Savitz, David A., et al., "Magnetic Field Exposure and Cardiovascular Disease Mortality among Electric Utility Workers," *American Journal of Epidemiology* 149, no. 2 (1999): 135–142.

Schmidt, T., et al., "Changes in Cardiovascular Risk Factors and Hormones during a Comprehensive Residential Three-Month Kriya Yoga Training and Vegetarian Nutrition," *Acta Physiol Scand Suppl* 640 (1997): 158–162.

Schlame, Michael, et al., "Solubilization, Purification, and Characterization of Cardiolipin Synthase from Rat Liver Mitochondria," *Journal of Biological Chemistry* 266, no. 33 (1991): 22938–22403.

Schlussel, E., et al., "Homocysteine-Induced Oxidative Damage: Mechanisms and Possible Roles in Neurodegenerative and Atherogenic Processes," *Journal of Biosciences* 50, nos. 9–10 (September/October 1995): 699–707.

Seckl, Jonathan R., et al., "Early Life Events and Later Development of Ischaemic Heart Disease," *The Lancet* 342 (November 13, 1993): 1236.

Segerstrom, S. C., et al., "Relationship of Worry to Immune Sequelae of the Northridge Earthquake," *J Behav Med* 21, no. 5 (October 1998): 433–450.

Semenkovich, Clay F., et al., "The Mystery of Diabetics and Atherosclerosis," *Diabetes* 46 (March 1997): 327–334.

Sgoutas-Emch, Sandra A., et al., "The Effects of an Acute Psychological Stressor on Cardiovascular, Endocrine, and Cellular Immune Response: A Prospective Study of Individuals High and Low in Heart Rate Reactivity," *Psychophysiology* 31 (1994): 264–271.

Sheline, Yvette I., et al., "How Safe Are Serotonin Reuptake Inhibitors for Depression in Patients with Coronary Heart Disease?" *American Journal of Medicine* 102, no. 1 (January 1997): 54–59.

Shimizu, K., et al., "Sympathetic Dysfunction in Heart Failure," *Bailieres Clinical Endocrinology and Metabolism* 7, no. 2 (April 1993): 439–463.

Simon, Dominique, et al., "Association between Plasma Total Testosterone and Cardiovascular Risk Factors in Healthy Adult Men: The Telecom Study," *Journal of Clinical Endocrinology and Metabolism* 82, no. 2 (1997): 682–685.

Skafar, Debra F., et al., "Female Sex Hormones and Cardiovascular Disease in Women," *Journal of Clinical Endocrinology and Metabolism* 82, no. 12 (1997): 3913–3918.

Snyman, C., et al., "Cellular Localization of Atrial Natriuretic Peptide and Tissue Kallilrein in the Human Hypothalamus," *Brazilian Journal of Medical and Biological Research* 27, no. 8 (August 1994): 1877–1883.

Solem, M. L., et al., "Modulation of Cardiac Ca2+ Channels by IGF1," *Biochemical and Biophysical Research Communications* 252, no. 1 (November 9, 1998): 151–155.

Solomon, G. F., et al., "Shaking Up Immunity: Psychological and Immunologic Changes After a Natural Disaster," *Psychosomatic Medicine* 59, no. 2 (March/April 1997): 114–127.

Sothern, R. B., et al., "Circadian Relationships between Circulating Atrial Natriuretic Peptides and Serum Sodium and Chloride and Healthy Humans," *Am J Nephrol* 16, no. 6 (1996): 462–470.

Sowers, James R., "Effects of Insulin and IGF-1 on Vascular Smooth Muscle Glucose and Cation Metabolism," *Diabetes* 45, suppl. 3 (July 1996): S47-S58.

Stacey, Michelle, "The Fall and Rise of Kilmer McCully," *The New York Times Magazine*, August 10, 1997, 25–29.

Stabler, Sally P., et al., "Elevation of Serum Cystathionine Levels in Patients with Cobalamin and Folate Deficiency," *Blood* 81, no. 12 (1993): 3404–3413.

Stampfer, Meir J., et al., "A Prospective Study of Plasma Homocysteine and Risk of Myocardial Infarction in U.S. Physicians," *Journal of the American Medical Association* 268, no. 7 (August 19, 1992): 877–881.

————, "Vitamin E Consumption and the Risk of Coronary Disease in Women," *New England Journal of Medicine* 328, no. 20 (May 20, 1993): 1444–1449.

Steinberg, Daniel, "Antioxidants and Atherosclerosis: A Current Assessment," *Circulation* 84, no. 3 (September 1991): 1420–1425.

Stern, M. D., et al., "Spontaneous Calcium Release from the Sarcoplasmic Reticulum in Myocardial Cells: Mechanisms and Consequences," *Cell Calcium* 9, nos. 5–6 (December 1988): 247–256.

Stone, Munshi M. N., et al., "Hyperhomocysteinemia Following a Methionine Load in Patients with Non-Insulin-Dependent Diabetes Mellitus and Macrovascular Disease," *Metabolism* 45, no. 1 (January 1996): 133–135.

Stout, Robert W., M.D., "Hyperinsulinemia and Atherosclerosis," *Diabetes* 45, suppl. 3 (1996): S45-S46.

————, "Insulin and Atheroma," *Diabetes* 13, no. 6 (1990): 631–654.

Strachan, David P., et al., "Relation of Chlamydia pneumoniae Serology to Mortality and Incidence of Ischaemic Heart Disease over 13 Years in the Caerphilly Prospective Heart Disease Study," *British Medical Journal* 318 (April 17, 1999): 1035–1040.

Sudhir, Krishnakutty, et al., "Endothelial Dysfunction in a Man with Disruptive Mutation in Oestrogen-Receptor Gene," *The Lancet* 349 (April 19, 1997): 1146–1147.

Sun, Y., et al., "Angiotensin II, Transforming Growth Factor-Beta 1 and Repair in the Infarcted Heart," *J Mol Cell Cardiol* 30, no. 8 (August 1998): 1559–1569.

Sung, C. P., et al., "Neuropeptide Y Upregulates the Adhesiveness of Human Endothelial Cells for Leukocytes," *Circ Res* 68, no. 1 (January 1991): 314–318.

Tamura, K., et al., "Chronotherapy for Coronary Heart Disease," *Japanese Heart Journal* 38, no. 5 (September 1997): 607–616.

Tavani, A., et al., "Margarine Intake and Risk of Nonfatal Acute Myocardial Infarction in Italian Women," *European Journal of Clinical Nutrition* 51, no. 1 (January 1997): 30–32.

Torgano, Giuseppe, M.D., et al., "Treatment of Helicobacter pylori and Chlamydia pneumoniae Infections Decreases Fibrinogen Plasma Level in Patients with Ischemic Heart Disease," *Circulation* 99 (1999): 1555–1559.

Tsutamoto, T., et al., "Interleukin-6 Spillover in the Peripheral Circulation Increases with the Severity of Heart Failure, and the High Plasma Level of Interleukin-6 Is an Important Prognostic Predictor in Patients with Congestive Heart Failure," *Journal of the American College of Cardiology* 31, no. 2 (February 1998): 391–398.

Tung, P., et al., "Nephropathy in Non-Insulin-Dependent Diabetes Mellitus," *Am J Med* 85, no. 5A (November 28, 1988): 131–136.

Tuomilehto, J., et al., "Effects of Calcium-Channel Blockade in Older Patients with Diabetes and Systolic Hypertension," *New England Journal of Medicine* 340, no. 9 (March 4, 1999): 677–684.

Tuomisto, Jouko, et al., "Decreased Uptake of 5-Hydroxytryptamine in Blood Platelets from Depressed Patients," *Nature* 262, no. 5569 (August 12, 1976): 596–598.

Ukkola, O., et al., "Apolipoprotein E Phenotype Is Related to Macro- and Microangiopathy in Patients with Non-Insulin-Dependent Diabetes Mellitus," *Atherosclerosis* 101, no. 1 (June 1993): 9–15.

Uvnas-Moberg, K., "Oxytocin Linked Antistress Effects—The Relaxation and Growth Response," *Acta Physiologica Scandinavica* 640, suppl. (1997): 38–42.

———, "Physiological and Endocrine Effects of Social Contact," *Annals of the New York Academy of Sciences* 807 (January 15, 1997): 146–163.

Van Cauter, Eve, et al., "Modulation of Glucose Regulation and Insulin Secretion by Circadian Rhythmicity and Sleep," *Journal of Clinical Investigation* 88 (September 1991): 934–942.

Van Den Berg, Maarten P., et al., "Atrial Natriuretic Peptide in Patients with Heart Failure and Chronic Atrial Fibrillation: Role of Duration of Atrial Fibrillation," *American Heart Journal* 135, no. 2, part 1 (February 1998): 242–244.

Van Der Put, N. M., et al., "Sequence Analysis of the Coding Region of Human Methionine Synthase: Relevance to Hyperhomocysteinaemia in Neural-Tube Defects and Vascular Disease," *QJM* 90, no. 8 (August 1997): 511–517.

Van Eck, M., et al., "The Effects of Perceived Stress, Traits, Mood States, and Stressful Daily Events on Salivary Cortisol," *Psychosomatic Medicine* 58, no. 5 (September 1996): 447–458.

Vesely, D. L., et al., "Circadian Relationships between Circulating Atrial Natriuretic Peptides and Serum Calcium and Phosphate in Healthy Humans," *Metabolism* 45, no. 8 (August 1996): 1021–1028.

Vogel, John H. K., M.D., "Learning the Signs of Heart Attack," *Santa Barbara News Press,* November 6, 1997, A13.

Wang, Hong, et al., "Inhibition of Growth and p21 Methylation in Vascular Endothelial Cells by Homocysteine but Not Cysteine," *Journal of Biological Chemistry* 272, no. 40 (October 3, 1997): 25380–25385.

Wang, S. Q., et al., "Dependence of Myocardial Hypothermia Tolerance on Sources of Activator Calcium," *Cryobiology* 35, no. 3 (November 1997): 193–200.

Warren, W. S., et al., "The Pineal Gland: Photoreception and Coupling of Behavioral, Metabolic, and Cardiovascular Circadian Outputs," *Journal of Biological Rhythms* 10, no. 1 (March 1995): 64–79.

———, "The Suprachiasmatic Nucleus Controls the Circadian Rhythm of Heart Rate via the Sympathetic Nervous System," *Physiology and Behavior* 55, no. 6 (June 1994): 1091–1099.

Watanabe, Y., et al., "Cross-Spectral Coherence between Geomagnetic Disturbance and Human Cardiovascular Variables at Non-Societal Frequencies," *Chronobiologia* 21, nos. 3–4 (July–December 1994): 265–272.

Webber, E. T., et al., "Nitric Oxide Synthase Inhibitor Blocks Light-Induced Phase Shifts of the Circadian Activity Rhythm, but Not c-Fos Expression in the Suprachiasmatic Nucleus of the Syrian Hamster," *Brain Research* 692, nos. 1–2 (September 18, 1995): 137–142.

Wehr, Thomas A., "Melatonin and Seasonal Rhythms," *Journal of Biological Rhythms* 12, no. 6 (December 1997): 518–527.

Welch, George N., M.D., et al., "Homocysteine and Atherothrombosis," *New England Journal of Medicine* 338, no. 15 (April 9, 1998): 1042–1050.

———, "Homocysteine-Induced Nitric Oxide Production in Vascular Smooth-Muscle Cells by NF-kappa B-Dependent Transcriptional Activation of Nos2," *Proc Assoc Am Physicians* 110, no. 1 (January 1998): 22–31.

"Weight Control: What Works and Why," *Mayo Clinic Health Letter,* suppl. (1994), 1–8.

Weiss, R. J., et al., "Platelet Activation and Myocardial Ischemia," *New England Journal of Medicine* 302, no. 23 (June 5, 1980): 1312.

Werner, O. R., et al., "Long-Term Endocrinologic Changes in Subjects Practicing the Transcendental Meditation and TM-Sidhi Program," *Psychosomatic Medicine* 48, nos. 1–2 (January/February 1986): 59–66.

Whitworth, J. A., et al., "Mechanisms of Cortisol-Induced Hypertension in Humans," *Steroids* 60, no. 1 (January 1995): 76–80.

Wick, M. J., et al., "Molecular Cross Talk between Epithelial Cells and Pathogenic Microorganisms," *Cell* 67, no. 4 (November 15, 1991): 651–659.

Wiegant, F. A. C., et al., "Stimulation of Cellular Self-Recovery by Application of the Similia Principle," *Alternative Therapies* 3, no. 2 (March 1997): 105–106.

Witt, D. M., "Oxytocin and Rodent Sociosexual Responses: From Behavior to Gene Expression," *Neuroscience and Biobehavioral Reviews* 19, no. 2 (Summer 1995): 315–324.

———, "Regulatory Mechanisms of Oxytocin-Mediated Sociosexual Behavior," *Annals of the New York Academy of Sciences* 807 (January 15, 1997): 287–301.

Wolfensberger, T. J., et al., "Natriuretic Peptides and Their Receptors in Human Neural Retina and Retinal Pigment Epithelium," *German Journal of Ophthalmology* 3, nos. 4–5 (August 1994): 248–252.

Woolf, Neville, et al., "Arterial Plaque and Thrombus Formation," *Scientific American Science and Medicine* (September/October 1994), 38–47.

Yanagimoto, M., et al., "Afferents Originating from the Dorsal Penile Nerve Excite Oxytocin Cells in the Hypothalamic Paraventricular Nucleus of the Rat," *Brain Research* 733, no. 2 (September 16, 1996): 292–296.

Young, L. J., et al., "Gene Targeting Approaches to Neuroendocrinology: Oxytocin, Maternal Behavior, and Affiliation," *Hormones and Behavior* 31, no. 3 (June 1997): 221–231.

Yudkin, John S., M.D., et al., "The Relationship of Concentrations of Insulin and Proinsulin-Like Molecules with Coronary Heart Disease Prevalence and Incidence," *Diabetes Care* 20, no. 7 (July 1997): 1093–1100.

Yudkin, John S., M.D., "Sucrose, Coronary Heart Disease, Diabetes, and Obesity: Do Hormones Provide a Link?" *American Heart Journal* 115 (February 1988): 493–498.

Zhalko-Tytarenko, O. V., et al., "The Investigation of the Long-Range Water Memory of Homeopathic Solutions Using NMR Relaxation," *Alternative Therapies* 3, no. 2 (March 1997): 106–107.

Zhong, H. H., et al., "Effects of Synergistic Signaling by Phytochrome A and Cryptochrome 1 on Circadian Clock-Regulated Catalase Expression," *Plant Cell* 9, no. 6 (June 1997): 947–955.

Zhou, Y. F., et al., "Association between Prior Cytomegalovirus Infection and the Risk of Restenosis After Coronary Atherectomy," *New England Journal of Medicine* 335, no. 9 (August 29, 1996): 624–630.

Ziegler, Dan, M.D., et al., "Effects of Treatment with the Antioxidant a-Lipoic Acid on Cardiac Autonomic Neuropathy in NIDDM Patients," *Diabetes Care* 20, no. 3 (March 1997): 369–373.

——, "A-Lipoic Acid in the Treatment of Diabetic Oeripheral and Cardiac Autonomic Neuropathy," *Diabetes* 46, suppl. 2 (September 1997): S62-S66.

Zureik, Mahmoud, et al., "Serum Cholesterol Concentration and Death from Suicide in Men: Paris Prospective Study I," *BMJ* 313 (September 14, 1996): 648–651.

Chapter Eight: Ten Seconds to Self-Destruct

Aakvaag, A., et al., "Growth Control of Human Mammary Cancer Cells in Culture: Effect of Estradiol and Growth Factors in Serum-Containing Medium," *Cancer Research* 50, no. 24 (December 15, 1990): 7806–7810.

Abbassy, A. A., et al., "Hyperprolactinaemia and Male Infertility," *Br J Urol* 54, no. 3 (June 1982): 305–307.

Ahmed, S. Ansar, et al., "Genetic Regulation of Testosterone-Induced Immune Suppression," *Cellular Immunology* 104 (1987): 91–98.

AinMelk, Y., et al., "Bromocriptine Therapy in Oligozoospermic Infertile Men," *Arch Androl* 8, no. 2 (March 1982): 135–141.

Alanko, A., et al., "Significance of Estrogen and Progesterone Receptors, Disease-Free Interval, and Site of First Metastasis on Survival of Breast Cancer Patients," *Cancer* 56, no. 7 (October 1, 1985): 1696–11700.

Ali, I. U., et al., "Lack of Evidence for the Prognostic Significance of c-erbB-2 Amplification in Human Breast Carcinoma," *Oncogene Res* 3, no. 2 (September 1988): 139–146.

Altman, Lawrence K., M.D., "Good News from the Front in the War against Cancer," *The New York Times,* May 26, 1998, B10.

Ambrosi, B., et al., "Effect of Bromocriptine and Metergoline in the Treatment of Hyperprolactinaemic States," *Acta Endocrinol (Copenh)* 100, no. 1 (May 1982): 10–17.

Ambrosini, Grazia, et al., "A Novel Anti-Apoptosis Gene, Survivin, Expressed in Cancer and Lymphoma," *Nature Medicine* 3, no. 8 (August 1997): 917–921.

Ames, Bruce N., et al., "The Causes and Prevention of Cancer," *Proceedings of the National Academy of Sciences (USA)* 92 (June 1995): 5258–5265.

Anderson, R. A., et al., "The Effects of Exogenous Testosterone on Sexuality and Mood of Normal Men," *Journal of Clinical Endocrinology and Metabolism* 75, no. 6 (December 1992): 1503–1507.

Ando, Sebastiano, et al., "Role of IRS-1 Signaling in Insulin-Induced Modulation of Estrogen Receptors in Breast Cancer Cells," *Biochemical and Biophysical Research Communications* 253 (1998): 315–319.

Antoniotti, S., et al., "Oestrogen and Epidermal Growth Factor Down-Regulate erbB-2 Oncogene Protein Expression in Breast Cancer Cells by Different Mechanisms," *British Journal of Cancer* 70, no. 6 (December 1994): 1095–1101.

————, "Tamoxifen Up-Regulates c-erbB-2 Expression in Oestrogen-Responsive Breast Cancer Cells In Vitro," *Eur J Cancer* 28, nos. 2–3 (1992): 318–321.

Aoyagi, H., "The Diverse Effects of Hormonal Therapeutic Agents on the Proliferation of Human Breast Cancer Cell Lines, MCF-7 and Its Variants," *Nippon Naibunpi Gakkai Zasshi, Folia Endocrinologica Japonica* 71, no. 1 (January 20, 1995): 39–52.

Arteaga, C. L., "Interference of the IGF System As a Strategy to Inhibit Breast Cancer Growth," *Breast Cancer Research and Treatment* 22, no. 1 (1992): 101–106.

Bammann, B. L., et al., "Total and Free Testosterone during Pregnancy," *Am J Obstet Gynecol* 137, no. 2 (June 1980): 293–298.

Bancroft, J., et al., "The Effects of Bromocriptine on the Sexual Behaviour of Hyperpro-lactinaemic Man: A Controlled Case Study," *Clin Endocrinol (Oxf)* 21, no. 2 (August 1984): 131–137.

Bartsch, C., et al., "Stage-Dependent Depression of Melatonin in Patients with Primary Breast Cancer: Correlation with Prolactin, Thyroid Stimulating Hormone, and Steroid Receptors," *Cancer* 64, no. 2 (July 15, 1989): 426–433.

Barr, S. I., et al., "Vegetarian vs. Nonvegetarian Diets, Dietary Restraint, and Subclinical Ovulatory Disturbances: Prospective Six-Month Study," *American Journal of Clinical Nutrition* 60, no. 6 (December 1994): 887–894.

Bechet, D., "Control of Gene Expression by Steroid Hormones," *Reprod Nutr Dev* 26, no. 5A (1986): 1025–1055.

Behre, H. M., et al., "Prostate Volume in Testosterone-Treated and Untreated Hypogonadal Men in Comparison to Age-Matched Normal Controls," *Clin Endocrinol (Oxf)* 40, no. 3 (March 1994): 341–349.

————, "Long-Term Effect of Testosterone Therapy on Bone Mineral Density in Hypogo-nadal Men," *Journal of Clinical Endocrinology and Metabolism* 82, no. 8 (August 1997): 2386–2390.

Berkhout, Ben, et al., "Identification of an Active Reverse Transcriptase Enzyme Encoded by a Human Endogenous HERV-K Retrovirus," *Journal of Virology* 73, no. 3 (March 1999): 2365–2375.

Berger, G. M., et al., "Marked Hyperinsulinaemia in Postmenopausal, Healthy Indian (Asian) Women," *Diabetic Medicine* 12, no. 9 (September 12, 1995): 788–795.

Berns, E. M., et al., "Prognostic Factors in Human Primary Breast Cancer: Comparison of c-myc and HER2/neu Amplification," *Journal of Steroid Biochemistry and Molecular Biology* 43, nos. 1–3 (September 1992): 13–19.

Bhatavdekar, J. M., et al, "Prognostic Significance of Plasma Prolactin in Breast Cancer: Comparison with the Expression of c-erbB-2 Oncoprotein," *Eur J Surg Oncol* 19, no. 5 (October 1993): 409–413.

Blask, D. E., et al., "Physiological Melatonin Inhibition of Human Breast Cancer Cell Growth In Vitro: Evidence for a Glutathione-Mediated Pathway," *Cancer Res* 57, no. 10 (May 15, 1997): 1909–1914.

————, "Effects of Melatonin on Cancer: Studies on MCF-7 Human Breast Cancer Cells in Culture," *J Neural Transm Suppl* 21 (1986): 433–449.

Bodnar, Andrea G., et al., "Extension of Life Span by Introduction of Telomerase into Normal Human Cells," *Science* 279 (January 16, 1998): 349–352.

Boman, K., M.D., et al., "The Influence of Progesterone and Androgens on the Growth of Endometrial Carcinoma," *Cancer* 71 (1993): 3565–3569.

Born, Jan, et al., "Effects of Sleep and Circadian Rhythm on Human Circulating Immune Cells," *Journal of Immunology* 158 (1997): 4454–4464.

Bridges, Bryn A., "Hypermutation under Stress," *Nature* 387 (June 5, 1997): 557–558.

Brinton, Louise A., "Hormones and Risk of Cancers of the Breast and Ovary," *Cancer Causes and Control* 7 (1996): 569–571.

Brody, Jane E., "Round Three in Cancer Battle: A Five-Year Drug Regimen," *The New York Times,* May 11, 1999, D7.

Brown, W. A., et al., "Serum Testosterone and Sexual Activity and Interest in Men," *Arch Sex Behav* 7, no. 2 (March 1978): 97–103.

Bruning, P. F., et al., "Body Measurements, Estrogen Availability and the Risk of Human Breast Cancer: A Case-Control Study," *International Journal of Cancer* 51 (1992): 14–19.

———, "Insulin Resistance and Breast-Cancer Risk," *International Journal of Cancer* 52, no. 4 (October 21, 1992): 511–516.

Bui, Thong T., et al., "Additional Bacillus Calmette-Guerin Therapy for Recurrent Transitional Cell Carcinoma After an Initial Complete Response," *Urology* 49 (1997): 687–691.

Bunk, Steve, "In Estrogen Research, Challenge Is to Cull Good from Bad," *The Scientist,* March 30, 1998, 10; 13.

Burkitt, Denis, M.D., "An Approach to the Reduction of the Most Common Western Cancers," *Archives of Surgery* 126 (March 1991): 345–347.

Burns-Cox, N., et al., "The Andropause: Fact or Fiction?" *Postgrad Med J* 73, no. 863 (September 1997): 553–556.

Butte, N. F., et al., "Leptin in Human Reproduction: Serum Leptin Levels in Pregnant and Lactating Women," *Journal of Clinical Endocrinology and Metabolism* 82, no. 2 (1997): 585–589.

Buvat, J., "Influence of Primary Hyperprolactinemia on Human Sexual Behavior," *Nouv Presse Med* 11, no. 48 (November 27, 1982): 3561–3563.

Cagnacci, A., et al., "Effects of Low Doses of Transdermal 17 Beta-Estradiol on Carbohydrate Metabolism in Postmenopausal Women," *Journal of Clinical Endocrinology and Metabolism* 74, no. 6 (June 1992): 1396–1400.

———, "Amplification of Pulsatile LH Secretion by Exogenous Melatonin in Women," *Journal of Clinical Endocrinology and Metabolism* 73, no. 1 (1991): 210–212.

Cappelletti, V., et al., "Effect of Progestin Treatment on Estradiol- and Growth Factor-Stimulated Breast Cancer Cell Lines," *Anticancer Research* 15 (November/December 1995): 2551–2555.

Chang, King-Jen, M.D., et al., "Influences of Percutaneous Administration of Estradiol and Progesterone on Human Breast Epithelial Cell Cycle In Vivo," *Fertility and Sterility* 63, no. 4 (April 1996): 785–790.

Chehab, Farid F., et al., "Early Onset of Reproductive Function in Normal Female Mice Treated with Leptin," *Science* 275 (January 3, 1997): 88–90.

Cini, G., et al., "Melatonin's Growth-Inhibitory Effect on Hepatoma AH 130 in the Rat," *Cancer Lett* 125, nos. 1–2 (March 13, 1998): 51–59.

Clarke, R. B., et al., "Type 1 Insulin-Like Growth Factor Receptor Gene Expression in Normal Human Breast Tissue Treated with Oestrogen and Progesterone," *British Journal of Cancer* 75, no. 2 (1997): 251–257.

Cohen, I. R., et al., "Effects of Estradiol on the Diurnal Rhythm of Serotonin Activity in Microdissected Brain Areas of Ovariectomized Rats," *Endocrinology* 122, no. 6 (June 1988): 2619–2625.

Cohen, Joel E., "Speculation on Population, Matters of Life and Death: Perspectives on Public Health, Molecular Biology, Cancer, and the Prospects for the Human Race," *Nature* 387 (June 5, 1997): 565–566.

Cohen, Michael, et al., "Hypotheses: Melatonin/Steroid Combination Contraceptives Will Prevent Breast Cancer," *Breast Cancer Research and Treatment* 33 (1995): 257–264.

Colditz, Graham A., M.D., "Postmenopausal Estrogens and Breast Cancer," *J Sos Gynecol Invest* 3, no. 2 (March/April 1996): 50–56.

Corpas, Emiliano, et al., "Human Growth Hormone and Human Aging," *Endocrine Reviews* 14, no. 1 (1993): 20–38.

Cos, S., et al., "Melatonin Modulates Growth Factor Activity in MCF-7 Human Breast Cancer Cells," *Journal of Pineal Research* 17, no. 1 (August 1994): 25–32.

———, "Melatonin Inhibition of MCF-7 Human Breast Cancer Cell Growth: Influence of Cell Proliferation Rate," *Cancer Lett* 93, no. 2 (July 13, 1995): 207–212.

———, "Melatonin Inhibits DNA Synthesis in MCF-7 Human Breast Cancer Cells In Vitro," *Life Sci* 58, no. 26 (May 24, 1996): 2447–2453.

Crespo, D., et al., "Interaction between Melatonin and Estradiol on Morphological and Morphometric Features of MCF-7 Human Breast Cancer Cells," *Journal of Pineal Research* 16, no. 4 (May 1994): 215–222.

Crook, David, Ph.D., et al., "Comparison of Transdermal and Oral Estrogen-Progestin Replacement Therapy: Effects of Serum Lipids and Lipoproteins," *Am J Obstet Gynecol* 166 (1992): 950–955.

Daan, S., et al., "An Effect of Castration and Testosterone Replacement on a Circadian Pacemaker in Mice (Mus musculus)," *Proceedings of the National Academy of Sciences (USA)* 72 (1975): 3744–3747.

Danforth, D. N., Jr., et al., "Melatonin Increases Oestrogen Receptor Binding Activity of Human Breast Cancer Cells," *Nature* 305, no. 5932 (September 22–28, 1983): 323–325.

Darrow, Janet M., et al., "Influence of Photoperiod and Gonadal Steroids on Hibernation in the European Hamster," *J Comp Physiol A* 163 (1988): 339–348.

Dati, C., et al., "C-erbB-2 and Ras Expression Levels in Breast Cancer Are Correlated and Show a Co-Operative Association with Unfavorable Clinical Outcome," *Int J Cancer* 47, no. 6 (April 1, 1991): 833–838.

———, "Inhibition of c-erbB-2 Oncogene Expression by Estrogens in Human Breast Cancer Cells," *Oncogene* 5, no. 7 (July 1990): 1001–1006.

————, "Expression of the erbB-2 Proto-Oncogene during Differentiation of the Mammary Gland in the Rat," *Cell Tissue Res* 285, no. 3 (September 1996): 403–410.

Dauchy, R. T., et al., "Light Contamination during the Dark Phase in 'Photoperiodically Controlled' Animal Rooms: Effect on Tumor Growth and Metabolism in Rats," *Laboratory Animal Sciences* 47, no. 5 (October 1997): 511–518.

Davidson, D. W., et al., "Increasing Circulating Androgens with Oral Testosterone Undecanoate in Eugonadal Men," *Journal of Steroid Biochemistry and Molecular Biology* 26, no. 6 (June 1987): 713–715.

Davidson, Michael H., et al., "Weight Control and Risk Factor Reduction in Obese Subjects Treated for Two Years with Orlistat," *Journal of the American Medical Association* 281, no. 3 (1999): 235–242.

Davis, S. N., et al., "Effects of Physiological Hyperinsulinemia on Counterregulatory Response to Prolonged Hypoglycemia in Normal Humans," *American Journal of Physiology* 267, no. 3 (September 1994): E402-E410.

Daws, M. R., et al., "Paradoxical Effects of Overexpression of the Type I Insulin-Like Growth Factor (IGF) Receptor on the Responsiveness of Human Breast Cancer Cells to IGFs and Estradiol," *Endocrinology* 137, no. 4 (April 1996): 1177–1186.

Demisch, K., et al., "Distribution of Testosterone in Plasma Proteins during Replacement Therapy with Testosterone Enanthate in Patients Suffering from Hypogonadism," *Andrologia* 15 (1983): 536–541.

Denner, Larry A., et al., "Regulation of Progesterone Receptor-Mediated Transcription by Phosphorylation," *Science* 250 (December 21, 1990): 1740–1743.

Denti, L., et al., "Effects of Aging on Dehydroepiandrosterone Sulfate in Relation to Fasting Insulin Levels and Body Composition Assessed by Bioimpedance Analysis," *Metabolism* 46, no. 7 (July 1997): 826–832.

De Pergola, G., et al., "Insulin-Like Growth Factor-1 (IGF-1) and Dehydroepiandrosterone Sulphate in Obese Women," *International Journal of Obesity and Related Metabolic Disorders* 17, no. 8 (August 1993): 481–483.

De Waard, F., et al., "A Unifying Concept of the Aetiology of Breast Cancer," *International Journal of Cancer* 41 (1988): 666–669.

Dineen, Sean, "Metabolic Effects of the Nocturnal Rise in Cortisol on Carbohydrate Metabolism in Normal Humans," *Journal of Clinical Investigation* 92, no. 5 (November 1993): 2283–2290.

Dufau, M. L., et al., "Mode of Secretion of Bioactive Luteinizing Hormone in Man," *Journal of Clinical Endocrinology and Metabolism* 57 (1983): 993–1000.

Earnest, D. J., et al., "Immortal Time: Circadian Clock Properties of Rat Suprachiasmatic Cell Lines," *Science* 283, no. 5402 (January 29, 1999): 693–695.

Ehrhard, P. B., et al., "Expression of Functional trk Protooncogene in Human Monocytes," *Proceedings of the National Academy of Sciences (USA)* 90, no. 12 (June 15, 1993): 5423–5427.

El-Tanani, M. K., et al., "Interaction between Estradiol and Growth Factors in the Regulation of Specific Gene Expression in MCF-7 Human Breast Cancer Cells," *Journal of Steroid Biochemistry and Molecular Biology* 60, nos. 5–6 (March 1997): 269–276.

————, "Insulin/IGF-1 Modulation of the Expression of Two Estrogen-Induced Genes in MCF-7 Cells," *Molecular and Cellular Endocrinology* 121, no. 1 (July 23, 1996): 29–35.

Esposti, D., et al., "The Pineal Gland-Opioid System Relation: Melatonin-Naloxone Interactions in Regulating GH and LH Releases in Man," *J Endocrinol Invest* 11 (1988): 103–106.

Evan, Gerard, "Cancer: A Matter of Life and Cell Death," *International Journal of Cancer* 71 (1997): 709–711.

Evans, D. G. R., et al., "Familial Breast Cancer," *BMJ* 308 (January 15, 1994): 183–187; 716.

Festing, Michael F. W., "Fat Rats and Carcinogenesis Screening," *Nature* 388 (July 24, 1997): 321–322.

Fisher, Bernard, et al., "Tamoxifen and Chemotherapy for Lymph Node-Negative, Estrogen Receptor-Positive Breast Cancer," *Journal of the National Cancer Institute* 89, no. 22 (November 19, 1997): 1673–1682.

Fletcher, Suzanne W., "Whither Scientific Deliberation in Health Policy Recommendations?" *New England Journal of Medicine* 336, no.16 (April 17, 1997): 1180–1183.

Flores, Juan Pablo, M.D., et al., "Elevated Interleukin-6 Levels in the Ovarian Hyperstimulation Syndrome: Ovarian Immmunohistochemical Localization of Interleukin-6 Signal," *Obstet Gynecol* 87, no. 4 (April 1996): 581–587.

Formby, Bent, "Immunologic Response in Pregnancy," *Endocrinology and Metabolism Clinics of North America* 24, no. 1 (March 1995): 187–205.

Formby, Bent, et al., "Progesterone Inhibits Growth and Induces Apoptosis in Breast Cancer Cells: Inverse Effects on Bcl-2 and p53," *Ann Clin Lab Sci* 28, no. 6 (November 1998): 360–369.

Fornander, T., et al., "Oestrogenic Effects of Adjuvant Tamoxifen in Postmenopausal Breast Cancer," *European Journal of Cancer* 29A, no. 4 (1993): 497–500.

Fossati, R., et al., "Cytotoxic and Hormonal Treatment for Metastatic Breast Cancer: A Systematic Review of Published Randomized Trials Involving 31,510 Women," *Journal of Clinical Oncology* 16, no. 10 (October 1998): 3439–3460.

Fox, Arnold, "Menopause Matters to Men, Too," *Doctor's Prescription for Healthy Living* 2, no. 3 (1998): 1; 14.

Franeschi, Silvia, et al., "Intake of Macronutrients and Risk of Breast Cancer," *The Lancet* 347 (May 18, 1996): 1352–1346.

Franschini, F., et al., "Melatonin Involvement in Immunity and Cancer," *Biol Signals* 7, no. 1 (January 1998): 61–72.

Gabler, S., et al., "E1B 55-Kilodalton-Associated Protein: A Cellular Protein with RNA-Binding Activity Implicated in Nucleocytoplasmic Transport of Adenovirus and Cellular mRNAs," *J Virol* 72, no. 10 (October 1998): 7960–7961.

Garnacho, Montero J., et al., "Lipids and Immune Function," *Nutricion Hospitalaria* 11, no. 4 (July/August 1996): 230–237.

Gaspardone, A., et al., "Enhanced Activity of Sodium-Lithium Countertransport in Patients with Cardiac Syndrome X: A Potential Link between Cardiac and Metabolic Syndrome X," *Journal of the American College of Cardiology* 32, no. 7 (December 1998): 2031–2034.

Geier, A., et al., "Serum and Insulin Inhibit Cell Death Induced by Cycloheximide in the Human Breast Cancer Cell Line MCF-7," *In Vitro Cellular and Developmental Biology* 28A, no. 6 (June 1992): 415–418.

Giesen, Holly A., et al., "Suppression of Men's Responses to Seasonal Changes in Day Length by Modern Artificial Lighting," *American Journal of Physiology* 269 (1995): R173–R178.

Gilad, Eli, et al., "Interplay between Sex Steroids and Melatonin in Regulation of Human Benign Prostate Epithelial Cell Growth," *Journal of Clinical Endocrinology and Metabolism* 82, no. 8 (August 1997): 2535–2541.

Giovannucci, E., "Insulin and Colon Cancer," *Cancer Causes and Control* 6, no. 2 (March 1995): 164–179.

Godden, J., et al., "The Response of Breast Cancer Cells to Steroid and Peptide Growth Factors," *Anticancer Research* 12, no. 5 (September/October 1992): 1683–1688.

Godo, G., "Hyperprolactinaemia and Female Infertility," *Acta Med Hung* 41, no. 4 (1984): 185–193.

Goldzieher, Joseph W., et al., "Selected Aspects of Polycystic Ovarian Disease," *Reproductive Endocrinology* 21, no. 1 (March 1992): 141–171.

Gompel, A., et al., "Epidermal Growth Factor Receptor and c-erbB-2 Expression in Normal Breast Tissue during the Menstrual Cycle," *Breast Cancer Research and Treatment* 38 (1996): 227–235.

Goode, Erica, "Insomnia in Aged Found Treatable," *The New York Times,* March 17, 1999, A17.

Gooren, L. J., "Androgen Levels and Sex Functions in Testosterone-Treated Hypogonadal Men," *Arch Sex Behav* 16, no. 6 (December 1987): 463–473.

Gottlieb, Scott, "Drug to Prevent Breast Cancer Near Approval," *BMJ* 317 (September 12, 1998): 697.

Granata, A. R., et al., "Relationship between Sleep-Related Erections and Testosterone Levels in Men," *J Androl* 18, no. 5 (September 1997): 522–527.

Grin, W., et al., "A Significant Correlation between Melatonin Deficiency and Endometrial Cancer," *Gynecol Obstet Invest* 45, no. 1 (1998): 62–65.

Grodum, E., et al., "Dopaminergic Inhibition of Pulsatile Luteinizing Hormone Secretion Is Abnormal in Regularly Menstruating Women with Insulin-Dependent Diabetes Mellitus," *Fertility and Sterility* 64, no. 2 (August 1995): 279–284.

Groopman, Jerome, "Decoding Destiny," *The New Yorker,* February 9, 1998, 42–47.

Guay, A. T., et al., "Effect of Raising Endogenous Testosterone Levels in Impotent Men with Secondary Hypogonadism: Double Blind Placebo-Controlled Trial with Clomiphene Citrate," *Journal of Clinical Endocrinology and Metabolism* 80, no. 12 (December 1995): 3546–3552.

Haffner, S. M., "Sex Hormone-Binding Protein, Hyperinsulinemia, Insulin Resistance and Noninsulin-Dependent Diabetes," *Hormone Research* 45, nos. 3–5 (1996): 233–237.

———, "Low Levels of Sex Hormone-Binding Globulin and Testosterone Are Associated with Smaller, Denser Low Density Lipoprotein in Normoglycemic Men," *Journal of Clinical Endocrinology and Metabolism* 81, no. 10 (1996): 3697–3701.

Hafner, F., et al., "Effect of Growth Factors on Estrogen Receptor Mediated Gene Expression," *Journal of Steroid Biochemistry and Molecular Biology* 58, no. 4 (July 1996): 385–393.

Haney, Daniel Q., "Breast Cancer Genes Linked to Mutations," *Santa Barbara News Press,* April 15, 1997, A4.

Hardy, K. J., et al., "Endocrine Assessment of Impotence—Pitfalls of Measuring Serum Testosterone without Sex-Hormone-Binding Globulin," *Postgrad Med J* 70, no. 829 (November 1994): 836–837.

Harte, J., et al., "Self-Similarity in the Distribution and Abundance of Species," *Science* 284 (April 9, 1999): 334–335.

Hayes, Frances J., et al., "Differential Control of Gonadotropin Secretion in the Human: Endocrine Role of Inhibin," *Journal of Clinical Endocrinology and Metabolism* 83, no. 6 (June 1998): 1835–1841.

He, L. W., "Prognostic Significance of Progesterone Receptor in Breast Cancer," *Chung Hua Chung Liu Tsa Chih* 11, no. 2 (March 1989): 121–123.

Heiss, Cindy J., et al., "Associations of Body Fat Distribution, Circulating Sex Hormones, and Bone Density in Postmenopausal Women," *Journal of Clinical Endocrinology and Metabolism* 80, no. 5 (1995): 1591–1596.

Helderman, J. Harold, "The Insulin Receptor on Activated Immunocompetent Cells," *Experimental Gerontology* 28 (1993): 323–327.

Henderson, Brian E., et al., "An Explanation for the Increasing Incidence of Testis Cancer: Decreasing Age at First Full-Term Pregnancy," *Journal of the National Cancer Institute* 89, no. 11 (June 4, 1997): 818–819.

Henderson, Craig, et al., "Are Breast Cancers in Young Women Qualitatively Distinct?" *The Lancet* 349 (May 24, 1997): 1488–1489.

Henry, J. P., "Biological Basis of the Stress Response." *Integral Physiological Behavioral Sciences* 27, no. 1 (January–March 1992): 66–83.

Hetts, Steven W., "To Die or Not to Die: An Overview of Apoptosis and Its Role in Disease," *Journal of the American Medical Association* 279, no. 4 (January 28, 1998): 300–307.

Hicks, B. H., et al., "Metergoline As an Alternative to Bromocriptine in Amenorrhoea," *Acta Endocrinol (Copenh)* 107, no. 4 (December 1984): 439–444.

Hill, S. M., et al., "Effects of the Pineal Hormone Melatonin on the Proliferation and Morphological Characteristics of Human Breast Cancer Cells (MCF-7) in Culture," *Cancer Res* 48, no. 21 (November 1, 1988): 6121–6126.

Holmberg, B., "Magnetic Fields and Cancer: Animal and Cellular Evidence—An Overview," *Environmental Health Perspectives* 103, suppl. 2 (March 1995): 63–67.

Horton, R., et al., "Androgen Induction of Steroid 5 Alpha-Reductase May Be Mediated via Insulin-Like Growth Factor-1," *Endocrinology* 133, no. 2 (August 1993): 447–451.

Hrushesky, William J. M., et al., "Evidence for an Ontogenic Basis for Circadian Coordination of Cancer Cell Proliferation," *Journal of the National Cancer Institute* 90, no. 19 (October 7, 1998): 1480–1484.

Hsu, D. S., et al., "Putative Human Blue-Light Photoreceptors hCRY1 and hCRY2 are Flavoproteins," *Biochemistry* 35, no. 44 (November 5, 1996): 13871–13877.

Inbal, Boaz, et al., "DAP Kinase Links the Control of Apoptosis to Metastasis," *Nature* 390 (November 13, 1997): 180–183.

Ishida, Hironori, M.D., et al., "The Prognostic Significance of p53 and bcl-1 Expression in Lung Adenocarcinoma and Its Correlation with Ki-67 Growth Fraction," *Cancer* 80, no. 6 (September 15, 1997): 1034–1045.

Ivanova, O. A., et al., "Steroid Hormone Receptors and Survival in Breast Cancer Patients," *Vopr Onkol* 32, no. 6 (1986): 71–76.

Jackson, James G., et al., "Insulin Receptor Substrate-1 Is the Predominant Signaling Molecule Activated by Insulin-Like Growth Factor-1, Insulin, and Interleukin-4 in Estrogen Receptor-Positive Human Breast Cancer Cells," *Journal of Biological Chemistry* 273, no. 16 (1998): 9994–10003.

Janczewski, Z., et al., "Clinical Andropause," *Pol Tyg Lek* 44, nos. 7–8 (February 13, 1989): 173–175.

Jang, Meishiang, et al., "Cancer Chemopreventive Activity of Resveratrol, a Natural Product Derived from Grapes," *Science* 275 (January 10, 1997): 218–223.

Jankun, Jerzy, et al., "Why Drinking Green Tea Could Prevent Cancer," *Nature* 387 (June 5, 1997): 561.

Jeng, M. H., et al., "Estrogenic Actions of RU486 in Hormone-Responsive MCF-7 Human Breast Cancer Cells," *Endocrinology* 132, no. 6 (June 1993): 2622–2630.

————, "Estrogenic Potential of Progestins in Oral Contraceptives to Stimulate Human Breast Cancer Cell Proliferation," *Cancer Research* 52, no. 23 (December 1, 1992): 6359–6546.

Jinno, Masao, et al., "A Therapeutic Role of Prolactin Supplementation in Ovarian Stimulation for In Vitro Fertilization: The Bromocriptine-Rebound Method," *Journal of Clinical Endocrinology and Metabolism* 82, no. 11 (1997): 3603–3611.

Johansson, G., et al., "Dietary Influence on Some Proposed Risk Factors for Colon Cancer: Fecal and Urinary Mutagenic Activity and the Activity of Some Intestinal Bacterial Enzymes," *Cancer Detect Prev* 21, no. 3 (1997): 258–266.

Johnson, R. W., et al., "Hormones, Lymphohemopoietic Cytokines and the Neuroimmune Axis," *Comparative Biochemistry and Physiology* 116A, no. 3 (1997): 183–201.

Kaaks, Rudolf, "Nutrition, Hormones, and Breast Cancer: Is Insulin the Missing Link?" *Cancer Causes and Control* 6 (November 7, 1996): 605–625.

Karalis, K., et al., "Cortisol Blockade of Progesterone: A Possible Molecular Mechanism Involved in the Initiation of Human Labor," *Nature Medicine* 2, no. 5 (May 1996): 556–560.

Karasek, M., et al., "Prolactinemia and Sexual Impotence: The Effects of Treatment with Bromocriptine," *Endokrynol Pol* 34, no. 6 (1983): 371–375.

Karlsson, C., et al., "Expression of Functional Leptin Receptors in the Human Ovary," *Journal of Clinical Endocrinology and Metabolism* 82, no. 12 (December 1997): 4144–4148.

Katzenellenbogen, B. S., et al., "Multihormonal Regulation of the Progesterone Receptor in MCF-7 Human Breast Cancer Cells: Interrelationships among Insulin/Insulin-Like Growth Factor-1, Serum, and Estrogen," *Endocrinology* 126, no. 2 (February 1990): 891–898.

Katzenellenbogen, B. S., "Biology and Receptor Interactions of Estriol and Estriol Derivatives In Vitro and In Vivo," *Journal of Steroid Biochemistry and Molecular Biology* 20, no. 4B (April 1984): 1033–1037.

Kauppila, Antti, et al., "Inverse Seasonal Relationship between Melatonin and Ovarian Activity in Humans in a Region with a Strong Seasonal Contrast in Luminosity," *Journal of Clinical Endocrinology and Metabolism* 65, no. 5 (1987): 823–828.

Keys, H. M., et al., "Cisplatin, Radiation, and Adjuvant Hysterectomy Compared with Radiation and Adjuvant Hysterectomy for Bulky Stage IB Cervical Carcinoma," *New England Journal of Medicine* 340, no. 15 (April 15, 1999): 1154–1161.

Klepsch, I., et al., "Clinical and Hormonal Effects of Testosterone Undecanoate (TU) in Male Sexual Impotence," *Endocrinologie* 20, no. 4 (October 1982): 289–293.

Kokko, E., et al., "Progesterone-Regulated Changes in Transcriptional Events in Rabbit Uterus," *Biochem Biophys Acta* 479, no. 3 (December 2, 1977): 354–366.

Kotulak, Ronald, "Cancer Drug Could Aid 29 Million U.S. Women," *Chicago Tribune*, April 7, 1998, A1.

Krause, W., "Effect of Bromocriptine in Oligozoospermic Men with Hyperprolactinaemia," *Reproduction* 4, no. 3 (July 1980): 241–246.

Krieg, Arthur M., "Human Endogenous Retroviruses," *Science and Medicine*, March/April 1997, 34–43.

Krieger, N., et al., "Race/Ethnicity, Social Class, and Prevalence of Breast Cancer Prognostic Biomarkers: A Study of White, Black, and Asian Women in the San Francisco Bay Area," *Ethn Dis* 7, no. 2 (Spring/Summer 1997): 137–149.

Kwan, M., et al., "The Nature of Androgen Action on Male Sexuality: A Combined Laboratory-Self-Report Study on Hypogonadal Men," *Journal of Clinical Endocrinology and Metabolism* 57, no. 3 (September 1983): 557–562.

La Torre, F., et al., "Role of Free Radicals, Telomeres, and Telomerases in Aging and Cancerogenesis," *Mol Med Today* 3, no. 5 (May 1997): 187.

Laughlin, G. A., et al., "Nutritional and Endocrine-Metabolic Aberrations in Women with Functional Hypothalamic Amenorrhea," *Journal of Clinical Endocrinology and Metabolism* 83, no. 1 (1998): 25–32.

———, "Hypoleptinemia in Women Athletes: Absence of Diurnal Rhythm with Amenorrhea," *Journal of Clinical Endocrinology and Metabolism* 82, no. 1 (1997): 318–321.

Lee, Adrian V., et al., "Enhancement of Insulin-Like Growth Factor Signaling in Human Breast Cancer: Estrogen Regulation of Insulin Receptor Substrate-1 Expression In Vitro and In Vivo," *Molecular Endocrinology* 10, no. 5 (1999): 787–796.

Leibenluft, Ellen, "Do Gonadal Steroids Regulate Circadian Rhythms in Humans?" *Journal of Affective Disorders* 29 (1993): 175–181.

Leibenluft, Ellen, et al., "Effects of Leuprolide-Induced Hypogonadism and Testosterone Replacement on Sleep, Melatonin, and Prolactin Secretion in Men," *Journal of Clinical Endocrinology and Metabolism* 82, no. 10 (1997): 3202–3207.

Lemus-Wilson, A., et al., "Melatonin Blocks the Stimulatory Effects of Prolactin on Human Breast Cancer Cell Growth in Culture," *British Journal of Cancer* 72, no. 6 (December 1995): 1435–1440.

Li, J. C., et al., "Influences of Light-Dark Shifting on the Immune System, Tumor Growth and Life Span of Rats, Mice and Fruit Flies As Well As on the Counteraction of Melatonin," *Biol Signals* 6, no. 2 (March 1997): 77–89.

Liautard, J., et al., "Specific Inhibition of IL-6 Signalling with Monoclonal Antibodies against the gp130 Receptor," *Cytokine* 9, no. 4 (April 1997): 233–241.

Lin, C., et al., "Enhancement of Blue-Light Sensitivity of Arabidopsis Seedlings by a Blue Light Receptor Cryptochrome 2," *Proceedings of the National Academy of Sciences (USA)* 95, no. 5 (March 3, 1998): 2686–2690.

Lloyd, J. M., et al., "Age-Related Changes in Proopiomelanocortin (POMC) Gene Expression in the Periarcuate Region of Ovariectomized Rats," *Endocrinology* 129, no. 4 (October 1991): 1896–1902.

Lovejoy, Jennifer C., et al., "Exogenous Androgens Influence Body Composition and Regional Body Fat Distribution in Obese Postmenopausal Women: A Clinical Research Center Study," *Journal of Clinical Endocrinology and Metabolism* 81, no. 6 (1996): 2198–2203.

Maas, D., et al., "Age-Related Changes in Male Gonadal Function: Implications for Therapy," *Drugs Aging* 11, no. 1 (July 1997): 45–60.

Maestronim, G. J., et al., "Melatonin in Human Breast Cancer Tissue: Association with Nuclear Grade and Estrogen Receptor Status," *Laboratory Investigation* 75, no. 4 (October 1996): 557–561.

Magnusson, Cecilia, et al., "Breast-Cancer Risk Following Long-Term Oestrogen- and Oestrogen-Progestin-Replacement Therapy," *Int J Cancer* 81 (1999): 339–344.

Malhotra, Khushbeer, et al., "Putative Blue-Light Photoreceptors from Arabidopsis thaliana and Sinapsis alba with a High Degree of Sequence Homology to DNA Photolyase Contain the Two Photolyase Cofactors but Lack DNA Repair Activity," *Biochemistry* 34, no. 20 (1995): 6892–6899.

Mandal, M., et al., "Bcl-2 Modulates Telomerase Activity," *Journal of Biological Chemistry* 272, no. 22 (May 30, 1997): 14183–14187.

Manier, Jeremy, " 'No Simple Answers' in Breast Cancer War," *Chicago Tribune*, April 7, 1998, A1.

Marin, Per, et al., "Assimilation and Mobilization of Triglycerides in Subcutaneous Abdominal and Femoral Adipose Tissue In Vivo in Men: Effects of Androgens," *Journal of Clinical Endocrinology and Metabolism* 80, no. 1 (1995): 239–243.

Martikainen, Hannu, M.D., et al., "Seasonal Changes in Pituitary Function: Amplification of Midfollicular Luteinizing Hormone Secretion during the Dark Season," *Fertility and Sterility* 65, no. 4 (April 1996): 718–720.

Martin, M. E., et al., "Adenovirus E1B 55K Represses p53 Activation In Vitro," *J Virol* 72, no. 4 (April 1998): 3146–3154.

Maugh II, Thomas H., "Men Who Want to Live Longer Will Love This Study," *Los Angeles Times*, January 26, 1998, S6.

McCurrach, M. E., et al., "Bax-Deficiency Promotes Drug Resistance and Oncogenic Transformation by Attenuating p53-Dependent Apoptosis," *Proceedings of the National Academy of Sciences (USA)* 94, no. 6 (March 18, 1997): 2345–2349.

McGuire, W. L., et al., "Role of Progesterone Receptors in Breast Cancer," *Semin Oncol* 12, suppl. 1 (1985): 12–16.

McKeown-Eyssen, G., "Epidemiology of Colorectal Cancer Revisited: Are Serum Triglycerides and/or Plasma Glucose Associated with Risk?" *Cancer Epidemiology, Biomarkers and Prevention* 3, no. 8 (December 3, 1994): 687–695.

McNeil, Caroline, "In Search of the Perfect SERM: Beyond Tamoxifen and Raloxifene," *Journal of the National Cancer Institute* 90, no. 13 (July 1, 1998): 956–957.

Meden, H., et al., "Elevated Serum Levels of a c-erbB-2 Oncogene Product in Ovarian Cancer Patients and in Pregnancy," *J Cancer Res Clin Oncol* 120, no. 6 (1994): 378–381.

Mellman, Michael J., et al., "Effect of Physiological Hyperinsulinemia on Counterregulatory Hormone Responses during Hypoglycemia in Humans," *Journal of Clinical Endocrinology and Metabolism* 75, no. 5 (1992): 1293–1297.

Messina, Frank, "As Family Struggles with Son's Cancer, Help Pours In," *Los Angeles Times,* June 5, 1998, A3.

Metherall, James E., et al., "Progesterone Inhibits Cholesterol Biosynthesis in Cultured Cells," *American Society for Biochemistry and Molecular Biology* 271, no. 5 (1996): 2627–2633.

Mielke, S., et al., "Expression of the c-erbB-2 Encoded Oncoprotein p185 (HER-2/neu) in Pregnancy As a Model for Oncogene-Induced Carcinogenesis," *Medical Hypotheses* 50, no. 5 (May 1998): 359–362.

———, "In Vivo Effects of Extrogens on c-erbB-2 Oncoprotein Levels in Chorionic Villous Tissue and Maternal Serum," *Gynecol Endocrinol* 11, no. 4 (August 1997): 237–241.

———, "Effects of Interfacing and Influencing Factors on the Analyses of p105 (c-erbB-2/HER-2) Oncoprotein Fragment in Serum," *Anticancer Research* 17, no. 4B (July/August 1997): 3125–3127.

Milazzo, Giovanni, et al., "High-Affinity Binding to an Atypical Insulin-Like Growth Factor-1 Receptor in Human Breast Cancer Cells," *Journal of Clinical Investigation* 89, no. 3 (March 1992): 899–908.

———, "Insulin Receptor Expression and Function in Human Breast Cancer Cell Lines," *Cancer Research* 52 (July 15, 1992): 3924–3930.

"Mineral May Cause Risk of Advanced Prostate Cancer, Study Says," *The New York Times,* August 19, 1998, A19.

Molis, T. M., et al., "Melatonin Modulation of Estrogen-Related Proteins, Growth Factors, and Proto-Oncogenes in Human Breast Cancer," *Journal of Pineal Research* 18, no. 2 (March 1995): 93–103.

———, "Modulation of Estrogen Receptor mRNA Expression by Melatonin in MCF-7 Human Breast Cancer Cells," *Mol Endocrinol* 8, no. 12 (December 1994): 1681–1690.

Mondaini, F., et al., "Sexuality Changes in a Hemodialysis Patient with Hyperprolactinemia: Therapeutic Possibilities," *Riv Ital Ginecol* 59 (1980): 93–96.

"Monounsaturates May Cut Breast Cancer Risk," *Health News,* February 17, 1998, 6.

Morley, J. E., et al., "Testosterone and Frailty," *Clin Geriatr Med* 13, no. 4 (November 1997): 685–695.

Morrow, David J., "Company Is Stopping Its Work on a Prominent Cancer Drug," *The New York Times*, February 10, 1999, A17.

Morrow, Linda A., et al., "Effects of Epinephrine on Insulin Secretion and Action in Humans," *Diabetes* 42 (February 1993): 307–315.

Motamedi, F., et al., "Bombesin-Induced Anorexia Requires Central Bombesin Receptor Activation: Independence from Interaction with Central Catecholaminergic Systems," *Psychopharmacology* 110, nos. 1–2 (1993): 193–197.

Muller, R. E., et al., "Interaction of Estradiol and Estriol with Uterine Estrogen Receptor In Vivo and in Excised Uteri or Cell Suspensions at 37°C.: Noncooperative Estradiol Binding and Absence of Estriol Inhibition of Estradiol-Induced Receptor Activation and Transformation," *Endocrinology* 117, no. 5 (November 1985): 1839–1847.

Mulligan, T., et al., "Testosterone for Erectile Failure," *J Gen Intern Med* 8, no. 9 (September 1993): 517–521.

Nagulesparen, M., et al., "Bromocriptine Treatment of Males with Pituitary Tumours, Hyperprolactinaemia, and Hypogonadism," *Clin Endocrinolo (Oxf)* 9, no. 1 (July 1978): 73–79.

Nakhla, Atif M., et al., "Estradiol Activates the Prostate Androgen Receptor and Prostate-Specific Antigen Secretion through the Intermediacy of Sex-Hormone-Binding Globulin," *Journal of Biological Chemistry* 272, no. 11 (March 14, 1997): 6838–6841.

Narod, Steven A., M.D., et al., "Oral Contraceptives and the Risk of Hereditary Ovarian Cancer," *New England Journal of Medicine* 339, no. 7 (August 13, 1998): 424–428.

Nasseri, Kiumarss, "Determinants of Breast Cancer Detection among Wisconsin (United States) Women, 1988–1990," *Cancer Causes and Control* 7 (1996): 626–627.

Neidhart, M., "Prolactin in Autoimmune Diseases," *Proc Soc Exp Biol Med* 217 (1998): 408–419.

Nelson, Randy J., et al., "Photoperiodic Effects on Tumor Development and Immune Function," *Journal of Biological Rhythms* 9, nos. 3–4 (1994): 233–249.

Nelson, J. Lee, "Microchimerism and Autoimmune," *New England Journal of Medicine* 338 (April 23, 1998): 1224–1225.

Nestler, John E., et al., "The Effects of Hyperinsulinemia on Serum Testosterone, Progesterone, Dehydroepiandrosterone Sulfate, and Cortisol Levels in Normal Women and in a Woman with Hyperandrogenism, Insulin Resistance, and Acanthosis nigricans," *Journal of Clinical Endocrinology and Metabolism* 64 (1987): 180.

———, "Insulin Stimulates Testosterone Biosynthesis by Human Thecal Cells from Women with Polycystic Ovary Syndrome by Activating Its Own Receptor and Using Inositolglycan Mediators As the Signal Transduction System," *Journal of Clinical Endocrinology and Metabolism* 83, no. 6 (1998): 2001–2005.

Nilsson, P. M., "Premature Ageing: The Link between Psychosocial Risk Factors and Disease," *Medical Hypotheses* 47, no. 1 (July 1996): 39–42.

Noguchi, M., et al., "Effects of Hormones on Tumor Growth and Immunoreactive Insulin-Like Growth Factor-1 of Estrogen Receptor-Positive Human Breast Cancer Transplanted in Nude Mice," *Japanese Journal of Cancer Research* 82, no. 11 (November 1991): 1199–1202.

Notides, A. C., et al., "Positive Cooperativity of the Estrogen Receptor," *Proceedings of the National Academy of Sciences (USA)* 78, no. 8 (August 1981): 4926–2930.

Nowak, Rachel, "Eunuchs Fight Back," *New Scientist,* December 1998/January 1999, 11.

Nuccitelli, R., et al., "Endogenous Ionic Currents and DC Electric Fields in Multicellular Animal Tissues," *Bioelectromagnetics,* suppl. 1 (1992): 147–157.

O'Carroll, R., et al., "Testosterone Therapy for Low Sexual Interest and Erectile Dysfunction in Men: A Controlled Study," *Br J Psychiatry* 145 (August 1984): 146–151.

O'Connell, Y., et al., "The Effect of Prolactin, Human Chorionic Gonadotropin, Insulin and Insulin-Like Growth Factor 1 on Adrenal Steroidogenesis in Isolated Guinea-Pig Adrenal Cells," *Journal of Steroid Biochemistry and Molecular Biology* 48, nos. 2–3 (February 1994): 235–240.

Ogasawara, Kouetsu, et al., "Requirement for IRF-1 in the Microenvironment Supporting Development of Natural Killer Cells," *Nature* 391, no. 6668 (February 12, 1998): 700–703.

Okulicz, W. C., et al., "Progesterone Regulation of the Occupied Form of Nuclear Estrogen Receptor," *Science* 213, no. 4515 (September 25, 1981): 1503–1505.

Orr-Weaver, Terry L., et al., "A Checkpoint on the Road to Cancer," *Nature* 392 (March 1998): 233–224.

Pal, B., et al., "Limitation of Joint Mobility and Shoulder Capsulitis in Insulin- and Non-Insulin-Dependent Diabetes Mellitus," *Br J Rheumatol* 25, no. 2 (May 1986): 147–151.

Panno, M. L., et al., "Effect of Oestradiol and Insulin on the Proliferative Pattern and on Oestrogen and Progesterone Receptor Contents in MCF-7 Cells," *Journal of Cancer Research and Clinical Oncology* 122, no. 12 (1996): 745–749.

Panzer, A., et al., "The Validity of Melatonin As an Oncostatic Agent," *Journal of Pineal Research* 22, no. 4 (May 1997): 184–202.

———, "Melatonin in Osteosarcoma: An Effective Drug?" *Medical Hypotheses* 48, no. 6 (June 1997): 523–525.

Papa, Vincenzo, et al., "Elevated Insulin Receptor Content in Human Breast Cancer," *Journal of Clinical Investigation* 86 (November 1990): 1503–1510.

Papanicolaou, Dimitris A., M.D., et al., "The Pathophysiologic Roles of Interleukin-6 in Human Disease," *Annals of Internal Medicine* 128, no. 2 (January 15, 1998): 127–137.

Parazzini, Fabio, et al., "Diabetes and Endometrial Cancer: An Italian Case-Control Study," *International Journal of Cancer* 81 (1999): 539–542.

Path, Gunter, et al., "Interleukin-6 and the Interleukin-6 Receptor in the Human Adrenal Gland: Expression and Effects on Steroidogeneses," *Journal of Clinical Endocrinology and Metabolism* 82, no. 7 (1997): 2343–2349.

Peifer, Mark, "B-Catenin As Oncogene: The Smoking Gun," *Science* 275 (March 21, 1997): 1752–1753.

Pennisi, Elizabeth, "New Tumor Suppressor Found—Twice," *Science* 275 (March 28, 1997): 1876–1878.

Perl, Anne-Karina, et al., "A Causal Role for E-Cadherin in the Transition from Adenoma to Carcinoma," *Nature* 392 (March 1998): 190.

Petridou, S., et al., "Light Induces Accumulation of Isocitrate Lyase mRNA in a Carotenoid-Deficient Mutant of Chlamydomonas reinhardtii," *Plant Mol Biol* 33, no. 3 (February 1997): 381–392.

Petterborg, L. J., et al., "Effect of Melatonin Replacement on Serum Hormone Rhythms in a Patient Lacking Endogenous Melatonin," *Brain Research Bulletin* 27 (1991): 181–185.

Pierce, L. J., et al., "Is c-erbB-2 a Predictor for Recurrent Disease in Early Stage Breast Cancer?" *Int J Radiat Oncol Biol Phys* 28, no. 2 (January 15, 1994): 395–403.

Pierini, A. A., et al., "Male Diabetic Sexual Impotence: Effects of Dopaminergic Agents," *Arch Androl* 6, no. 4 (June 1981): 347–350.

Plymate, S. R., et al., "Circadian Variation in Testosterone, Sex Hormone-Binding Globulin, and Calculated Non-Sex-Hormone-Binding Globulin Bound Testosterone in Healthy Young and Elderly Men," *J Androl* 10 (1989): 366–371.

Rakic, Z., et al., "Testosterone Treatment in Men with Erectile Disorder and Low Levels of Total Testosterone in Serum," *Arch Sex Behav* 26, no. 5 (October 1997): 495–504.

Ram, P. T., et al., "Estrogen Receptor Transactivation in MCF-7 Breast Cancer Cells by Melatonin and Growth Factors," *Mol Cell Endocrinol* 141, nos. 1–2 (June 25, 1998): 53–64.

Rao, K., et al., "Serum Prolactin Levels in Male Patients with Erectile Dysfunction," *Indian J Med Res* 74 (September 1981): 412–414.

Rao, L., et al., "The E1B 19K Protein Associates with Lamins In Vivo and Its Proper Localization Is Required for Inhibition of Apoptosis," *Oncogene* 15, no. 13 (September 25, 1997): 1587–1597.

Rea, D., "Effects of an Exon 5 Variant of the Estrogen Receptor in MCF-7 Breast Cancer Cells," *Cancer Research* 56, no. 7 (April 1, 1996): 1556–1563.

Reber, Paul M., "Prolactin and Immunomodulation," *American Journal of Medicine* 95 (December 1993): 637–644.

Reiter, R. J., "Melatonin Suppression by Static and Extremely Low Frequency Electromagnetic Fields: Relationship to the Reported Increased Incidence of Cancer," *Rev Environ Health* 10, nos. 3–4 (July 1994): 171–186.

Riddle, Donald L., "A Message from the Gonads," *Nature* 399 (May 27, 1999): 308–309.

Riis, Bente J., M.D., et al., "The Effect of Percutaneous Estradiol and Natural Progesterone on Postmenopausal Bone Loss," *Am J Obstet Gynecol* 156 (1987): 61–65.

Robbins, Mark, "All Stressed Out," *Nature* 389 (September 25, 1997): 331–332.

Ronco, A. L., et al., "The Pineal Gland and Cancer," *Anticancer Research* 16, no. 4A (July 1996): 2033–2039.

Roth, J. A., et al., "Melatonin Suppression of PC12 Cell Growth and Death," *Brain Research* 768, nos. 1–2 (September 12, 1997): 63–70.

Ruder, A. M., et al., "Estrogen and Progesterone Receptors in Breast Cancer Patients: Epidemiologic Characteristics and Survival Differences," *Cancer* 64, no. 1 (July 1, 1989): 196–202.

Saad, Zahida, et al., "Expression of Genes That Contribute to Proliferative and Metastatic Ability in Breast Cancer Resected during Various Menstrual Phases," *The Lancet* 351 (1998): 1170–1173.

Saceda, Miguel, et al., "Regulation of Estrogen Receptor Concentration and Activity by an erbB/HER Ligand in Breast Carcinoma Cell Lines," *Endocrinology* 137, no. 10 (1996): 4322–4330.

Saegusa, M., et al., "Bcl-2 Expression Is Correlated with a Low Apoptotic Index and Associated with Progesterone Receptor Immunoreactivity in Endometrial Carcinomas," *J Pathol* 180, no. 3 (November 1996): 275–282.

———, "Bcl-2 Is Closely Correlated with Favorable Prognostic Factors and Inversely Associated with p53 Protein Accumulation in Endometrial Carcinomas: Immunohistochemical and Polymerase Chain Reaction/Loss of Heterozygosity Findings," *J Cancer Res Clin Oncol* 123, no. 8 (1997): 429–434.

———, "Progesterone Therapy for Endometrial Carcinoma Reduces Cell Proliferation but Does Not Alter Apoptosis," *Cancer* 83, no. 1 (July 1, 1998): 111–121.

Salmimies, P., et al., "Effects of Testosterone Replacement on Sexual Behavior in Hypogonadal Men," *Arch Sex Behav* 11, no. 4 (August 1982): 345–353.

Sasson, Shlomo, et al., "Estriol and Estrone Interaction with the Estrogen Receptor: II. Estriol and Estrone-Induced Inhibition of the Cooperative Binding of [3H] Estradiol to the Estrogen Receptor," *Journal of Biological Chemistry* 258, no. 13 (July 10, 1983): 8118–8122.

———, "Inability of [3H] Estriol to Induce Maximal Cooperativity of the Estrogen Receptor," *Journal of Steroid Biochemistry and Molecular Biology* 20, no. 4B (April 1984): 1027–1032.

———, "The Estriol-Induced Inhibition of the Estrogen Receptor's Positive Cooperativity," *Journal of Steroid Biochemistry and Molecular Biology* 20, no. 4B (April 1984): 1021–1026.

Sattar, Naveed, et al., "Insulin-Sensitising Agents in Polycystic-Ovary Syndrome," *The Lancet* 351 (January 31, 1998): 305–306.

Schaefer, Ernst J., et al., "Changes in Plasma Lipoprotein Concentrations and Composition in Response to a Low-Fat, High-Fiber Diet Are Associated with Changes in Serum Estrogen Concentrations in Premenopausal Women," *Metabolism: Clinical and Experimental* 44, no. 6 (June 6, 1995): 749–756.

Schiavi, R. C., et al., "Effect of Testosterone Administration on Sexual Behavior and Mood in Men with Erectile Dysfunction," *Arch Sex Behav* 26, no. 3 (June 1997): 231–241.

Schoonen, W. G., et al., "Effects of Two Classes of Progestagens, Pregnane and 19-Nortestosterone Derivatives, on Cell Growth of Human Breast Tumor Cells: I. MCF-7 Cell Lines," *Journal of Steroid Biochemistry and Molecular Biology* 55, nos. 3–4 (December 1995): 423–427.

Schreiber-Agus, Nicole, et al., "Role of Mxi1 in Ageing Organ Systems and the Regulation of Normal and Neoplastic Growth," *Nature* 393 (June 4, 1998): 483–489.

Schwartz, M. F., et al., "Plasma Testosterone Levels of Sexually Functional and Dysfunctional Men," *Arch Sex Behav* 9, no. 5 (October 1980): 355–366.

Schwartz, Michael W., et al., "Leptin Increases Hypothalamic Pro-opiomelanocortin mRNA Expression in the Rostral Arcuate Nucleus," *Diabetes* 46 (December 1997): 2119–2123.

Seal, B. S., et al., "Phylogenetic Relationships among Highly Virulent Newcastle Disease Virus Isolates Obtained from Exotic Birds and Poultry from 1989 to 1996," *J Clin Microbiol* 36, no. 4 (April 1998): 1141–1145.

See, R. H., et al., "Adenovirus E1B 19,000-Molecular-Weight Protein Activates c-Jun N-Terminal Kinase and c-Jun-Mediated Transcription," *Mol Cell Biol* 18, no. 7 (July 1998): 4012–4022.

Sharpe, Richard M., "Do Males Rely on Female Hormones?" *Nature* 390 (December 4, 1997): 447–450.

Shen, Kuo-Liang, M.D., et al., "The Extent of Proliferative and Apoptotic Activity in Intraductal and Invasive Ductal Breast Carcinomas Detected by Ki-67 Labeling and Terminal Deoxynucleotidyl Transferase-Mediated Digoxigenin-11-dUTP Nick End Labeling," *Cancer* 82, no. 12 (June 15, 1998): 2373–2381.

Simko, M., et al., "Effects of 50 EMF Exposure on Microneucleus Formation and Apoptosis in Transformed and Nontransformed Human Cell Lines," *Bioelectromagnetics*, 19, no. 2 (1998): 85–91.

Simon, Dominique, et al., "Association between Plasma Total Testosterone and Cardiovascular Risk Factors in Healthy Adult Men: The Telecom Study," *Journal of Clinical Endocrinology and Metabolism* 82, no. 2 (1997): 682–685.

Simpson, R. J., et al., "Interleukin-6: Structure-Function Relationships," *Protein Science* 6, no. 5 (May 1997): 929–955.

Singh, J., et al., "Dietary Fat and Colon Cancer: Modulating Effect of Types and Amount of Dietary Fat on Ras-p21 Function during Promotion and Progression Stages of Colon Cancer," *Cancer Research* 57, no. 2 (January 14, 1997): 253–258.

Sinha, M. K., et al., "Nocturnal Rise of Leptin in Lean, Obese, and Non-Insulin-Dependent Diabetes Mellitus Subjects," *Journal of Clinical Investigation* 97, no. 5 (March 1, 1996): 1344–1347.

Skakkebaek, N. E., et al., "Androgen Replacement with Oral Testosterone Undecanoate in Hypogonadal Men: A Double Blind Controlled Study," *Clin Endocrinol (Oxf)* 14, no. 1 (January 1981): 49–61.

Smanik, E. J., et al., "Effect of Progesterone on the Activity of Occupied Nuclear Estrogen Receptor In Vitro," *Mol Cell Endocrinol* 64, no. 1 (June 1989): 111–117.

Sokol, R. Z., et al., "Comparison of the Kinetics of Injectable Testosterone in Eugonadal and Hypogonadal Men," *Fertility and Sterility* 37, no. 3 (March 1982): 425–430.

Spicer, L. J., et al., "Adipose Obese Gene Product, Leptin, Inhibits Bovine Ovarian Thecal Cell Steroidogenesis," *Biol Reprod* 58, no. 1 (January 1998): 207–212.

Sprangers, S. A., et al., "Chronic Underfeeding Increases the Positive Feedback Efficacy of Estrogen on Gonadotropin Secretion," *PSEBM* 216 (1997): 398–403.

Sporn, Michael B., "The War on Cancer," *The Lancet* 347 (May 18, 1996): 1377–1381.

Steegenga, W. T., et al., "The Large E1B Protein Together with the E4 or f6 Protein Target p53 for Active Degradation in Adenovirus Infected Cells," *Oncogene* 16, no. 3 (January 22, 1998): 349–357.

Stegmayr, B., et al., "Hyperprolactinaemia and Testosterone Production: Observations in Two Men on Long-Term Dialysis," *Horm Res* 21, no. 4 (1985): 224–228.

Stewart, A. J., et al., "Modulation of the Proliferative Response of Breast Cancer Cells to Growth Factors by Oestrogen," *British Journal of Cancer* 66, no. 4 (October 1992): 640–648.

Stoll, B. A., et al., "New Hormone-Related Markers of High Risk to Breast Cancer," *Annals of Oncology* 3, no. 6 (June 1992): 435–438.

Strohl, Lydia, "Trace Your Family (Health) Tree," *USA Weekend*, April 9–11, 1999, 30.

Sugaya, A., et al., "Glucose Transporter 4 (GLUT4) mRNA Abundance in the Adipose Tissue and Skeletal-Muscle Tissue of Ovariectomized Rats Treated with 17 Beta-Estradiol or Progesterone," *J Obstet Gynaecol Res* 25, no. 1 (February 1999): 9–14.

Suwa, H., et al., "Effect of Estradiol on 5 Alpha-Reductase Activity in Osteoblast-Like Cell," *Nippon Naibunpi Gakkai Zasshi, Folia Endocrinologica Japonica* 71, no. 5 (July 20, 1995): 651–658.

Svetec, D. A., et al., "The Effect of Parenteral Testosterone Replacement on Prostate Specific Antigen in Hypogonadal Men with Erectile Dysfunction," *J Urol* 158, no. 5 (November 1997): 1775–1777.

Swanek, George E., et al., "Covalent Binding of the Endogenous Estrogen 16a-Hydroxyestrone to Estradiol Receptor in Human Breast Cancer Cells: Characterization and Intranuclear Localization," *Proceedings of the National Academy of Sciences (USA)* 85 (November 1988): 7831–7835.

Swerdloff, R. S., et al., "Androgen Deficiency and Aging in Men," *West J Med* 159, no. 5 (November 1993): 579–585.

Swerdlow, A. J., et al., "Risks of Breast and Testicular Cancers in Young Adult Twins in England and Wales: Evidence on Prenatal and Genetic Aetiology," *The Lancet* 350 (1997): 1723–1728.

Tamaya, Teruhiko, et al., "Effects of Estradiol-17B and Estradiol on Their Binding Sites in the Rabbit Uterus," *Comp Biochem Physiol* 95B, no. 2 (1990): 415–418.

Tanaka, Nobuyuki, et al., "Cooperation of the Tumor Suppressors IRF-1 and p53 in Response to DNA Damage," *Nature* 382 (August 29, 1996): 816–818.

Tenover, J. L., "Testosterone and the Aging Male," *J Androl* 18, no. 2 (March 1997): 103–106.

Tenover, J. S., "Effects of Testosterone Supplementation in the Aging Male," *Journal of Clinical Endocrinology and Metabolism* 75, no. 4 (1992): 1092–1098.

Thomas, A., et al., "Suppression of the p300-Dependent mdm2 Negative-Feedback Loop Induces the p53 Apoptotic Function," *Genes Dev* 12, no. 13 (July 1, 1998): 1975–1985.

Thorner, M. O., et al., "Bromocriptine Treatment of Hyperprolactinaemic Hypogonadism," *Acta Endocrinol Suppl (Copenh)* 216 (1978): 131–146.

Ticher, A., et al., "The Pattern of Hormonal Circadian Time Structure (Acrophase) As an Assessor of Breast-Cancer Risk," *International Journal of Cancer* 65, no. 5 (March 1, 1996): 591–593.

Tiniakos, D. G., et al., "C-erbB-2 and p53 Expression in Breast Cancer Fine Needle Aspirates," *Cytopathology* 7, no. 3 (June 1996): 178–186.

Tonolo, G., et al., "Cyclical Variation of Plasma Lipids, Apolipoproteins, and Lipoprotein(a) during Menstrual Cycle of Normal Women," *American Journal of Physiology* 269, no. 6 (December 1995): E1101-E1105.

Travis, A., et al., "C-erbB-3 in Human Breast Carcinoma: Expression and Relation to Prognosis and Established Prognostic Indicators," *British Journal of Cancer* 74, no. 2 (July 1996): 229-233.

Trichopoulos, Dimitrios, "Hypothesis: Does Breast Cancer Originate In Utero?" *The Lancet* 335 (1990): 939-940.

Tsigos, C., et al., "Dose Effects of Recombinant Human Interleukin-6 on Pituitary Hormone Secretion and Energy Expenditure," *Neuroendocrinology* 66, no. 1 (July 1997): 54-62.

Tsutamoto, T., et al., "Interleukin-6 Spillover in the Peripheral Circulation Increases with the Severity of Heart Failure, and the High Plasma Level of Interleukin-6 Is an Important Prognostic Predictor in Patients with Congestive Heart Failure," *Journal of the American College of Cardiology* 31, no. 2 (February 1998): 391-398.

Turnbull, Andrew V., et al., "Corticotropin-Releasing Factor (CRF) and Endocrine Responses to Stress: CRF Receptors, Binding Protein, and Related Peptides," *PSEBM* 215 (1997): 1-10.

Uusitupa, Matti, et al., "Effects of Two High-Fat Diets with Different Fatty Acid Compositions on Glucose and Lipid Metabolism in Healthy Young Women," *American Journal of Clinical Nutrition* 59 (1994): 1310-1316.

Van Cauter, Eve, et al., "Modulation of Glucose Regulation and Insulin Secretion by Circadian Rhythmicity and Sleep," *Journal of Clinical Investigation* 88 (September 1991): 934-942.

Vance, Mary Lee, M.D., "Hypopituitarism," *New England Journal of Medicine* 330, no. 23 (June 9, 1994): 1651-1662.

Vermeulen, A., "Biological Manifestations of the Andropause," *Fiziol Zh* 36, no. 5 (September 1990): 90-93.

——, "The Male Climacterium," *Ann Med* 25, no. 6 (December 1993): 531-534.

Vicburger, M. I., et al., "Testosterone Levels After Bromocriptine Treatment in Patients Undergoing Long-Term Hemodialysis," *J Androl* 6, no. 2 (March 1985): 113-116.

Von Treuer, K., et al., "Overnight Human Plasma Melatonin, Cortisol, Prolactin, TSH, under Conditions of Normal Sleep, Sleep Deprivation, and Sleep Recovery," *Journal of Pineal Research* 20, no. 1 (January 1996): 7-14.

Waldstreicher, Joanne, et al., "Gender Differences in the Temporal Organization of Prolactin (PRL) Secretion: Evidence for a Sleep-Independent Circadian Rhythm of Circulating PRL Levels—A Clinical Research Center Study," *Journal of Clinical Endocrinology and Metabolism* 81, no. 4 (1996): 1483-1487.

Wang, C., et al., "Androgen Replacement Therapy," *Ann Med* 29, no. 5 (October 1997): 365-370.

Wang, F., et al., "Identification of a Functional Imperfect Estrogen-Responsive Element in the 5'-Promoter Region of the Human Cathepsin D Gene," *Biochemistry* 36, no. 25 (June 24, 1997): 77793-77801.

Watson, Patrice, et al., "Prognosis of BRCA1 Hereditary Breast Cancer," *The Lancet* 351 (January 31, 1998): 304–305.

Watts, C. K., et al., "Oestrogen Receptor Gene Structure and Function in Breast Cancer," *Journal of Steroid Biochemistry and Molecular Biology* 41, nos. 3–8 (March 1992): 529–536.

Wehr, Thomas A., et al., "Suppression of Men's Responses to Seasonal Changes in Day Length by Modern Artificial Lighting," *American Journal of Physiology* 269, no. 38 (1995): R173-R178.

Weiderpass, Elisabete, et al., "Risk of Endometrial and Breast Cancer in Patients with Diabetes Mellitus," *International Journal of Cancer* 71 (1997): 360–363.

Weiland, N. G., et al., "Aging Abolishes the Estradiol-Induced Suppression and Diurnal Rhythm of Proopiomelanocortin Gene Expression in the Arcuate Nucleus," *Endocrinology* 131, no. 6 (December 1992): 2959–2964.

Weise, T. E., et al., "Optimization of Estrogen Growth Response in MCF-7 Cells," *In Vitro Cellular and Developmental Biology* 28A, nos. 9–10 (September/October 1992): 595–602.

Wijngaarden, T. Vink-van, et al., "Inhibition of Insulin and Insulin-Like Growth Factor I Stimulated Growth of Human Breast Cancer Cells by 1,25-Dihydroxyvitamin D_3 and the Vitamin D_3 Analogue EB1089," *European Journal of Cancer* 32A, no. 5 (1996): 842–848.

Williamson, David F., Ph.D., "Pharmacotherapy for Obesity," *Journal of the American Medical Association* 281, no. 3 (January 20, 1999): 278–280.

Willett, W. C., "Specific Fatty Acids and Risks of Breast and Prostate Cancer: Dietary Intake," *American Journal of Clinical Nutrition* 66, suppl. 6 (December 1997): 1557S-1563S.

Wilson, Sean T., et al., "Melatonin Augments the Sensitivity of MCF-7 Human Breast Cancer Cells to Tamoxifen In Vitro," *Journal of Clinical Endocrinology and Metabolism* 75, no. 2 (1992): 669–670.

Winters, S. J., et al., "Altered Pulsatile Secretion of Luteinizing Hormone in Hypogonadal Men with Hyperprolactinaemia," *Clin Endocrinol (Oxf)* 21, no. 3 (September 1984): 257–263.

Wolk, Alocja, Ph.D., et al., "A Prospective Study of Association of Monounsaturated Fat and Other Types of Fat with Risk of Breast Cancer," *Arch Intern Med* 158 (January 12, 1998): 41–45.

Wu, F. C., et al., "The Behavioural Effects of Testosterone Undecanoate in Adult Men with Klinefelter's Syndrome: A Controlled Study," *Clin Endocrinol (Oxf)* 16, no. 5 (May 1982): 489–497.

Wutz, Anton, et al., "Imprinted Expression of the Igf2r Gene Depends on an Intronic CpG Island," *Nature* 389 (October 16, 1997): 745.

Ying, S. W., et al., "Human Malignant Melanoma Cells Express High-Affinity Receptors for Melatonin: Antiproliferative Effects of Melatonin and 6-Chloromelatonin," *Eur J Pharmacol* 246, no. 2 (July 15, 1993): 89–96.

Yu, W. H., et al., "Role of Leptin in Hypothalamic-Pituitary Function," *Proceedings of the National Academy of Sciences (USA)* 94 (February 1997): 1023–1028.

Zava, D. T., et al., "Estrogenic Activity of Natural and Synthetic Estrogens in Human Breast Cancer Cells in Culture," *Environmental Health Perspectives* 105, suppl. 3 (April 1997): 637–645.

————, "Estrogen and Progestin Bioactivity of Foods, Herbs, and Spices," *Proc Soc Exp Biol Med* 217, no. 3 (March 1998): 369–378.

Zelissen, P. M., "Drug Treatment of Sex Disorders in Men," *Ned Tijdschr Geneeskd* 140, no. 50 (December 14, 1996): 2528.

Zgliczynski, S., et al., "Effect of Testosterone Replacement Therapy on Lipids and Lipoproteins in Hypogonadal and Elderly Men," *Atherosclerosis* 121, no. 1 (March 1996): 35–43.

Zhang, Yuqing, et al., "Alcohol Consumption and Risk of Breast Cancer: The Framingham Study Revisited," *American Journal of Epidemiology* 149, no. 2 (January 15, 1999): 93–101.

Zhong, H. H., et al., "Effects of Synergistic Signaling by Phytochrome A and Cryptochrome 1 on Circadian Clock-Regulated Catalase Expression," *Plant Cell* 9, no. 6 (June 1997): 947–955.

Zhou, Jian, et al., "Anatomy of the Human Ovarian Insulin-Like Growth Factor System," *Biology of Reproduction* 48 (1993): 467–482.

PART IV ONLY THE PARANOID SURVIVE
Chapter Nine: Damage Control

Abbasi, A. A., et al., "Experimental Zinc Deficiency in Man: Effect on Spermatogenesis," *Trans Assoc Am Physicians* 92 (1979): 292–302.

Albrink, Margaret J., M.D., "Dietary Fiber, Plasma Insulin, and Obesity," *American Journal of Clinical Nutrition* 31 (October 1978): S277–S279.

Alexander, R. McNeill, "News of Chews: The Optimization of Mastication," *Nature* 391 (January 22, 1998): 329.

Almendingen, K., et al., "Influence of the Diet on Cell Proliferation in the Large Bowel and the Rectum: Does a Strict Vegetarian Diet Reduce the Risk of Intestinal Cancer?" *Tidsskr Nor Laegeforen* 115, no. 18 (August 10, 1995): 2252–2256.

Ameer, B., et al., "Drug Interactions with Grapefruit Juice," *Clinical Pharmacokinetics* 33, no. 2 (August 1997): 103–121.

"Are You Myth-Informed about Milk?" *Illinois Country Living*, August 1996, 8.

Ball, D., et al., "Blood and Urine Acid-Base Status of Premenopausal Omnivorous and Vegetarian Women," *Br J Nutr* 78, no. 5 (November 1997): 683–693.

Bang, H. O., et al., "Plasma Lipid and Lipoprotein Pattern in Greenlandic West-Coast Eskimos," *The Lancet* 1 or 7, (June 5, 1971): 1143–1146.

Barr, S. I., et al., "Vegetarian vs. Nonvegetarian Diets, Dietary Restraint, and Subclinical Ovulatory Disturbances: Prospective Six-Month Study," *American Journal of Clinical Nutrition* 60, no. 6 (December 1994): 887–894.

Bederova, A., et al., "Lipid and Antioxidant Blood Levels in Vegetarians," *Nahrung* 40, no. 1 (February 1996): 17–20.

Bengmark, S., et al., "Gastrointestinal Surface Protection and Mucosa Reconditioning," *JPEN J Parenter Enteral Nutr* 19, no. 5 (September/October 1995): 410–415.

Berger, R. J., et al., "Energy Conservation and Sleep," *Behavioural Brain Research* 69, nos. 1–2 (July/August 1995): 65–73.

Berry, Elliot M., et al., "Effects of Diets Rich in Monounsaturated Fatty Acids on Plasma Lipoproteins—the Jerusalem Nutrition Study: II. Monounsaturated Fatty Acids vs. Carbohydrates 1–3," *American Journal of Clinical Nutrition* 56 (1992): 394–403.

Blackburn, Henry, M.D., "Sounding Board: Olestra and the FDA," *New England Journal of Medicine* 334 (April 11, 1996): 984–986.

Borchers, Andrea T., et al., "Complementary Medicine: A Review of Immunomodulatory Effects of Chinese Herbal Medicines 1–3," *American Journal of Nutrition* 66 (1997): 1303–1312.

Brandao-Neto, J., et al., "Zinc: An Inhibitor of Prolactin (PRL) Secretion in Humans," *Horm Metab Res* 21, no. 4 (April 1989): 203–206.

———, "Endocrine Interaction between Zinc and Prolactin: An Interpretative Review," *Biol Trace Elem Res* 49, nos. 2–3 (August 1995): 139–149.

Brenner, I. K., et al., "The Impact of Heat Exposure and Repeated Exercise on Circulating Stress Hormones," *European Journal of Applied Physiology and Occupational Physiology* 76, no. 5 (1997): 445–454.

Breslow, R. A., et al., "Telomerase and Early Detection of Cancer: A National Cancer Institute Workshop," *Journal of the National Cancer Institute* 89, no. 9 (May 7, 1997): 618–623.

Brestrich, M., et al., "Lactovegetarian Diet: Effect on Changes in Body Weight, Lipid Status, Fibrinogen and Lipoprotein (a) in Cardiovascular Patients during Inpatient Rehabilitation Treatment," *Z Kardiol* 85, no. 6 (June 1996): 418–427.

Brody, Jane E., "Milk Fat As Cancer Fighter," *The New York Times*, June 25, 1997, B10.

———, "Avoiding Confusion on Serving Size Is Key to Food Pyramid," *The New York Times*, April 13, 1999, D6.

———, "Americans Gamble on Herbs As Medicine," *The New York Times*, February 9, 1999, D1.

Cahill, D. J., et al., "Multiple Follicular Development Associated with Herbal Medicine," *Human Reproduction* 9, no. 8 (August 1994): 1469–1470.

Caticha, O., et al., "Total Body Zinc Depletion and Its Relationship to the Development of Hyperprolactinemia in Chronic Renal Insufficiency," *J Endocrinol Invest* 19, no. 7 (July 1996): 441–448.

Chalmers, R. A., et al., "Mitochondrial Carnitine-Acylcarnitine Translocase Deficiency Presenting As Sudden Neonatal Death," *J Pediatr* 131, no. 2 (August 1997): 220–225.

Coghlan, Andy, "A Plateful of Medicine," *New Scientist*, November 2, 1996, 12–13.

Connor, William E., M.D., et al., "Should a Low-Fat, High-Carbohydrate Diet Be Recommended for Everyone?" *New England Journal of Medicine* 337 (August 21, 1997): 562–563.

Curran-Celentano, Joanne, et al., "Alterations in Vitamin A and Thyroid Hormone Status in Anorexia Nervosa and Associated Disorders," *The American Journal of Clinical Nutrition*, 42, no. 6 (December 1985): 1183–1191.

Dahse, R., et al., "Telomeres and Telomerase: Biological and Clinical Importance," *Clin Chem* 43, no. 5 (May 1997): 708–714.

Damayanti, M., et al., "Effect of Plant Extracts and Systemic Fungicide on the Pineapple Fruit-Rotting Fungus, Ceratocystis paradoxa," *Cytobios* 86, no. 346 (1996): 155–165.

Da Silva, Wilson, "A Steady Heart," *New Scientist,* August 1, 1997, 12.

Davidson, Michael H., et al., "Weight Control and Risk Factor Reduction in Obese Subjects Treated for Two Years with Orlistat," *Journal of the American Medical Association* 281, no. 3 (1999): 235–242.

De Masters, B. K., et al., "Differential Telomerase Expression in Human Primary Intracranial Tumors," *Am J Clin Pathol* 107, no. 5 (May 1997): 548–554.

Demmelmair, H., et al., "Trans Fatty Acid Contents in Spreads and Cold Cuts Usually Consumed by Children," *Zeitschrift fur Ernahrungswissenschaft* 35, no. 3 (September 1996): 235–240.

Dorgan, J. F., et al., "Effects of Dietary Fat and Fiber on Plasma and Urine Androgens and Estrogens in Men: A Controlled Feeding Study," *American Journal of Clinical Nutrition* 64, no. 6 (December 1996): 850–855.

During, Matthew J., et al., "Glucose Modulates Rat Substantia Nigra GABA Release In Vivo via ATP-Sensitive Potassium Channels," *Journal of Clinical Investigation* 95 (May 1995): 2403–2408.

Endres, Stefan, et al., "The Effect of Dietary Supplementation with n-3 Polyunsaturated Fatty Acids on the Synthesis of Interleukin-1 and Tumor Necrosis Factor by Mononuclear Cells," *New England Journal of Medicine* 320, no. 5 (February 2, 1989): 265–271.

Engler, Marguerite M., et al., "Effects of Dietary y-Linolenic Acid on Blood Pressure and Adrenal Angiotensin Receptors in Hypertensive Rats," *GAMMA* (1998): 234–237.

Favaretto, A. L., et al., "Oxytocin Releases Atrial Natriuretic Peptide from Rat Atria In Vitro That Exerts Negative Inotropic and Chronotropic Action," *Peptides* 18, no. 9 (1997): 1377–1381.

Feldman, Elaine B., et al., "How Grapefruit Juice Potentiates Drug Bioavailability," *Nutrition Reviews* 55 (November 1997): 398–400.

———, "Position Paper on Trans Fatty Acids 1–3," *American Journal of Clinical Nutrition* 63 (1996): 663–670.

Fernstrom, J. D., et al., "Effect of Chronic Corn Consumption on Serotonin Content of Rat Brain," *Nature: New Biology* 234, no. 45 (November 10, 1971): 62–64.

"Fiber Bounces Back," *Consumer Reports on Health* 7, no. 3 (March 1995): 25–28.

Frentzel-Beyme, R., et al., "Vegetarian Diets and Colon Cancer: The German Experience," *American Journal of Clinical Nutrition* 59 (May 1994): 1143S–1152S.

Fu, Y. K., et al., "Growth Hormone Augments Superoxide Anion Secretion of Human Neutrophils by Binding to the Prolactin Receptor," *Journal of Clinical Investigation* 89, no. 2 (February 1992): 451–457.

Gannage, M. H., et al., "Ostomalacia Secondary to Celiac Disease, Primary Hyperparathyroidism, and Graves' Disease," *Am J Med Sci* 315, no. 2 (February 1998): 136–139.

Gates, J. R., et al., "Association of Dietary Factors and Selected Plasma Variables with Sex Hormone-Binding Globulin in Rural Chinese Women," *American Journal of Clinical Nutrition* 63, no. 1 (January 1996): 22–31.

Gegax, T. Trent, "Fast-Food Fast Tracker," *Newsweek,* May 26, 1997, 57.

Ghatei, M. A., et al., "Fermentable Dietary Fibre, Intestinal Microflora and Plasma Hormones in the Rat," *Clinical Science* 93, no. 2 (August 1997): 109–112.

Gibson, Glenn, et al., "Dietary Modulation of the Human Colonic Microbiota: Introducing the Concept of Prebiotics," *J Nutr* 125 (1995): 1401–1412.

Gillman, M. W., et al., "Margarine Intake and Subsequent Coronary Heart Disease in Men," *Epidemiology* 8, no. 2 (March 1997): 144–149.

Gordon, J. I., et al., "Epithelial Cell Growth and Differentiation: III. Promoting Diversity in the Intestine—Conversations between the Microflora, Epithelium, and Diffuse GALT," *Am J Physiol* 273, no. 3 (September 1997): G565–G570.

Gurney, James G., et al., "Aspartame Consumption in Relation to Childhood Brain Tumor Risk: Results from a Case-Control Study," *Journal of the National Cancer Institute* 89, no. 14 (July 16, 1997): 1072–1074.

Haanwinckel, M. A., et al., "Oxytocin Mediates Atrial Natriuretic Peptide Release and Natriuresis After Volume Expansion in the Rat," *Proceedings of the National Academy of Sciences (USA)* 92, no. 17 (August 15, 1995): 7902–7906.

Haugen, B. R., et al., "Telomerase Activity in Benign and Malignant Thyroid Tumors," *Thyroid* 7, no. 3 (June 1997): 337–342.

Himelstein, Victoria, "Cancer Experts Say Linda Did All the Right Things . . . But Even Paul's $ Millions Couldn't Save Her," *Star,* May 5, 1998, 41.

Hirobe, C., et al., "Cytotoxic Flavonoids from Vitex Agnus-Castus," *Phytochemistry* 46, no. 3 (October 1997): 521–524.

Holzapfel, Wilhelm H., et al., "Overview of Gut Flora and Probiotics," *International Journal of Food Microbiology* 41 (1998): 85–101.

"How Fat Affects Arteries," *Health News,* December 30, 1997, 1–8.

"How Much Can Diet Lower Cholesterol?" *Health News,* February 11, 1997, 5.

Igisu, H., et al., "Protection of the Brain by Carnitine," *Sangyo Eiseigaku Zasshi* 37, no. 2 (March 1995): 75–82.

Jackson, A. A., et al., "Urinary Excretion of 5-L-Oxoproline (Pyroglutamic Acid) Is Increased in Normal Adults Consuming Vegetarian or Low Protein Diets," *J Nutr* 126, no. 11 (November 1996): 2813–2822.

Jacob, S., et al., "Enhancement of Glucose Disposal in Patients with Type II Diabetes by Alpha-Lipoic Acid," *Arzneimittel-Forschung* 45, no. 8 (August 1995): 872–874.

Jacobson, Michael, et al., "Snack Attack: Olestra," *Nutrition Action,* March 1998, 1–7.

Jacobson, Michael, "Liquid Candy: How Soft Drinks Are Harming Americans' Health," *Center for Science in the Public Interest* 26, no. 3 (April 1999): 1–9.

Jakobs, B. S., et al., "Fatty Acid Beta-Oxidation in Peroxisomes and Mitochondria: The First Unequivocal Evidence for the Involvement of Carnitine in Shuttling Propionyl-CoA from Peroxisomes to Mitochondria," *Biochemical and Biophysical Research Communications* 213, no. 3 (August 24, 1995): 1035–1041.

Jenkins, David J., M.D., et al., "Decrease in Postprandial Insulin and Glucose Concentrations by Guar and Pectin," *Annals of Internal Medicine* 86 (1977): 20–23.

———, "Metabolic Effects of Non-Absorbable Carbohydrates," *Scand J Gastroenterol* 222 (1997): 10–13.

Jibrin, Janis, "How Sweet It Is? Here's the Real Scoop on Sugar," *American Health*, December 1995, 58–61.

Johansson, G., et al., "Dietary Influence on Some Proposed Risk Factors for Colon Cancer: Fecal and Urinary Mutagenic Activity and the Activity of Some Intestinal Bacterial Enzymes," *Cancer Detect Prev* 21, no. 3 (1997): 258–266.

Johnson, Greg, "Chips Are Down in Marketing Olestra," *Los Angeles Times*, March 10, 1998, A1.

Kahler, W., et al., "Diabetes Mellitus—A Free Radical-Associated Disease: Results of Adjuvant Antioxidant Supplementation," *Zeitschrift fur die Gesamte Innere medizin und Ihre Grenzgebiete* 48, no. 5 (May 1993): 223–232.

Kannan, S., et al., "Telomerase Activity in Premalignant and Malignant Lesions of Human Oral Mucosa," *Cancer Epidemiol Biomarkers Prev* 6, no. 6 (June 1997): 413–420.

Katan, Martijn B., et al., "Beyond Low-Fat Diets," *New England Journal of Medicine* 337, no. 8 (August 21, 1997): 563–566.

———, "High-Oil Compared with Low-Fat, High-Carbohydrate Diets in the Prevention of Ischemic Heart Disease," *American Journal of Clinical Nutrition* 66 (1997): 974S-979S.

Keillor, Garrison, "In Autumn We All Get Older Again," *Time*, November 6, 1995, 90.

Kern, Fred, Jr., M.D., "Normal Plasma Cholesterol in an 88-Year-Old Man Who Eats 25 Eggs a Day," *New England Journal of Medicine* 324, no. 13 (March 28, 1991): 896–899.

Key, T. J., et al., "Dietary Habits and Mortality in 11,000 Vegetarians and Health-Conscious People: Results of a 17-Year Follow-Up," *BMJ* 313, no. 7060 (September 28, 1996): 775–779.

Khamaisi, M., et al., "Lipoic Acid Reduces Glycemia and Increases Muscle GLUT4 Content in Streptozotocin-Diabetic Rats," *Metabolism: Clinical and Experimental* 46, no. 7 (July 1997): 763–768.

Kinoshita, H., et al., "Detection of Telomerase Activity in Exfoliated Cells in Urine from Patients with Bladder Cancer," *Journal of the National Cancer Institute* 89, no. 10 (May 21, 1997): 724–730.

Kiritsy, P. J., et al., "Acute Effects of Aspartame on Systolic Blood Pressure in Spontaneously Hypertensive Rats," *Journal of Neural Transmission* 66, no. 2 (1986): 121–128.

Kjeldsen-Kragh, J., et al., "Changes in Laboratory Variables in Rheumatoid Arthritis Patients during a Trial of Fasting and One-Year Vegetarian Diet," *Scand J Rheumatol* 24, no. 2 (1995): 85–93.

———, "Inhibition of Growth of Proteus mirabilis and Escherichia coli in Urine in Response to Fasting and Vegetarian Diet," *APMIS (AMS)* 103, no. 11 (November 1995): 818–822.

Kleiner, Kurt, "Fake Fat Leaks Fuels Funding Fury," *New Scientist*, December 13, 1997, 15.

Koike, K., et al., "Purification and Characterization of Rabbit Small Intestinal Cytochromes P450 Belonging to CYP2J and CYP4A Subfamilies," *Biochemical and Biophysical Research Communications* 232, no. 3 (March 27, 1997): 643–647.

Kontessis, P. A., et al., "Renal, Metabolic, and Hormonal Responses to Proteins of Different Origin in Normotensive, Nonproteinuric Type I Diabetic Patients," *Diabetes Care* 18, no. 9 (September 1995): 1233.

Krajlcovilcovla-Kudllalckovla, M., et al., "Lipid and Antioxidant Blood Levels in Vegetarians," *Nahrung* 40, no. 1 (February 1996): 17–20.

———, "Selected Vitamins and Trace Elements in the Blood of Vegetarians," *Ann Nutr Metab* 39, no. 6 (1995): 334–339.

———, "The Plasma Profile of Fatty Acids in Vegetarians," *Bratisl Lek Listy* 98, no. 1 (January 1997): 23–27.

———, "Influence of Vegetarian and Mixed Nutrition on Selected Haematological and Biochemical Parameters in Children," *Nahrung* 41, no. 5 (October 1997): 311–314.

———, "Selected Parameters of Lipid Metabolism in Young Vegetarians," *Ann Nutr Metab* 38, no. 6 (1994): 331–335.

Kyo, S., et al., "Application of Telomerase Assay for the Screening of Cervical Lesions," *Cancer Research* 57, no. 10 (May 15, 1997): 1863–1867.

———, "Telomerase Activity in Human Urothelial Tumors," *Am J Clin Pathol* 107, no. 5 (May 1997): 555–560.

Lang, C. C., et al., "Decreased Intestinal CYP3A in Celiac Disease: Reversal After Successful Gluten-Free Diet—A Potential Source of Interindividual Variability in First-Pass Drug Metabolism," *Clinical Pharmacology and Therapeutics* 59, no. 1 (January 1996): 41–46.

Leung, L. H., "Pantothenic Acid As a Weight-Reducing Agent: Fasting without Hunger, Weakness, and Ketosis," *Medical Hypotheses* 44 (1995): 403–405.

Ley, Beth M., "The Potato Antioxidant: Alpha Lipoic Acid," A Health Learning Handbook. BL Publications Aliso Viejo, CA, 1996.

Metherall, James E., et al., "Progesterone Inhibits Cholesterol Biosynthesis in Cultured Cells," *American Society for Biochemistry and Molecular Biology* 271, no. 5 (1996): 2627–2633.

Liebman, Bonnie, et al., "Hot Cereals: An End to Breakfast Boredom," *Nutrition Action*, March 1998, 1–6.

Liu, Y., et al., "Prolactin and Testosterone Regulation of Mitochondrial Zinc in Prostate Epithelial Cells," *Prostate* 30, no. 1 (January 1997): 26–32.

Lorenson, M. Y., et al., "Prolactin (PRL) Is a Zinc-Binding Protein: I. Zinc Interactions with Monomeric PRL and Divalent Cation Protection of the Intragranular PRL Cysteine Thiols," *Endocrinology* 137, no. 3 (March 1996): 808–816.

Loughran, O., et al., "Evidence for the Inactivation of Multiple Replicative Lifespan Genes in Immortal Human Squamous Cell Carcinoma Keratinocytes," *Oncogene* 14, no. 16 (April 24, 1997): 1955–1964.

Low, Phillip A., et al., "The Roles of Oxidative Stress and Antioxidant Treatment in Experimental Diabetic Neuropathy," *Diabetes* 46, suppl. 2 (September 2, 1997): S38-S42.

Lown, K. S., et al., "Grapefruit Juice Increases Felodipine Oral Availability in Humans by Decreasing Intestinal CYP3A Protein Expression," *Journal of Clinical Investigation* 99, no. 10 (May 15, 1997): 2545–2553.

Lundahl, J., et al., "Effects of Grapefruit Juice Ingestion—Pharmacokinetics and Haemodynamics of Intravenously and Orally Administered Felodipine in Healthy Men," *European Journal of Clinical Pharmacology* 52, no. 2 (1997): 139–145.

Lundahl, J., et al., "Relationship between Time of Intake of Grapefruit and Its Effect on Pharmacokinetics and Pharmacodynamics of Felodipine in Healthy Subjects," *European Journal of Clinical Pharmacology* 49, nos. 1–2 (1995): 61–67.

MacLean, C. R., et al., "Effects of the Transcendental Meditation Program on Adaptive Mechanisms: Changes in Hormone Levels and Responses to Stress After Four Months of Practice," *Psychoneuroendocrinology* 22, no. 4 (May 1997): 277–295.

Maher, T. J., et al., "Possible Neurologic Effects of Aspartame, a Widely Used Food Additive," *Environmental Health Perspectives* 75 (November 1987): 53–57.

Malinow, Manuel R., et al., "Reduction of Plasma Homocysteine Levels by Breakfast Cereal Fortified with Folic Acid in Patients with Coronary Heart Disease," *New England Journal of Medicine* 338, no. 15 (April 9, 1998): 1009–1051.

Mandal, M., et al., "Bcl–2 Modulates Telomerase Activity," *Journal of Biological Chemistry* 272, no. 22 (May 30, 1997): 14183–14187.

Mantzoros, C. S., et al., "Zinc May Regulate Serum Leptin Concentrations in Humans," *J Am Coll Nutr* 17, no. 3 (June 1998): 270–275.

Marston, Wendy, "Gut Reactions," *Newsweek,* November 17, 1997, 95–99.

Medkova, I. L., et al., "The Results of Exposure to an Antisclerotic Vegetarian Diet Enriched with Soy-Based Products on Patients in the Secondary Prevention of Ischemic Heart Disease," *Ter Arkh* 69, no. 9 (1997): 52–55.

————, "Balanced Vegetarian Diet in Combined Rehabilitation of Patients Suffering from Ischemic Heart Disease," *Klin Med* 75, no. 1 (1997): 28–31.

Meydani, Mohsen, "Vitamin E," *The Lancet* 345 (January 21, 1995): 170–175.

Michels, Karin, et al., "Trans Fatty Acids in European Margarines," *New England Journal of Medicine* 332 (February 23, 1995): 541–542.

Milewicz, A., et al., "Vitex Agnus Castus Extract in the Treatment of Luteal Phase Defects Due to Latent Hyperprolactinemia: Results of a Randomized Placebo-Controlled Double-Blind Study," *Arzneimittel-Forschung* 43, no. 7 (July 1993): 752–756.

Miller, Debra L., et al., "Effect of Fat-Free Potato Chips with and without Nutrition Labels on Fat and Energy Intakes," *American Journal of Clinical Nutrition* 68 (1998): 282–290.

Miller, J. C. Brand, et al., "The Carnivore Connection: Dietary Carbohydrate in the Evolution of NIDDM," *Diabetologia* 37 (1994): 1280–1286.

Mills, P. J., et al., "Beta-Adrenergic Receptor Sensitivity in Subjects Practicing Transcendental Meditation," *Journal of Psychosomatic Research* 34, no. 1 (1990): 29–33.

Mirsky, Steve, "Chewing the Fat," *Scientific American,* January 1997, 31.

Monmaney, Terrence, "Adding Fiber Cuts Heart Attack Risk, Study Finds," *Los Angeles Times,* February 14, 1996, A1.

Morgan, S. A., et al., "A Low-Fat Diet Supplemented with Monosaturated Fat Results in Less HDL-C Lowering than a Very-Low-Fat Diet," *Journal of the American Dietetic Association* 97, no. 2 (February 1997): 151–156.

Mulvad, G., et al., "The Inuit Diet: Fatty Acids and Antioxidants, Their Role in Ischemic Heart Disease, and Exposure to Organochlorines and Heavy Metals—An International Study," *Arctic Medical Research* 55, suppl. 1 (1996): 20–24.

Nagamatsu, M., et al., "Lipoic Acid Improves Nerve Blood Flow, Reduces Oxidative Stress, and Improves Distal Nerve Conduction in Experimental Diabetic Neuropathy," *Diabetes Care* 18, no. 8 (August 1995): 1160–1167.

Nair, P., et al., "Vegetarianism, Dietary Fibre and Gastro-Intestinal Disease," *Dig Dis* 12, no. 13 (May/June 1994): 177–185.

Nawaz, S., et al., "Telomerase Expression in Human Breast Cancer with and without Lymph Node Metastases," *Am J Clin Pathol* 107, no. 5 (May 1997): 542–547.

Nelson, Gary J., et al., "Low-Fat Diets Do Not Lower Plasma Cholesterol Levels in Healthy Men Compared to High-Fat Diets with Similar Fatty Acid Composition at Constant Caloric Intake," *Lipids* 30, no. 11 (1995): 969–976.

Okawa, M., et al., "Vitamin B_{12} Treatment for Sleep-Wake Rhythm Disorders," *Biological Psychiatry* 29 (1991): 41S.

Olney, J. W., et al., "Increasing Brain Tumor Rates: Is There a Link to Aspartame?" *Journal of Neuropathology and Experimental Neurology* 55, no. 11 (November 1996): 1115–1123.

Omura, Y., et al., "Non-Invasive Evaluation of the Effects of Opening and Closing of the Eyes, and of Exposure to a Minute Light Beam, As Well As to Electrical or Magnetic Field, on the Melatonin, Serotonin, and Other Neuro-Transmitters of Human Pineal Gland Representation Areas and the Heart," *Acupuncture and Electro-Therapeutics Research* 18, no. 2 (April-June 1993): 125–151.

Ornish, Dean, M.D., "Can Lifestyle Changes Reverse Coronary Heart Disease?" *World Review of Nutrition and Dietetics* 72 (1993): 38–48.

———, "Low-Fat Diets," *New England Journal of Medicine* 338, no. 2 (1998): 127.

Orth-Gomer, K., et al., "Fresh Start After Heart Disease: Changed Life Style Is an Important Part of Rehabilitation," *Lakartidningen* 91, no. 5 (February 2, 1994): 379–384.

Ovesen, L., et al., "Fatty Acid Composition of Danish Margarines and Shortenings, with Special Emphasis on Trans Fatty Acids," *Lipids* 31, no. 9 (September 1996): 971–975.

Packer, Lester, et al., "Alpha-Lipoic Acid As a Biological Antioxidant," *Free Radical Biology and Medicine* 19, no. 2 (August 1995): 227–250.

———, "Neuroprotection by the Metabolic Antioxidant Alpha-Lipoic Acid," *Free Radical Biology and Medicine* 22, nos. 1–2 (1997): 359–378.

Packer, Lester, "Antioxidant Properties of Lipoic Acid and Its Therapeutic Effects in Prevention of Diabetes Complications and Cataracts," *Annals of the New York Academy of Sciences* 738 (1995): 257–264.

Pagliassotti, Michael J., et al., "Increased Net Hepatic Glucose Output from Gluconeogenic Precursors After High-Sucrose Diet Feeding in Male Rats," *American Journal of Physiology* 272 (1997): R526-R531.

Palinski, Wulf, et al., "Low-Density Lipoprotein Undergoes Oxidative Modification In Vivo," *Proceedings of the National Academy of Sciences (USA)* 86 (February 1989): 1372–1376.

Pao, C. C., et al., "Differential Expression of Telomerase Activity in Human Cervical Cancer and Cervical Intraepithelial Neoplasia Lesions," *J Clin Oncol* 15, no. 5 (May 1997): 1932–1937.

Papaconstantinou, H. T., et al., "Glutamine Deprivation Induces Apoptosis in Intestinal Epithelial Cells," *Surgery* 124, no. 2 (August 1998): 152–159.

Pasolini, G., et al., "Effects of Aging on Dehydroepiandrosterone Sulfate in Relation to Fasting Insulin Levels and Body Composition Assessed by Bioimpedance Analysis," *Metabolism* 46, no. 7 (July 1997): 826–832.

Peltonen, R., et al., "Faecal Microbial Flora and Disease Activity in Rheumatoid Arthritis during a Vegan Diet," *Br J Rheumatol* 36, no. 1 (January 1997): 64–68.

Pendergast, D. R., et al., "The Role of Dietary Fat on Performance, Metabolism, and Health," *American Journal of Sports Medicine* 24, no. 6 (1996): S53-S58.

Pinto, J. M., et al., "Administration of Aspartame Potentiates Pentylenetetrazole- and Fluorothyl-Induced Seizures in Mice," *Neuropharmacology* 27, no. 1 (January 1998): 51–55.

Plioplys, A. V., et al., "Amantadine and L-Carnitine Treatment of Chronic Fatigue Syndrome," *Neuropsychobiology* 35, no. 1 (1997): 16–23.

Prasad, A. S., "Zinc Deficiency in Human Subjects," *Prog Clin Biol Res* 129 (1983): 1–33.

Prasad, A. S., et al., "Zinc Status and Serum Testosterone Levels of Healthy Adults," *Nutrition* 12, no. 5 (May 1996): 344–348.

Raben, A., et al., "Decreased Postprandial Thermogenesis and Fat Oxidation but Increased Fullness After a High-Fiber Meal Compared with a Low-Fiber Meal," *American Journal of Clinical Nutrition* 59, no. 6 (June 1994): 1386–1394.

Rao, Ramachandra M., Ph.D., et al., "Anti-Diabetic Effects of Dietary Supplement 'Pancreas Tonic,' " *Journal of the National Medical Association* 90, no. 10 (October 1998): 614–618.

Reaven, Gerald M., M.D., et al., "Comparison of Plasma Glucose and Insulin Responses to Mixed Meals of High-, Intermediate-, and Low-Glycemic Potential," *Diabetes Care* 11, no. 4 (April 1988): 323–329.

———, "Effect of a High Carbohydrate Diet on Insulin Binding to Adipocytes and on Insulin Action In Vivo in Man," *Diabetes* 28 (August 1979): 731–736.

———, "Studies of the Mechanism of Fructose-Induced Hypertriglyceridemia in the Rat," *Metabolism* 31, no. 11 (November 1982): 1077–1083.

Reaven, Peter, et al., "Effects of Oleate-Rich and Linoleate-Rich Diets on the Susceptibility of Low Density Lipoprotein to Oxidative Modification in Mildly Hypercholesterolemic Subjects," *Journal of Clinical Investigation* 91 (February 1993): 668–676.

Reddy, S., et al., "The Influence of Material Vegetarian Diet on Essential Fatty Acid Status of the Newborn," *Eur J Clin Nutr* 48, no. 5 (May 1994): 358–368.

Reimer, R. A., et al., "Dietary Fiber Modulates Intestinal Proglucagon Messenger Ribonucleic Acid and Postprandial Secretion of Glucagon-Like Peptide-1 and Insulin in Rats," *Endocrinology* 137, no 9 (September 1996): 3948–3956.

Reiser, Sheldon, et al., "Isocaloric Exchange of Dietary Starch and Sucrose in Humans," *American Journal of Clinical Nutrition* 32 (August 1979): 1659–1669.

Rimm, E. B., et al., "Vegetable, Fruit, and Cereal Fiber Intake and Risk of Coronary Heart Disease among Men," *Journal of the American Medical Association* 275, no. 6 (February 14, 1996): 447–451.

Ritter, M. M., et al., "Effects of a Vegetarian Life Style on Health," *Fortschr Med* 113, no. 16 (June 10, 1995): 239–242.

Roberts, Paul, "The New Food Anxiety," *Psychology Today* 31, no. 2 (March/April 1998): 30–38; 74.

Rogers, Adam, "Miracles That May Keep You Going," *Newsweek,* June 30, 1997, 59.

Roy, S., et al., "Modulation of Cellular Reducing Equivalent Homeostasis by Alpha-Lipoic Acid: Mechanisms and Implications for Diabetes and Ischemic Injury," *Biochemical Pharmacology* 53, no. 3 (February 7, 1997): 393–399.

Saarela, S., et al., "Function of Melatonin in Thermoregulatory Processes," *Life Sciences* 54, no. 5 (1994): 295–311.

Salmeron, Jorge, M.D., et al., "Dietary Fiber, Glycemic Load, and Risk of Non-Insulin-Dependent Diabetes Mellitus in Women," *Journal of the American Medical Association* 277, no. 6 (February 12, 1997): 472–477.

Schaefer, Ernst J., et al., "Changes in Plasma Lipoprotein Concentrations and Composition in Response to a Low-Fat, High-Fiber Diet Are Associated with Changes in Serum Estrogen Concentrations in Premenopausal Women," *Metabolism: Clinical and Experimental* 44, no. 6 (June 6, 1995): 749–756.

Schmidt, T., et al., "Changes in Cardiovascular Risk Factors and Hormones during a Comprehensive Residential Three-Month Kriya Yoga Training and Vegetarian Nutrition," *Acta Physiol Scand Suppl* 640 (1997): 158–162.

Selvendran, Robert R., Ph.D., "The Plant Cell Wall As a Source of Dietary Fiber: Chemistry and Structure," *American Journal of Clinical Nutrition* 39 (February 1984): 320–337.

Seung-Yeol, Nah, et al., "A Trace Component of Ginseng That Inhibits Ca2+ Channels through a Pertussis Toxin-Sensitive G Protein," *Proceedings of the National Academy of Sciences (USA)* 92 (September 1995): 8739–8743.

Shankar, Anuraj H., et al., "Zinc and Immune Function: The Biological Basis of Altered Resistance to Infection," *American Journal of Clinical Nutrition* 68 (1998): 447S–463S.

Sheehan, John P., et al., "Effect of High Fiber Intake in Fish Oil-Treated Patients with Non-Insulin-Dependent Diabetes Mellitus," *American Journal of Clinical Nutrition* 66 (1997): 1183–1187.

Sido, B., et al., "Glutamine Deficiency of the Intestine in Crohn Disease: Basic Principles for Substitution Therapy," *Langenbecks Arch Chir Suppl Kongressbd* 114 (1997): 653–656.

Simon, G. L., et al., "The Human Intestinal Microflora," *Dig Dis Sci* 31, suppl. 9 (September 1986): 147S–162S.

Sliutz, G., et al., "Agnus Castus Extracts Inhibit Prolactin Secretion of Rat Pituitary Cells," *Hormone and Metabolic Research* 25, no. 5 (May 1993): 253–255.

Soneru, I. L., et al., "Acetyl-L-Carnitine Effects on Nerve Conduction and Glycemic Regulation in Experimental Diabetes," *Endocr Res* 23, nos. 1–2 (February 1997): 27–36.

Spiller, Gene A., et al., "Guar Gum and Plasma Cholesterol," *Arteriosclerosis and Thrombosis* 11 (1991): 1204–1208.

Stoppler, H., et al., "The Human Papillomavirus Type 16 E6 and E7 Oncoproteins Dissociate Cellular Telomerase Activity from the Maintenance of Telomere Length," *Journal of Biological Chemistry* 272, no. 20 (May 16, 1997): 13332–13337.

Sun, Z., et al., "Inefficient Secretion of Human H27A-Prolactin, a Mutant That Does Not Bind Zn2+," *Mol Endocrinol* 11, no. 10 (September 1997): 1544–1551.

Tillakaratne, N. J., et al., "Gamma-Aminobutyric Acid (GABA) Metabolism in Mammalian Neural and Nonneural Tissues," *Comparative Biochemistry and Physiology* 112, no. 2 (October 1995): 247–263.

Travaglini, P., et al., "Effect of Oral Zinc Administration on Prolactin and Thymulin Circulating Levels in Patients with Chronic Renal Failure," *Journal of Clinical Endocrinology and Metabolism* 68, no. 1 (January 1989): 186–190.

———, "Zinc and Bromocriptine Long-Term Administration in Patients with Prolactinomas: Effects on Prolactin and Thymulin Circulating Levels," *Int J Neurosci* 59, nos. 1–3 (July 1991): 119–125.

Tremel, Harald, et al., "Glutamine Dipeptide-Supplemented Parenteral Nutrition Maintains Intestinal Function in the Critically Ill," *Gastroenterology* 107 (1994): 1595–1601.

Umbricht, C. B., et al., "Telomerase Activity: A Marker to Distinguish Follicular Thyroid Adenoma from Carcinoma," *Cancer Research* 57, no. 11 (June 1, 1997): 2144–2147.

Uvnas-Moberg, K., "Physiological and Endocrine Effects of Social Contact," *Annals of the New York Academy of Sciences* 807 (January 15, 1997): 146–163.

Van Der Hulst, Rene R. W. J., et al., "Glutamine and the Preservation of Gut Integrity," *The Lancet* 341 (May 29, 1993): 1363–1365.

———, "Glutamine Extraction by the Gut Is Reduced in Depleted Cancer," *Ann Surg* 225, no. 1 (January 1997): 112–121.

Van Eck, M., et al., "The Effects of Perceived Stress, Traits, Mood States, and Stressful Daily Events on Salivary Cortisol," *Psychosomatic Medicine* 58, no. 5 (September 1996): 447–458.

Vlachokosta, Frederika V., et al., "Dietary Carbohydrate, a Big Mac, and Insulin Requirements in Type I Diabetes," *Diabetes Care* 11, no. 4 (April 1988): 330–336.

Walter, Paul, et al., "Effects of Vegetarian Diets on Aging and Longevity," *Nutrition Reviews* 55 (January 1997): 1–6.

Wasa, M., et al., "Glutamine As a Regulator of DNA and Protein Biosynthesis in Human Solid Tumor Cell Lines," *Ann Surg* 224, no. 2 (August 1996): 189–197.

Werner, O. R., et al., "Long-Term Endocrinologic Changes in Subjects Practicing the Transcendental Meditation and TM-Sidhi Program," *Psychosomatic Medicine* 48, nos. 1–2 (January/February 1986): 59–66.

Williams, Stephen, "A Six Pack of Stout and a Coffin to Go," *Newsweek*, October 20, 1997, 76.

Williamson, David F., Ph.D., "Pharmacotherapy for Obesity," *Journal of the American Medical Association* 281, no. 3 (January 20, 1999): 278–280.

Wilson, B. E., et al., "Effects of Chromium Supplementation on Fasting Insulin Levels and Lipid Parameters in Healthy, Non-Obese Young Subjects," *Diabetes Research and Clinical Practice* 28, no. 3 (June 1995): 179–184.

Wood, Diana, "Sugarland Express: Beware! Your Favorite Foods Could Be Raising Your Insulin Level to Dizzying Heights," *W*, October 1997, 159–160.

Wurtman, Richard J., et al., "Effects of Oral Aspartame on Plasma Phenylalanine in Humans and Experimental Rodents," *Journal of Neural Transmission* 70, nos. 1–2 (1987): 169–173.

———, "Daily Rhythms in the Concentrations of Various Amino Acids in Human Plasma," *New England Journal of Medicine* 279 (1968): 171–175.

Wurtman, Richard J., "Daily Rhythms in Mammalian Protein Metabolism," *Mammalian Protein Metabolism* 4 (1970): 445–479.

Yerboeket-van de Venne, W. P., et al., "Effects of Dietary Fat and Carbohydrate Exchange on Human Energy Metabolism," *Appetite* 26, no. 3 (June 1996): 287–300.

Yudkin, John, M.D., "Sucrose, Coronary Heart Disease, Diabetes, and Obesity: Do Hormones Provide a Link?" *American Heart Journal* 115, no. 2 (February 1988): 493–498.

Zeldin, D. C., et al, "CYP2J Subfamily Cytochrome P450s in the Gastrointestinal Tract: Expression, Localization, and Potential Functional Significance," *Molecular Pharmacology* 51, no. 6 (June 1997): 931–943.

Zeng, X., et al., "Chemical Constituents of the Fruits of Vitex trifolia L.," *Chung-Kuo Chung Yao Tsa Chih: China Journal of Chinese Materia Medica* 21, no. 3 (March 1996): 167–168; 191.

Ziegler, Dan, M.D., et al., "Effects of Treatment with the Antioxidant a-Lipoic Acid on Cardiac Autonomic Neuropathy in NIDDM Patients," *Diabetes Care* 20, no. 3 (March 1997): 369–373.

———, "Treatment of Symptomatic Diabetic Peripheral Neuropathy with the Anti-Oxidant Alpha-Lipoic Acid: A Three-Week Multicentre Randomized Controlled Trial (ALADIN Study)," *Diabetologia* 38, no. 12 (December 1995): 1425–1433.

Zumbach, M. S., et al., "Tumor Necrosis Factor Increases Serum Leptin Levels in Humans," *Journal of Clinical Endocrinology and Metabolism* 82, no. 12 (December 1997): 4080–4082.

Chapter Ten: Be Afraid, Be Very Afraid

Bardasano, J., L., et al., "Metabolic Treatment and Magnetic Fields, Department of Medical Specialties, University of Alcala de Henares, P-258-C, 310.

Bartsch, C., et al., "Stage-Dependent Depression of Melatonin in Patients with Primary Breast Cancer: Correlation with Prolactin, Thyroid Stimulating Hormone, and Steroid Receptors," *Cancer* 64, no. 2 (July 15, 1989): 426–433.

Blomer, U., et al., "Bcl-xL Protects Adult Septal Cholinergic Neurons from Axotomized Cell Death," *Neurobiology* 95, no. 5 (March 3, 1998): 2603–2608.

Bodnar, Andrea G., et al., "Extension of Life Span by Introduction of Telomerase into Normal Human Cells," *Science* 279 (January 16, 1998): 349–352.

Cadossi, R., Hentz, V. R., Kipp, J., Iverson, R., Ceccherelli, G., Zucchini, P., Emilia, G., Torelli, G., Franceschi, C., et al., "Effect of Low Frequency Low Energy Pulsing Electromagnetic Field (PEMF) on X-Ray-Irradiated Mice," *Exp Hematol*, no. 2 (February 17, 1989): 88–95. Published erratum appears in *Exp Hematol*, no. 8 (September 17, 1989): 922.

Dandona, P., et al., "Oxidative Damage to DNA in Diabetes Mellitus," *The Lancet* 347 (February 17, 1996): 444–445.

Dauchy, R. T., et al., "Light Contamination during the Dark Phase in 'Photoperiodically Controlled' Animal Rooms: Effect on Tumor Growth and Metabolism in Rats," *Laboratory Animal Sciences* 47, no. 5 (October 1997): 511–518.

Finch, Caleb E., et al., "Genetics of Aging," *Science* 278 (October 17, 1997): 407–411.

Garcia-Maurino, Sofia, et al., "Melatonin Enhances IL-2, IL-6, and IFN-y Production by Human Circulating CD4+ Cells," *Journal of Immunology* 159 (1997): 574–581.

"Glenn Cut from Test on Melatonin," *Santa Barbara News Press,* October 21, 1998, A6.

Halliwell, Barry, "Free Radicals, Antioxidants, and Human Disease: Curiosity, Cause, or Consequence?" *The Lancet* 344 (September 10, 1994): 721–724.

Jacob, Robert A., et al., "Oxidative Damage and Defense 1–3," *American Journal of Clinical Nutrition* 63 (1996): 985S-990S.

Kluger, Jeffrey, "Can We Stay Young?" *Time,* November 25, 1996, 89–98.

Kolata, Gina, "Doctors Debate Use of Drug to Help Women's Sex Lives," *The New York Times,* April 25, 1998, A7.

Kumei, Y., et al., "Microgravity Induces Prostaglandin E2 and Interleukin-6 Production in Normal Rat Osteoblasts: Role in Bone Demineralization," *J Biotechnol* 47, nos. 2–3 (June 27, 1996): 313–324.

La Torre, F., et al., "Role of Free Radicals, Telomeres, and Telomerases in Aging and Cancerogenesis," *Mol Med Today* 3, no. 5 (May 1997): 187.

Linnane, Anthony W., et al., "Mitochondrial DNA Mutations As an Important Contributor to Aging and Degenerative Diseases," *The Lancet* 1 (March 25, 1989): 642–645.

Mandal, M., et al., "Bcl-2 Modulates Telomerase Activity," *Journal of Biological Chemistry* 272, no. 22 (May 30, 1997): 14183–14187.

McNeil, Donald G., Jr., "In Bushmanland, Hunters' Tradition Turns to Dust," *The New York Times,* November 13, 1997, A3.

Miller, Martin, "Ageless Quest for Fountain of Youth Is Alive and Well," *Los Angeles Times,* April 9, 1998, E1.

Millington, W. R., et al., "A Diurnal Rhythm in Proopiomelanocortin Messenger Ribonucleic Acid That Varies Concomitantly with the Content and Secretion of beta-Endorphin in the Intermediate Lobe of the Rat Pituitary," *Endocrinology* 118, no. 2 (February 1986): 829–834.

Morris, Jason Z., et al., "A Phosphatidylinositol-3-OH Kinase Family Member Regulating Longevity and Diapause in Caenorhabditis elegans," *Nature* 382 (August 8, 1996): 536–538.

Moss, Robert, "The Problem with Evolution: Where Have We Gone Wrong?" *The Scientist,* October 13, 1997, 7.

O'Connell, Y., et al., "The Effect of Prolactin, Human Chorionic Gonadotropin, Insulin and Insulin-Like Growth Factor 1 on Adrenal Steroidogenesis in Isolated Guinea-Pig Adrenal Cells," *Journal of Steroid Biochemistry and Molecular Biology* 48, nos. 2–3 (February 1994): 235–240.

Papanicolaou, Dimitris A., M.D., et al., "The Pathophysiologic Roles of Interleukin-6 in Human Disease," *Annals of Internal Medicine* 128, no. 2 (January 15, 1998): 127–137.

Path, Gunter, et al., "Interleukin-6 and the Interleukin-6 Receptor in the Human Adrenal Gland: Expression and Effects on Steroidogeneses," *Journal of Clinical Endocrinology and Metabolism* 82, no. 7 (1997): 2343–2349.

Pennisi, Elizabeth, "Do Fateful Circles of DNA Cause Cells to Grow Old?" *Science* 279 (January 2, 1998): 34.

Quinn, Graham E., et al., "Myopia and Ambient Lighting at Night," *Nature* 399 (May 13, 1999): 113.

Radov, Daniel B., "Electromagnetic Alchemy," *American Scientist* 87 (March/April 1999): 123–124.

Sen, Chandan K., et al., "Antioxidant and Redox Regulation of Gene Transcription," *FASEB* 10 (1996): 709–720.

Schneider, David, "Some Levity in Physics," *American Scientist* 87 (March/April 1999): 122–123.

Schreiber-Agus, Nicole, et al., "Role of Mxi1 in Ageing Organ Systems and the Regulation of Normal and Neoplastic Growth," *Nature* 393 (June 4, 1998): 483–489.

Skulachev, V. P., "Aging Is a Specific Biological Function Rather than the Result of a Disorder in Complex Living Systems: Biochemical Evidence in Support of Weismann's Hypothesis," *Biochemistry (Mosc)* 62, no. 11 (November 1997): 1191–1195.

Thornhill, Alan, "Aborigines Became 'Poachers' in Their Native Land," *Santa Barbara News Press,* December 7, 1997, A14.

Tsigos, C., et al., "Dose Effects of Recombinant Human Interleukin-6 on Pituitary Hormone Secretion and Energy Expenditure," *Neuroendocrinology* 66, no. 1 (July 1997): 54–62.

Victoria, Ann, "World's Oldest Human Celebrates 141st Year!" *Weekly World News,* April 7, 1998, 22.

Vines, Gail, "Into the Dark: Does the Strange Decline of Amphibian Populations Hold a Sinister Message for Us All?" *New Scientist,* June 13, 1998, 48.

Von Treuer, K., et al., "Overnight Human Plasma Melatonin, Cortisol, Prolactin, TSH, under Conditions of Normal Sleep, Sleep Deprivation, and Sleep Recovery," *Journal of Pineal Research* 20, no. 1 (January 1996): 7–14.

Westerlind, K. C., et al., "The Skeletal Effects of Space Flight in Growing Rats: Tissue-Specific Alterations in mRNA Levels for TGF-beta," *J Bone Miner Res* 10, no. 6 (June 1995): 843–848.

Xu, Lin, et al., "Glucocorticoid Receptor and Protein/RNA Synthesis-Dependent Mechanisms Underlie the Control of Synaptic Plasticity by Stress," *Neurobiology* 95, no. 6 (March 17, 1998): 3204–3208.

BIBLIOGRAPHY AND SUGGESTED READING

Abbas, Abul K., et al. *Cellular and Molecular Immunology.* Philadelphia, Pa.: W. B. Saunders Company, 1994.

Ackerman, Diane. *A Natural History of the Senses.* New York: Vintage Books, 1990.

Aldridge, Susan. *Magic Molecules.* Cambridge: Cambridge University Press, 1998.

Alvarez, A. *Night.* New York: W. W. Norton & Company, 1995.

Anderson, Harvey G., et al. *Energy and Macronutrient Intake Regulation: Independent or Interrelated Mechanisms,* "Fuel Homeostasis and the Nervous System," 1991.

Atkins, Robert C., M.D. *Dr. Atkins' New Diet Revolution.* New York: Avon Books, 1992.

———. *Dr. Atkins' Vita-Nutrient Solution.* New York: Simon & Schuster, 1998.

Baker, Robin, Ph.D. *Sperm Wars.* New York: Basic Books, 1996.

Baggish, Jeff, M.D. *How Your Immune System Works.* Los Angeles: Ziff-Davis Press, 1994.

———. *Making the Prostate Therapy Decision.* Los Angeles: Lowell House, 1996.

Balin, Arthur K., M.D., Ph.D., et al. *The Life of the Skin.* New York: Bantam Books, 1997.

Bazell, Robert. *Her 2.* New York: Random House, 1998.

Becker, Robert O., M.D., et al. *The Body Electric.* New York: William Morrow, 1985.

Behe, Michael J. *Darwin's Black Box.* New York: The Free Press, 1996.

Benjamin, B., et al. *Mortality on the Move.* Oxford: Actuarial Education Services, 1997.

Benson, Herbert, M.D., et al. *Relaxation Response.* New York: Wing Books, 1975.

Biddle, Wayne. *A Field Guide to Germs.* New York: Henry Holt and Company, 1995.

Black, Ira B. *Information in the Brain.* Cambridge, Mass.: The MIT Press, 1994.

Bloom, Howard. *The Lucifer Principle.* New York: The Atlantic Monthly Press, 1995.

Blum, Deborah, et al. *A Field Guide for Science Writers.* New York: Oxford University Press, 1997.

Booth, Martin. *A Biography of Arthur Conan Doyle.* London: Hodder and Stoughton, 1997.

Borbely, Alexander. *Secrets of Sleep.* New York: Basic Books, 1984.

Boune, Jean Marie, M.D. *Brainfood.* Boston: Little, Brown and Company, 1990.

Bratman, Steven, M.D. *Beat Depression with St. John's Wort.* Rocklin, CA.: Prima Publishing, 1997.

Breggin, Peter R., M.D., et al. *Talking Back to Prozac.* New York: St. Martin's Press, 1994.

Brownlee, Harriet. *The Low-Carbohydrate Gourmet.* New York: William Morrow, 1974.

Burkholz, Herbert. *The FDA Follies.* New York: Basic Books, 1994.

Buss, David M. *The Evolution of Desire.* New York: Basic Books, 1994.

Cairns-Smith, A. G. *Evolving the Mind.* New York: Cambridge University Press, 1996.

Calvin, William H. *How Brains Think.* New York: Basic Books, 1996.

Campbell, Bernard G., et al. *Humankind Emerging.* New York: HarperCollins Publishers, 1996.

Cannon, Geoffrey, et al. *Dieting Makes You Fat.* New York: Pocket Books, 1987.

Capra, Fritjof. *The Tao of Physics.* London: Flamingo, 1982.

————. *The Web of Life.* London: Flamingo, 1997.

Cavalli-Sforza, Luca L., et al. *The History and Geography of Human Genes.* Princeton, N.J.: Princeton University Press, 1994.

Chopra, Deepak, M.D. *Quantum Healing.* New York: Bantam Books, 1990.

Clark, Hulda Regehr, Ph.D., N.D. *The Cure for All Diseases.* San Diego: New Century Press, 1995.

Clark, William R. *Sex & The Origins of Death.* New York: Oxford University Press, 1996.

Cooper, Jack R., et al. *The Biochemical Basis of Neuropharmacology.* New York: Oxford University Press, 1996.

Coren, Stanley. *Sleep Thieves.* New York: The Free Press, 1997.

Crossen, Cynthia. *Tainted Truth.* New York: Simon & Schuster, 1994.

Csermely, Peter. *Stress of Life from Molecules to Man.* New York: The New York Academy of Sciences, 1998.

Cummings, Stephen, M.D., et al. *Homeopathic Medicines.* New York: Jeremy P. Tarcher/Perigee, 1991.

Davis-Floyd, Robbie, et al. *From Doctor to Healer.* New Brunswick, N.J.: Rutgers University Press, 1998.

DeGregorio, Michael W., et al. *Tamoxifen and Breast Cancer.* New Haven: Yale University Press, 1994.

DeLillo, Don. *White Noise.* Penguin Books, 1991.

Deutsch, David. *The Fabric of Reality.* New York: Penguin Books, 1997.

De Waal, Frans. *Good Natured.* Cambridge, Mass.: Harvard University Press, 1996.

Diamond, Harvey and Marilyn. *Fit for Life.* New York: Warner Books, 1985.

Diamond, Jared. *The Third Chimpanzee.* New York: Harper Perennial, 1992.

Doyle, Arthur Conan. *The Sign of the Four.* London: Music for Pleasure, Ltd., 1981.

————. *The Five Orange Pips of Sherlock Holmes.* Providence, R.I.: Jamestown, 1976.

Drickamer, Lee C., et al. *Animal Behavior.* Dubuque, IA: William. C. Brown Publishers, 1996.

Dufty, William. *Sugar Blues.* New York: Warner Books, 1975.

Eades, Michael R., M.D., et al. *Protein Power.* New York: Bantam Books, 1996.

Eaton, S. Boyd, M.D., et al. *The Paleolithic Prescription.* New York: Harper & Row, 1988.

Ekeland, Ivar. *Mathematics and the Unexpected.* Chicago and London: The University of Chicago Press, 1988.

Erdmann, Robert, Ph.D. *Fats That Can Save Your Life.* Meirion Jones, 1995.

Fabris, N., et al. *Ontogenetic and Phylogenetic Mechanisms of Neuroimmunomodulation.* New York: The New York Academy of Sciences, 1991.

Fabian, Andrew C., *Society, Science, & the Universe. Evolution.* Cambridge: Cambridge University Press, 1998.

Ferris, Timothy. *The Whole Shebang.* New York: Touchstone, 1997.

Feynman, Richard P. *The Meaning of It All.* London: Allen Lane, 1998.

Fienup-Riordan, Ann. *Eskimo Essays.* New Brunswick, N. J.: Rutgers University Press, 1990.

Fishman, Alfred P., M.D. *The Myocardium—Its Biochemistry and Biophysics.* New York: New York Heart Association, Inc., 1960.

Leffert, H. L. *Growth Regulation by Ion Fluxes.* New York: The New York Academy of Sciences, 1980.

Fraser, J. T. *The Voices of Time.* New York: George Braziller, 1966.

Frazer, Alan, et al. *Biological Bases of Brain Function and Disease.* New York: Raven Press, 1994.

Fussell, Betty. *The Story of Corn.* New York: Alfred A. Knopf, 1994.

Ganong, William F. *Review of Medical Physiology.* Norwalk, CT: Appleton & Lange, 1993.

Gass, George H., et al. *Handbook of Endocrinology.* New York: CRC Press, 1996.

Gerber, Richard, M.D. *Vibrational Medicine.* Santa Fe: Bear & Company, 1988.

Gershon, Michael D., M.D. *The Second Brain.* New York: HarperCollins Publishers, 1998.

Globe Digest. *Fat, Sodium & Cholesterol Counter.* New York: Globe Communications Corp., 1997.

Godagama, Shantha, M.D. *The Handbook of Ayurveda.* Boston: Journey Editions, 1998.

Goldberg, Burton. *Heart Disease.* Tiburon, CA: Future Medicine Publishing, 1998.

Gordon, Richard. *The Literary Companion to Medicine.* New York: St. Martin's Press, 1993.

Gosden, Roger. *Cheating Time.* New York: W. H. Freeman and Company, 1996.

Gratzer, Walter. *A Bedside Nature.* New York: W. H. Freeman and Company, 1998.

Hallowell, Edward M., M.D., et al. *Driven to Distraction.* New York: Simon & Schuster, 1994.

Haraway, Donna. *Primate Visions.* New York: Routledge & Kegan Paul, 1989.

Hudler, George W. *Magical Mushrooms, Mischievous Molds.* Princeton, N.J.: Princeton University Press, 1998.

Hughes, Ted. *Tales from Ovid.* New York: Farrar, Straus and Giroux, 1997.

Huxley, Aldous. *Brave New World.* Leicester: Charnwood, 1983.

Jeans, Allene, et al. *Physiological Effects of Food Carbohydrates.* Washington, D.C.: American Chemical Society, 1975.

Jonsson, Gudrun. *Gut Reaction.* London: Random House, 1998.

Julien, Robert M., M.D., Ph.D. *A Primer of Drug Action.* New York: W. H. Freeman and Company, 1995.

Kaplan, Bert. *The Inner World of Mental Illness.* New York: Harper & Row, 1964.

Kesey, Ken. *One Flew Over the Cuckoo's Nest.* New York: Samuel French, 1974.

Klass, Perri. *A Not Entirely Benign Procedure.* New York: Plume, 1994.

Kogelman, Stanley, M.D., et al. *Mind over Math.* New York: McGraw-Hill, 1978.

Kotulak, Ronald. *Inside the Brain.* Kansas City, Missouri: Andrews & McMeel, 1996.

Lamm, Steven, M.D. *Thinner at Last.* New York: Simon & Schuster, 1995.

Langone, John. *Harvard MED.* Holbrook, Mass.: Adams Media Corporation, 1995.

Levine, Arnold J. *Viruses.* New York: Scientific American Library, 1992.

Liberman, Jacob, M.D., Ph.D. *Medicine of the Future.* Santa Fe: Bear & Company, 1991.

Lightman, Alan. *Einstein's Dreams.* New York: Warner Books, 1994.

Livingston-Wheeler, Virgina, M.D., et al. *The Conquest of Cancer.* New York: Franklin Watts, 1984.

Lowe, Ernest, et al. *Diabetes: A Guide to Living Well.* Minneapolis: Chronimed Publishing, 1992.

Lovelock, James. *Gaia.* Oxford: Oxford University Press, 1979.

McGee, Harold. *On Food and Cooking.* New York: Collier Books, 1984.

———. *The Curious Cook.* Toronto: Maxwell Macmillan Canada, 1990.

Mackarness, Richard, M.D. *Eat Fat and Grow Slim.* New York: Doubleday & Company, Inc., 1959.

Margulis, Lynn. *Symbiotic Planet.* New York: Basic Books, 1998.

Marsden, Kathryn. *Food Combing Diet.* London: HarperCollins Publishers, 1993.

Martin, Emily. *Flexible Bodies.* Boston: Beacon Press, 1994.

Maxmen, Jerrold S., M.D., et al. *Psychotropic Drugs Fast Facts.* 2nd ed. New York and London: W. W. Norton & Company, 1995.

Mayer, Jean. *A Diet for Living.* New York: David McKay Company, Inc., 1975.

Mayr, Ernst. *Toward a New Philosophy of Biology.* Cambridge, Mass.: Harvard University Press, 1988.

Medina, John J. *The Clock of Ages.* New York: Cambridge University Press, 1996.

Miller, Jonathan, et al. *Darwin for Beginners.* New York: Pantheon Books, 1982.

Mithen, Steven. *The Prehistory of the Mind.* New York: Thames and Husdon, 1996.

Modrow, John. *How to Become a Schizophrenic.* Washington: Apollyon Press, 1992.

Mohrman, David E., et al. *Cardiovascular Physiology.* New York: McGraw-Hill, 1991.

Moir, Anne, et al. *Brainsex.* London: Arrow Books, 1998.

Moore, Thomas J. *Deadly Medicine.* New York: Simon & Schuster, 1995.

Moore, W. Tabb, et al. *Diagnostic Endocrinology.* St. Louis, Missouri: Mosby, 1996.

Moore-Ede, Martin, M.D., Ph.D., et al. *The Complete Idiot's Guide to Getting a Good Night's Sleep.* New York: Alpha Books, 1998.

Morgan, Elaine. *The Aquatic Ape Hypothesis.* London: Souvenir Press, Ltd., 1997.

———. *The Scars of Evolution.* New York: Oxford University Press, 1990.

Morrison, Philip and Phylis. *The Ring of Truth.* New York: Random House, 1987.

Moyers, Bill. *Healing and the Mind.* New York: Doubleday & Company, Inc., 1993.

Nesse, Randolph M., M.D., and George C. Williams. *Why We Get Sick.* New York: Random House, 1994.

Newsom-Davis, John, et al. *Brain*. Oxford: Oxford University Press, 1998.

Nuland, Sherwin B. *How We Die*. New York: Vintage Books, 1995.

Null, Gary, Ph.D. *Healing with Magnets*. New York: Carroll & Graf Publishers, Inc., 1998.

Novabiochem International. *A Complete Catalog and Scientific Reference Guide*. Cambridge, Mass: 1996.

Opie, Lionel H. *The Heart Physiology: From Cell To Circulation*. Philadelphia, Pa.: Lippincott-Raven Publishers, 1998.

Ornish, Dean. *Love & Survival*. New York: HarperCollins Publishers, Inc., 1997.

Ortiz de Montellano, Bernard R. *Aztec Medicine, Health, and Nutrition*. London: Rutgers University Press, 1990.

Paungger, Johanna, et al. *Moon Time*. Munich: Saffron Walden, 1993.

Pearsall, Paul, Ph.D. *The Heart's Code*. New York: Broadway Books, 1998.

Pert, Candace B., Ph.D. *Molecules of Emotion*. New York: Scribner, 1997.

Pinker, Steven. *How the Mind Works*. New York: W. W. Norton & Company, 1997.

Plotkin, Henry. *Darwin Machines*. Cambridge, Mass.: Harvard University Press, 1994.

Proctor, Robert N. *Cancer Wars*. New York: Basic Books, 1995.

Ratey, John J., M.D., et al. *Shadow Syndromes*. New York: Pantheon Books, 1997.

Raymo, Chet. *Skeptics and True Believers*. New York: Walker & Company, 1998.

Regelson, William, M.D., et al. *The Superhormone Promise*. New York: Simon & Schuster, 1996.

Reiter, Russel J. *Melatonin*. New York: Bantam Books, 1995.

Restak, Richard, M.D. *Brainscapes*. New York: Hyperion, 1995.

Rhodes, Richard. *Deadly Feasts*. New York: Simon & Schuster, 1997.

Ridley, Matt. *The Red Queen*. New York: Macmillan Publishing Company, 1993.

Rinzler, Carol Ann. *Feed a Cold Starve a Fever*. New York: Ballantine Books, 1979.

Roberts, Jenny. *Bible Facts*. New York: Barnes & Noble Books, 1997.

Rosenberg, Charles E., et al. *Framing Disease*. New Brunswick, N.J.: Rutgers University Press, 1992.

Rothman, David J., et al. *Medicine and Western Civilization*. New Brunswick, N.J.: Rutgers University Press, 1995.

Roueche, Berton. *The Medical Detectives*. New York: Truman Talley Books/Plume, 1991.

Ruden, Ronald, M.D. *The Craving Brain*. New York: HarperCollins Publishers, Inc., 1997.

Sandblom, Philip, M.D., Ph.D. *Creativity and Disease*. New York: Marion Boyars, 1992.

Schwartz, Erika, M.D., et al. *Natural Energy.* New York: G. P. Putnam's Sons, 1998.

Scientific American. *Life, Death and the Immune System.* New York: W. H. Freeman and Company, 1994.

Sears, Barry, Ph.D. *The Anti-Aging Zone.* New York: HarperCollins Publishers, Inc., 1999.

———. *Enter the Zone.* New York: HarperCollins Publishers, Inc., 1995.

Sipple, Horace L., et al. *Sugars in Nutrition.* New York: Academic Press, 1974.

Small, Meredith F. *What's Love Got to Do with It?* New York: Anchor Books, 1995.

Snyder, Solomon H. *Drugs and the Brain.* New York: Scientific American Library, 1996.

Stabiner, Karen. *To Dance with the Devil: The New War on Breast Cancer.* New York: Bantam Doubleday Dell Publishing Group, Inc., 1997.

Starr, Paul. *The Social Transformation of American Medicine.* New York: Basic Books, 1982.

Stein, Philip L., et al. *Physical Anthropology.* New York: McGraw-Hill, 1982.

Steward, H. Leighton, et al. *Sugar Busters.* New York: Ballantine Books, 1995.

Stillman, Irwin Maxwell, M.D., et al. *The Doctor's Quick Weight Loss Diet.* New Jersey: Prentice Hall, 1967.

Stocking, George W., Jr. *Victorian Anthropology.* New York: The Free Press, 1987.

Stringer, Christopher, et al. *African Exodus.* New York: Henry Holt and Company, 1996.

Stryer, Lubert. *Biochemistry.* New York: W. H. Freeman and Company, 1975.

Sullivan, Lawrence E. *Healing and Restoring.* New York: Macmillan Publishing Company, 1989.

Sylvia, Claire, et al. *A Change of Heart.* New York: Warner Books, 1997.

Talbot, Michael. *The Holographic Universe.* New York: HarperCollins Publishers, Inc., 1991.

Taller, Herman, M.D. *Calories Don't Count.* New York: Simon & Schuster, 1961.

Taylor, Timothy. *The Prehistory of Sex.* New York: Bantam Books, 1996.

The Naturopathic Handbook of Herbal Formulas. Cambridge, Mass.: Herbal Research Publications, Inc., 1995.

Theodosakis, Jason, M.D., et al. *The Arthritis Cure.* New York: St. Martin's Press, 1997.

Thomas, Paul J., et al. *Comets and the Origin and Evolution of Life.* New York: Springer, 1997.

Time-Life Books. *Mysteries of Mind, Space & Time—The Unexplained.* New York: Websters Unified, 1992.

Timiras, Paola S., M.D., Ph.D., et al. *Hormones and Aging.* Boca Raton, FL.: CRC Press, 1995.

Tourney, Christopher P. *Conjuring Science.* New Brunswick, NJ: Rutgers University Press, 1996.

Trefil, James. *Are We Unique?* New York: John Wiley & Sons, Inc., 1997.

Twain, Mark. *Life on the Mississippi.* WANT/Thirteen Nebraska TV and Great Amwell Co., 1980. Videocassette.

Veggeberg, Scott K. *Medication of the Mind.* New York: Henry Holt and Company, 1996.

Villoldo, Alberto, Ph.D., et al. *Healing States.* New York: Simon & Schuster, 1987.

Volk, Tyler. *Gaia's Body.* New York: Copernicus, 1998.

Von Bingen, Hildegard. *Mystical Visions.* Santa Fe: Bear & Company, 1986.

Waldrop, M. Mitchell. *Complexity.* New York: Simon & Schuster, 1992.

Warrier, Gopi, et al. *Ayurveda.* Dorset, England: Element Books Limited, 1997.

Watson, Lyall. *Dark Nature.* New York: HarperCollins Publishers, Inc. 1996.

Weil, Andrew. *The Natural Mind.* Boston, Mass.: Houghton Mifflin Company, 1986.

Weiner, Annette B. *The Sexual Life of Savages.* Boston, MA: Beacon Press, 1987.

Wells, H. G. *The Definitive Time Machine.* Bloomington, IN: IU Press, 1987.

Wiederholt, Wigbert C. *Neurology for Non-Neurologists.* Philadelphia, PA: W. B. Saunders Company, 1995.

Williams, Guy. *The Age of Agony.* Chicago: Academy Chicago Publishers, 1986.

Williams, Tom, Ph.D. *Chinese Medicine.* Dorset, England: Element Books, 1996.

Wilson, Edward O. *Consilience: The Unity of Knowledge.* New York: Alfred A. Knopf, 1998.

Wolfson, Richard, et al. *Physics.* HarperCollins Publishers, 1990.

Wolinsky, Stephen. *Quantum Consciousness.* Norfolk, CT: Bramble Books, 1993.

Wolpoff, Milfred, et al. *Race and Human Evolution.* New York: Simon & Schuster, 1997.

Wood, Lawrence C., M.D., et al. *Your Thyroid.* New York: Ballantine Books, 1995.

Wright, Jonathan V., M.D. *Natural Hormone Replacement.* Petaluma, CA: Smart Publications, 1997.

Zimmerman, Barry E., et al. *Killer Germs.* Chicago: Contemporary Books, 1996.

GLOSSARY

adaptation: In evolutionary biology, any structure, physiological process, or behavioral trait that makes an animal better able to survive and reproduce compared to conspecifics. Also used to describe the process of evolutionary change leading to the formation of such a trait.

adaptive behavior: Behavior patterns that make an organism more fit to survive and reproduce in comparison with other members of the same species.

adhesion: The molecular force of attraction in the area of contact between unlike substances.

adipose tissue: Fat cells.

adrenal glands: Paired endocrine glands, located next to the kidneys in the abdomen. The adrenal cortex produces steroid hormones involved in water balance, glucose metabolism, and electrolyte balance. The adrenal medulla produces adrenaline and noradrenaline, which are involved in glucose metabolism, heart rate, and blood pressure.

albedo effect: The reflection of a portion of solar radiation by the atmosphere.

alleles: Genes occupying equivalent positions in paired chromosomes, yet producing different effects in the phenotype when they are homozygous. They are alternative states of a gene, originally produced by mutation.

amino acids: A group of organic compounds that act as building blocks for proteins.

amylase: Any enzyme that digests starch.

androgen: A generic term for male sex hormones, e.g., testosterone.

ANF: Atrial Natriuretic Factor, a peptide or substance secreted from the atrium of the heart that conveys information immediately from the heart to various organs of the body, including the endocrine organs and the brain.

antagonism: The condition of being an opposing principle, force, or factor, as when two hormones have opposite effects on target tissues.

anthropology: The science of humankind; the systematic study of human evolution, human variability, and human behavior, past and present.

antibiotic: Any of a large number of substances, produced by various microorganisms and fungi, capable of inhibiting or killing bacteria and usually not harmful to higher organisms; for example, penicillin, streptomycin.

313

antibody: A protein produced as a defense mechanism to attack a foreign substance invading the body.

antigens: Any organic substances recognized by the body as foreign that stimulate the production of an antibody.

arteriosclerosis: Inelasticity and thickening of the arterial walls.

artery: A vessel carrying blood away from the heart and toward a capillary bed.

atherosclerosis: Narrowing of the arteries.

atom: The smallest indivisible unit of an element still retaining the element's characteristics.

ATP (adenosinetriphosphate): A ubiquitous small molecule involved in many biological energy exchange reactions, consisting of the nitrogenous base adenine, the sugar ribose, and three phosphate residues.

atrium: Also called the auricle, either of the two upper chambers of the heart, each of which receives blood from veins and, in turn, forces it into the corresponding ventricle.

Australopithecus afarensis: A gracile australopithecine species that inhabited East Africa between four and 2.5 million years ago; if the Lothagam jaw is included in the species, it goes back to 5.6 million years ago.

autoimmune disease: A disease in which an organism's immune system attacks and destroys one or more of the organism's own tissues.

bacterium: Any of numerous prokaryotic organisms.

bark: The portion of a stem outside the wood (xylem), consisting of cambium, phloem, cortex, epidermis, cork cambium, and cork; everything from the vascular cambium outward.

basal metabolic rate (BMR): The rate at which energy is released within the body under conditions of minimal activity.

behavioral ecology: A subdiscipline within animal behavior that deals with the ways in which animals interact with their environment and the survival value of behavior as well as its contribution to reproductive success.

behavior genetics: The study of the role that genes play in controlling behavior.

beta cells: Cells that make insulin. These cells are found in the islets of Langerhans in the pancreas.

biological clock: An internal timing mechanism that involves both an internal self-sustaining pacemaker and cyclic environmental synchronizers.

biological rhythm: A cyclical pattern of behavior, occurring at some regular period.

biomass: The total weight of living material of a species or population.

biosphere: The entire part of the earth's land, soil, waters, and atmosphere in which living organisms are found.

biotic control: Population control by living factors, including both intraspecific and interspecific influences. Compare abiotic control.

bipedal: Moving erect on the hind limbs only.

blood-brain barrier: In the brain, state of highly selective permeability to many substances that readily move into or out of other tissues, attributed in part to lack of the usual looseness of capillary structure.

bone: The hard connective tissue forming the skeleton of most vertebrates, consisting primarily of a collagen matrix impregnated with calcium phosphate.

bottleneck: Also called a population bottleneck, denoting a relatively short period of time during which the size of a population becomes unusually small, resulting in a random change in gene frequencies.

brain: 1. In vertebrates, the anterior enlargement of the central nervous system, encased in the cranium. 2. In invertebrates, any anterior concentration of neurons more or less corresponding in function to the vertebrate brain.

calorie: 1. Also called a small calorie (calorie proper), the amount of heat (or equivalent chemical energy) needed to raise the temperature of 1 gram of water by 1°C. 2. Also called a large calorie, or kilocalorie, the heat needed to raise the temperature of 1 kilogram of water by 1°C.; 1000 small calories.

capillary: The smallest of blood vessels; the fine channel between the arteriole and venule.

carbohydrate: Class of organic compounds with multiple hydroxyl side groups and an aldehyde or ketone group, including sugars, starches, cellulose, and chitin, having the empirical formula $(CH_2O)n$.

cardiac: pertaining to the heart; near or toward the heart.

cardiac coherence: A state of cardiovascular and neurophysiological balance indicated by smooth, steady cardiac tracings as measured by electrocardiographs administered by the Heart Math Institute.

cardiac conduction system: Cardiology's name for the complex bundle of fibers relaying information and energy within and from the heart.

carnivorous: Flesh-eating.

cartilage: A firm, elastic, flexible, translucent type of connective tissue; in development, a precursor of bone formation.

cell: 1. The structural unit of plant and animal life, consisting of cytoplasm and a nucleus, enclosed in a semipermeable membrane. 2. Any similar organization, as that of a protist or prokaryotic organism.

cell-mediated response: The response of activated cytotoxic T cells, which includes the identification of, binding to, and lysis of cancerous and virus-infected cells.

cell respiration: The energy-yielding metabolism of foods in which oxygen is used.

cell theory: The universally accepted proposal that cells are the functional units of organization in living organisms and that all cells today come from pre-existing cells.

cellular memory: The theory that each of the 75 trillion cells in the body has various levels of stored information left there by the heart's conduction of L energy, which can be retrieved by focusing less on the brain and more on the heart. The impact of cellular memory is illustrated by the recall of heart transplant recipients of various forms of their donor's memories. Since information is a form of energy and, like matter, energy can not be destroyed, cellular memories are infinite.

central nervous system (CNS): that part of the nervous system that is condensed and centrally located; for example, the brain and spinal cord of vertebrates and the brain and ganglia of insects.

cerebral cortex: The outermost region of the cerebrum, also called the gray matter, consisting of several dense layers of neural cell bodies and including numerous conscious centers, as well as regions specializing in voluntary movement and sensory reception.

chakra: From the Sanskrit word meaning "wheel," chakras, according to Indian yogic teachings, are the body's energy centers, resembling whirling vortices of subtle energy. There are seven chakras, the fourth being the central, or "heart," chakra. These energy centers relate to the levels of flowing Qi (pronounced "chee") referred to in the two-thousand-year-old system of Chinese medicine.

chemical reaction: The reciprocal action of chemical agents on one another; chemical change.

chemical synapse: Synapses between neurons involving a space, the synaptic cleft, across which neurotransmitters must pass for a neural impulse to begin in the second neuron.

chlorophyll: A green photosynthetic pigment found in chloroplasts, cyanobacteria, and chloroxybacteria. It occurs in several forms, such as chlorophyll a, b, and c.

cholesterol: A lipid molecule that is needed for making parts of the cell fabric as well as steroid hormones but that also, if deposited in artery walls, leads to atherosclerosis.

chromatin: The substance of chromosomes, a molecular complex consisting of DNA, histones, nonhistone chromosomal proteins, and usually some RNA of unknown function.

chromosomal mutation: A massive change in DNA, usually referring to breakage involving a whole chromosome that has not been repaired or has been repaired improperly.

chromosomes: Coiled, threadlike structures of DNA, bearing the genes and found in the nucleis of all plant and animal cells.

circadian rhythm: A biological rhythm of about a day in length or period.

circannual rhythm: A biological rhythm of about a year in length or period.

citric acid cycle: Also called tricarboxylic acid cycle, a cyclic series of chemical transformations in the mitochondrion by which pyruvate is degraded to carbon dioxide, NAD and FAD are reduced to NADH and $FADH_2$, and ATP is generated.

closed circulatory system: A system in which blood is enclosed within arteries, veins, and capillaries and is not in direct contact with cells other than those lining these vessels.

codon: 1. A series of three nucleotides in mRNA specifying a specific amino acid. 2. The colinear, complementary series of three nucleotides or nucleotide pairs in the DNA from which mRNA codon is transcribed.

coenzyme: A small organic molecule required for an enzymatic reaction.

coevolution: The change in gene frequencies resulting from two species acting as strong selective forces on one another.

cognition: The processes in the minds of animals that govern their general mental functions, including perception, representation, and memory.

cohesion: The attraction between the molecules of a single substance.

collagen: In animals, a widely distributed fibrous protein of connective tissue that forms much of the structure of tendons and ligaments.

colon: In mammals, the large intestine from the cecum to the rectum; including the ascending, transverse, descending, and sigmoid regions and the rectum.

colony: 1. A group of animals or plants of the same kind living in a close semidependent association. 2. An aggregation of bacteria growing together as the descendants of a single individual, usually on a culture plate.

common descent: Descent of two or more species (or individuals) from a common ancestor; for example, the similarity in blood chemistry of apes and humans is due to their common descent.

competition: The attempt of two or more organisms to utilize the same resource.

competitive inhibition: Enzyme inhibition involving molecules, similar to the substrate, that compete for the active site.

complete digestive tract: A tubular digestive tract with an anal as well as an oral opening.

connective tissue: A principal type of vertebrate supporting tissue, often with an extracellular matrix of collagen. Included are bone, cartilage, ligaments, and blood.

corpus callosum: A broad, white neural tract in the mammalian brain that connects the cerebral hemispheres and correlates their activities.

corpus luteum: A structure forming from a collapsed follicle after ovulation that produces progesterone in the second half of the menstrual cycle.

cortex: 1. The outer layer or rind of an organ, such as the adrenal cortex and kidney cortex. 2. The portion of a plant stem between the epidermis and the vascular tissue.

corticosteroid: A steroid hormone produced by the adrenal glands.

counterregulatory (stress) hormones: hormones released during stressful situations. These hormones include glucagon, epinephrine (adrenaline), norepinephrine, cortisol, and growth hormone. They cause the liver to release glucose and the cells to release fatty acids for extra energy. If there's not enough insulin present in the body, these extra fuels can lead to hyperglycemia and ketoacidosis.

cultural evolution: Changes in human culture resulting from the accumulated experience of humankind. Cultural evolution can produce adaptations to the environment faster than organic evolution can.

culture: Humans' systems of learned behavior, symbols, customs, beliefs, institutions, artifacts, and technology, characteristic of a group and transmitted by its members to their offspring.

cycle: Repeating units that make up a pattern of biological rhythms.

Cyclic AMP (cAMP): Adenosine monophosphate in which the phosphate is linked between the 3rd and 5th carbons of the ribose group; serves as an intracellular gene regulator under a variety of circumstances.

death rate: In human populations, the number of deaths per 1,000 people per year.

dendrites: The fine extensions from a nerve cell body, usually providing the main receptive area of the cell for synaptic contacts.

depolarized: Having had a reduction in the difference in charge (potential) between the outside and inside of a membrane.

diabetes mellitus: A genetic disease of carbohydrate metabolism characterized by abnormally high levels of glucose in the blood and urine, and the inadequate secretion or utilization of insulin.

differentiation: In development, the process whereby a cell or cell line becomes morphogically, developmentally, or physiologically specialized.

dihydrotestosterone: A derivative of testosterone that is more potent, molecule for molecule, than testosterone but does not act equally on all androgen-sensitive tissues.

direct fitness: A measure of an individual's potential to contribute genes to future generations via personal reproduction.

disaccharide: A carbohydrate consisting of two simple sugar subunits.

diurnal: Pertaining to an animal with an activity period during the light portion of the daily cycle.

diversity: 1. Variety; variability. 2. The range of types in a major taxon: plant diversity. 3. In ecology, a measure of the number of species coexisting in a community.

DNA (deoxyribonucleic acid): Chemical substance found in chromosomes and mitochondria that reproduces itself and carries the genetic code.

DNA replication: The semiconservative synthesis of DNA in which the double helix opens, the two strands separate, and each is used as a template for producing a new opposing strand.

dominant: Describes a trait that is expressed in the phenotype even when the organism is carrying only one copy of the underlying hereditary material (one copy of the responsible gene).

double helix: The configuration of the native DNA molecule, which consists of two antiparallel strands wound helically around each other.

drift: 1. The chance fluctuation of allele frequencies from generation to generation in a finite population. 2. The long-term consequences of such fluctuations, such as the loss or fixation of selectively neutral alleles.

ecological niche: The range of ecological variables (e.g., temperature, moisture, etc.) in which a species can exist and reproduce.

ecosystem: Ecological system; the interacting community of all the organisms in an area and their physical environment, together with the flow of energy among the system's components.

effector: A tissue or organ that responds to an action potential or a hormone.

electroreceptor: Sensory receptors that detect electric fields.

electrical synapse: Contact between neurons formed by gap junctions, in which an action potential passes directly from one neuron to the next.

element: A substance that cannot be separated into simpler substances by purely chemical means.

endocrine glands: A series of ductless glands in both invertebrates and vertebrates that release hormones into the body through blood or lymph.

endocrine hormone: A hormone that acts at some distance from its source cell and is usually transported in the blood, as opposed to paracrine hormones, which act on neighboring cells, and autocrine hormones, which remain within the producing cell.

endocrine system: The endocrine glands taken together, as well as their hormonal actions and interactions.

endocrinology: The science of hormone production, action, and control.

endogenous: Processes within an animal; used here with particular reference to the internal, genetically based, components of biological rhythms.

endogenous clock mechanism: Any internal processes that are genetically based and that play a role in setting or regulating biological rhythms.

endorphins: Neuropeptides synthesized in the central nervous system of vertebrates that produce morphinelike effects.

endothelium: An epithelial tissue that forms the inner lining of blood and lymph vessels.

entrainment: The process by which a biological clock is set or reset by synchronizing with an external, environmental stimulus.

entropy: In thermodynamics, the amount of energy in a closed system that is not available for doing work; also defined as a measure of the randomness or disorder of such a system.

environment: The surrounding conditions, influences, or forces that influence or modify an organism, population, or community.

enzyme: A protein that converts a molecule to a different product rapidly and with high specificity.

epithelium: A tissue consisting of tightly adjoining cells that cover a surface or line a canal or cavity, and that serves to enclose and protect.

essential amino acid: One of the amino acids that the body cannot synthesize and thus must be provided by the diet if dietary diseases are to be avoided.

essential fatty acid: One of the fatty acids that the body cannot synthesize and thus must be provided by the diet if dietary diseases are to be avoided.

estrogen: The female sex hormone, which is mainly produced by the ovaries.

estrous cycle: The period of behavioral and physiological changes from one ovulatory event to another.

estrus: The day of the fertility cycle when an animal is sexually receptive.

evolution: A change in the frequency of alleles in a population over generations. The change is caused by natural selection and/or genetic drift.

exchanges: Food groups used by the American Diabetes Association and the American Dietetic Association's exchange lists for meal planning. There are seven basic groups: starch, other carbohydrates, meat and meat substitutes, vegetable, fruit, milk, and fat. Any food in a given group can be exchanged for any other food in that group in the appropriate amount.

excitatory synapse: A synapse in which the secretion of a neurotransmitter stimulates neural impulses in the receiving neuron.

excretion: The removal of metabolic wastes, particularly nitrogenous wastes, from the body.

extinction: The loss of a species due to the death of all its members.

extracellular: Outside, between, or among cells.

fats: The most concentrated source of calories in the diet. Saturated fats are found primarily in animal products. Unsaturated fats mainly come from plants and can be monounsaturated (olive or canola oil) or polyunsaturated (corn and other oils). Excess intake of fat, especially saturated fat, can cause elevated blood cholesterol, increasing the risk of heart disease and stroke.

fatty acid: An organic acid consisting of a linear hydrocarbon "tail" and one terminal carboxyl group.

feedback: Process by which a change in one component in a system affects other components, which in turn bring about changes in the first component.

fertility rate: The number of births per 1,000 women who are between 15 and 44 years of age; a clearer indicator of reproductive activity in a population than the birth rate.

fiber: The parts of plants that the body can't digest, such as fruit and vegetable skins. Fiber aids in the normal functioning of the digestive system, specifically the intestinal tract.

fibrinogen: A globular blood protein that is converted into fibrin by the action of thrombin as part of the normal blood clotting process.

fitness: The potential for an individual to contribute genes to future generations as a function of its adaptive traits.

food chain: A sequence of organisms in an ecological community, each of which is food for the next higher organism, from the primary producer to the top predator.

food web: A group of interacting food chains; all the feeding relations of a community taken together; the flow of chemical energy among organisms.

forebrain: 1. The anterior of the three primary divisions of the vertebrate brain. 2. The parts of the brain developed from the embryonic forebrain.

fossil: The remains of an organism, or direct evidence of its presence, preserved in rock. Generally only the hard parts of animals—teeth and bones—are preserved.

free radical: An often highly reactive agent that can damage the cell fabric and other molecules.

free-running rhythm: The activity cycle that an animal exhibits when placed in a constant environment; its period is different from any known cyclic environmental variable.

frontal lobe: An anterior division of the cerebral hemisphere, believed to be the site of higher cognition.

fruit: The seed-bearing ovary of a flowering plant.

functional neuroanatomy: The study of the size, structure, and arrangement of cells within the nervous system, particularly the brain.

gastrointestinal tract: The entire digestive tube, from the mouth to the anus.

gene: Primarily, a functional unit of the chromosomes in cell nuclei that controls the coding and inheritance of phenotypic traits; some genes also occur in a closed loop in the mitochondria.

gene flow: Transmission of genes between populations through exogamy, which increases the variety of genes available to each and creates or maintains the genetic makeup of the populations.

gene pool: All the genes of a population available at a given time (summing genes within a species yields the species' gene pool).

gene replacement therapy: In medicine, the use of recombinant DNA to substitute for a gene that causes a condition needing correction.

gene sequencing: Determining the specific sequence of nucleotides in a gene.

gene splicing: The use of recombinant DNA techniques to form covalent bonds between DNA from different sources.

genetic code: The chemical code based on four nucleotides, carried by DNA and RNA, that specifies amino acids in sequence for protein synthesis.

genetic drift: Genetic changes in populations caused by random phenomena rather than by natural selection.

genetic engineering: The manipulation of genes through recombinant DNA techniques.

genetic equilibrium: The state of a population in which the frequency of certain alleles remains constant generation after generation.

genetic load: Recessive genes in a population that are harmful when expressed in a rare homozygous condition.

genetic variability: A broad term indicating the presence of different genetic constitutions in a population or populations.

genetics: 1. The science of heredity, dealing with the resemblances and differences of related organisms resulting from the interaction of their genes and the environment. 2. The study of the structure, function, and transmission of genes.

genome: The totality of DNA unique to a particular organism or species.

genotype: The genetic makeup of a plant or animal; all information contained in each gene of the organism.

gestational diabetes: Diabetes that develops during pregnancy. The mother's blood glucose rises due to hormones secreted during pregnancy, and the mother cannot produce enough insulin to handle the higher blood glucose levels. Although gestational diabetes usually goes away after pregnancy, about 60 percent of women who've had gestational diabetes eventually develop Type II diabetes.

germ cell: The egg or sperm cell.

glial cells: Supportive cells that are closely associated with neurons.

glucagon: A polypeptide hormone secreted by the pancreatic islets of Langerhans, the action of which increases the blood glucose level by stimulating the breakdown of glycogen in the liver.

glucose: Also called dextrose, blood sugar, corn sugar, and grape sugar, a six-carbon sugar occurring in an open chain form or either of two ring forms, the subunits of which the polysaccharides starch, glycogen, and cellulose are composed. Glucose is a constituent of most other polysaccharides and disaccharides.

glycerol: A triple alcohol component of neutral fats and of phospholipids.

glycogen: A highly complex polysaccharide consisting of alpha glucose subunits; a carbohydrate storage material in the liver, muscle, and other animal tissues.

glycolysis: A biochemical process involving the enzymatic, anaerobic breakdown of glucose in cells, yielding ATP pyruvate and NADH.

glycoprotein: A compound containing polypeptide and carbohydrate subunits.

gonads: Glands responsible for the production of gametes in which certain gonadal hormones are produced. These consist of ovaries in females and the testes in males.

heart disease: A condition in which the heart cannot efficiently pump blood. Coronary artery disease is the most common form of heart disease. It occurs when the arteries that nourish the heart muscle narrow or become blocked. People with diabetes have a higher risk than the general population of developing heart disease.

heritability: A property of phenotypic traits; the proportion of a trait's interindividual variance that is due to genetic variance.

hibernation: A condition of deep sleep and reduced metabolic activity observed in some animals, particularly during the winter months.

homeobox: A region within homeotic or control genes consisting of some 100 nucleotides, the base sequence of which is very similar in a variety of organisms. Homeoboxes are thought to play a key role in the activation of control genes.

homeostasis: A tendency toward a stable or equilibrium state with respect to the internal physiological conditions of an animal.

hominids: Living or fossil members of the primate family Hominidae, which includes *Homo sapiens,* earlier species of the genus Homo, Australopithecus, and Paranthropus.

hominoid: A primate group composed of humans, apes, and related extinct forms.

homology: A similarity between two structures that is due to inheritance from a common ancestor.

Homo erectus: Hominid species that inhabited much of the Old World 1.8 to 0.3 million years ago; successor to "early Homo."

Homo sapiens: among living primates, the scientific name for modern humans; archaic members of the species first appeared about 400,000 years ago.

hormones: Chemical products of ductless glands that are carried by the circulatory system and that influence various physiological processes in the body.

hormone replacement therapy (HRT): A chemical formulation of estrogen or estrogen and progesterone for treating postmenopausal women.

human immunodeficiency virus (HIV): The retrovirus responsible for AIDS (acquired immune deficiency syndrome).

hyperglycemia: A condition in which blood glucose levels are too high (.250 mg/dl). Symptoms include frequent urination, increased thirst, and weight loss.

hyperphagia: A condition in which an animal does not stop eating when it normally would.

hyperpolarized: A description for a membrane whose polarity is greater than its typical resting potential.

hypoglycemia: Also called insulin reaction, a condition in which blood glucose levels drop too low (generally, below 70 mg/dl). Symptoms include moodiness, numbness in the arms and hands, confusion, and shakiness or dizziness.

When left untreated, this condition can become severe and lead to unconsciousness.

hypophagia (aphagia): A condition in which an animal does not eat as much as it normally would.

hypothalamus: The part of the brain that, inter alia, controls the pituitary gland.

hypothesis: A proposition set forth as an explanation for a specified group of phenomena, either asserted merely as a provisional conjecture to guide investigation or accepted as highly probable in the light of established facts.

immune response: The entire array of physiological and development responses involving specific protective actions against a foreign substance; including phagocytosis, the production of antibodies, complement fixation, lysis, agglutination, and inflammation.

immune system: In invertebrates, widely dispersed tissues that respond to the presence of the antigens of invading microorganisms or foreign chemical substances.

immunosuppression: Suppression of the immune system. People who receive kidney or pancreas transplants take immunosuppressive drugs to prevent the immune system from attacking the new organ.

imprinting: A process that occurs when an animal learns to make a particular response to only one type of animal or object. The sensory modes used for establishing such a connection can be visual, auditory, olfactory, or some combination of these, depending upon the animal.

impulse: A neural impulse; a wave of excitement transmitted through a neuron.

inborn error of metabolism: A genetic defect in which an individual lacks one of the enzymes of biochemical pathway.

inducer: 1. In molecular genetics, a small molecule that triggers the activity of an inducible enzyme. 2. In embryology, a substance that stimulates the differentiation of cells or the development of a particular structure.

inflammatory response: A nonspecific immune reaction brought on by the release of kinins, histamine, and other agents that increases permeability of nearby capillaries and causes redness and swelling of tissue.

inhibitory block: According to the classical definition of instinct, the neurological inhibitors of behavior that are selectively removed by the perception of the appropriate releaser.

inhibiting hormone: Any of several hypothalamic neurosecretions targeted for the adenohypophysis, which responds by slowing the release of one of its hormones.

inhibitory synapse: A synapse in which the secretion of a neurotransmitter increases the threshold voltage requirement of the receiving neuron, thereby inhibiting it.

innate: Behavior that has either a fixed genetic basis or a high degree of genetic preprogramming.

instinct: Innate behavior involving appetitive and consummatory phases.

insulin: A hormone produced by the pancreas that helps the body use glucose. It is the "key" that unlocks the "doors" to cells and allows glucose to enter. The glucose then fuels the cells.

insulin resistance: A condition in which the body does not respond to insulin properly. This is the most common cause of Type II diabetes.

intelligence: A collection of mental capacities including imagination, problem-solving ability, memory, the ability to use information gained from past experiences, perceptiveness, and behavioral flexibility. It is the processes by which animals obtain information about their environment, retain it, and use the information to make decisions during the course of their behavioral activities.

interbreeding: 1. Commonly breeding together. 2. Hybridizing.

interglacial: A period in which glaciers retreat and the climate warms.

interleukin-1 through -15L: Chemical messengers released by antigen-presenting cells and helper T cells that stimulate cell division in aroused T and B lymphocytes.

interneuron: A neuron that connects two or more separate neurons.

interstitial cells: Cells of the testis that have an endocrine function.

intracellular: Within cells.

intron: A region of DNA separating two parts of a structural gene; it is transcribed but later removed from mRNA during posttranscriptional modification.

in vitro: The test tube or any other artificial environment.

in vivo: In the living body of a plant or animal.

ion: Any electrostatically charged atom or molecule.

ion channel: In the neural membrane, sodium and potassium channels that, through the opening and closing of gates, selectively admit or reject ions.

irritability: The ability of a cell to undergo a change in membrane potential.

islets of Langerhans: The beta, alpha, and delta endocrine cells within the pancreas that secrete the hormones insulin, glucagon, and somatostatin, respectively.

ketoacidosis: Also called diabetic coma, a severe condition caused by a lack of insulin or an elevation in stress hormones. It is marked by high blood glucose levels and ketones in the urine, and occurs almost exclusively in those with Type I diabetes.

ketones: Acids produced when the body breaks down fat for fuel. This occurs when there is not enough insulin to permit glucose to enter the cells and fuel them or when there are too many stress hormones.

kidney: 1. In vertebrates, one of a pair of ducted excretory organs situated in the body cavity beneath the dorsal peritoneum, serving to excrete nitrogenous wastes and to regulate the balance of body ions and fluids. 2. Any analogous organ in invertebrate metazoans.

knockout gene: A genetically engineered mutant gene that is introduced into an embryo to study the specific effects of that gene.

knuckle walking: Quadrupedal walking on the knuckles of the hands and the soles of the feet, used by Bonobos, chimpanzees, and gorillas.

laws of thermodynamics: In physics, laws governing the interconversions of energy.

lesion: An area of tissue that has been destroyed by an agent such as electric current or a chemical.

leukocyte: A vertebrate white blood cell, including eosinophils, neutrophils, basophils, monocytes, and lymphocytes.

ligament: A tough, flexible, but inelastic band of connective tissue that connects bones or that supports an organ in place.

ligase: An enzyme that heals nicks in DNA.

light-harvesting complex: A cluster of photosynthetic pigments that receives energy from photons and transfers that energy to a single reaction center.

light reaction: That part of photosynthesis directly dependent on the capture of photons; specifically, the photolysis of water, the thylakoid electron transport system, and the chemiosmotic synthesis of ATP and NADPH.

limbic system: The emotional brain; a group of structures in the brain important in regulating behavior such as eating, drinking, aggression, sexual activity, and expressions of emotion. Proportionately smaller in humans than in other primates, it operates below the level of consciousness.

lipase: Any fat-digesting enzyme.

lipid: Fat molecule.

liposome: A spherical bilayer of phospholipids that forms spontaneously in water.

liver: In vertebrates, a large, glandular, highly vascular organ that serves many metabolic functions, including detoxification, the production of blood proteins, food storage, the biochemical alteration of food molecules, and the production of bile.

locus: The specific place on a chromosome where a gene is located.

longevity: Maximum life span recorded for a species.

long-term memory: 1. Learning that persists for more than a few hours, the memory trace of which is physically located in a different part of the brain from short-term memory. 2. The part of the brain and the general neural function with which such persistent memory traces are associated.

luteinizing hormone (LH): A pituitary gonadotropin that causes follicles to ovulate, corpora lutea to secrete progesterone, and Leydig cells to secrete testosterone.

lymph node: A rounded, encapsulated mass of lymphoid tissue through which lymph ducts drain, consisting of a fibrous mesh containing numerous lymphocytes and phagocytes.

lymphatic system: The system of lymphatic vessels, lymph nodes, lymphocytes, the thoracic duct, and the thymus, which together serve to drain body tissues of excess fluids and to combat infections.

lymphoid tissue: Tissue in which lymphocytes are activated and aggregate.

lymphocyte: Any of several varieties of similar-appearing leukocytes involved in the production of antibodies and in other aspects of the immune response.

lysis: The destruction of lysing of a cell by rupture of the plasma membrane.

lysosome: A small membrane-bounded cytoplasmic organelle, generally containing strong digestive enzymes or other cytotoxic materials.

macrophage: A large phagocyte that forms from a monocyte.

major histocompatibility complex (MHC): Genes that code for cell surface proteins and glycoproteins and that make individuals biochemically unique.

mating system: The species-typical pattern of mate finding, reproduction, and parenting of offspring.

melanin: The characteristic animal surface pigmentation; also found in plants.

melatonin: A hormone, produced by the pineal gland during the hours of darkness, that affects diurnal body rhythms.

meme: A small mental representation of cultural information, such as a commercial jingle, car design, clothing fashion, dance step, or simple phrase. The "science" of memetics studies the ways in which memes can act as "brain viruses" and "infect" our consciousness by becoming annoying, dominating, distracting memories.

memory: The capacity of an organism to form lasting connections based on past experiences; the ability to store and use information.

menopause: In human females, (1) the cessation of menstruation, usually occurring between the ages of 45 and 50; (2) the whole group of physical, physiological, and behavioral occurrences and changes associated with the cessation of menstruation.

menses: The period of shedding of the lining (endometrium) of the uterus and associated fluids if an ovum is not fertilized, most notably in primates.

menstrual cycle: The period from the end of one ovulatory cycle, as demarcated by menstrual flow, to the end of the next cycle in female primates.

menstruation: In nonpregnant females of the human species only, the periodic discharge of blood, secretion, and tissue debris resulting from the normal, temporary breakdown of the uterine mucosa in the absence of implantation following ovulation.

messenger RNA (mRNA): 1. In prokaryotes, RNA directly transcribed from an operation or structural gene containing one or more contiguous regions specifying a polypeptide sequence. 2. In eukaryotes, RNA transcribed from a structural gene tailored and usually capped and polyadenylated in the nucleus, transported to the cytoplasm, and containing a single contiguous region specifying a polypeptide sequence as well as leader and follower sequences.

metabolic pathway: An orderly series or progression of enzyme-mediated chemical reactions leading to a final product, each step catalyzed by its own specific enzyme.

metabolism: The total chemical changes and processes of living cells.

metabolite: 1. A metabolic waste, especially one that is toxic. 2. An intermediate in a biochemical pathway.

microorganism: Any organism too small to be seen readily without the aid of a microscope, such as bacterium, protist, or yeast.

midbrain: The middle of the three divisions of the vertebrate embryonic brain; the adult structures derived from the embryonic midbrain.

mitochondria: Granular or rod-shaped bodies in the cytoplasm of cells that function in the metabolism of fat and proteins; probably of bacterial origin.

molecular biology: A branch of biology concerned with the ultimate physico-chemical organization of living matter; the study of biological systems using biochemical methods.

molecule: A unit of chemical substance consisting of atoms bound to one another by covalent bonds.

monkey: Usually a small or medium-sized, long-tailed, arboreal, quadrupedal, vegetarian primate. There are two groups: New World monkeys and Old World monkeys.

monogamy: A mating system in which a male and female bond for some period of time and share in the rearing of offspring.

monosaccharide: A sugar not composed of smaller sugar subunits (for example, glucose and fructose).

mortality rate: The number of deaths per unit of time occurring among a specified number of individuals in a given area or population.

motor neuron: A neuron that synapses with a muscle membrane.

mDNA: genetic material found in the mitochondria of cells.

mucosa: The highly glandular mucous membrane lining an organ.

multicellular: Consisting of a number of specialized cells that cooperatively carry out the functions of life.

mutagen: A chemical or physical agent that causes mutations.

mutate: 1. To alter, cause a change, or cause a mutation or DNA change to occur; to mutagenize. 2. To change in state or genetic condition, to become altered, to undergo a mutation.

mutation: Generally, spontaneous change in the chemistry of a gene that can alter its phenotypic effect. The accumulation of such changes may contribute to the evolution of a new species of animal or plant.

mutation rate: The rate at which new mutations occur, generally in terms of mutations per locus per gamete per generation.

myelin sheath: Fatty sheath surrounding the axons of many vertebrate neurons.

natural killer (NK) cell: A free-roving lymphocyte that identifies, binds to, and lyses cancerous and virus-infected cells as part of the nonspecific immune response.

natural selection: The disproportionate survival and reproductive success of organisms that possess certain alleles as a result of the influence of those alleles.

negative feedback: An automated control mechanism in which an action, brought about by a chemical or physical stimulus, directly or indirectly reduces that stimulus. Such an inhibiting effect constitutes a negative feedback loop.

nerve: 1. A filamentous band of nerve cell axons and dendrites and protective and supporting tissue that connects parts of the nervous system with other parts of the body. 2. Pertaining to the nerve or nervous system; for example, nerve cell, nerve net, nerve fiber.

nerve cell body: The largest part of a neuron, which typically contains the nucleus.

neural impulse: A transient membrane depolarization, followed by immediate repolarization, traveling in a wave-like manner along a neuron.

neurocardiology: The field that studies the heart as a neurohormonal organ.

neurons: Nerve cells; the basic units of the nervous system.

neuropathy: Damage to the nerves. Neuropathies are often broken down into two categories. Peripheral neuropathies affect the nerves controlling sensation (and, less commonly, muscles) in the feet, hands, and joints. Autonomic neuropathies affect the nerve function of various organs, including those of the digestive system and urinary tract.

neuropeptides: Neurotransmitters made up of amino acids that are active not only in the brain but also, like microcosmic keys fitting into tiny keyholes in the cells of the body, act as "bits of brain" that float throughout the body and help unlock a cell's memory.

neurotransmitter: A chemical released by the presynaptic membrane of a synapse that attaches to receptor molecules on the postsynaptic membrane and causes a change in the permeability of that membrane.

neutrophil: The most common mammalian phagocytic leukocyte.

nocturnal: Pertaining to animals whose primary activity occurs during the dark portion of the daily cycle.

nonlocality: The quantum physics principle that holds that distance and barriers of time and space are illusions of the materialistic, substantiality-oriented brain and that there are no limits of distance, time, or barriers in the transmission of energy, as illustrated by prayer, remote viewing, and other so-called psychic phenomena.

nucleic acid: Either DNA or RNA, DNA being a double polymer of deoxynucleotides and RNA being a polymer of nucleotides.

nucleotide: A compound consisting of a nitrogenous base and a phosphate group linked to the 1st and 5th carbons or ribose, respectively; the repeating subunit of DNA and RNA.

nucleus: The sac within each cell that contains the chromosomes.

nutrition: The process of being nourished, particularly the steps through which an organism obtains food and uses it for bodily processes.

obesity: An abnormal and excessive amount of body fat. Most obese people are significantly overweight. However, obesity also occurs in people who are not overweight, but have more body fat than muscle. Obesity is considered a chronic illness. It is on the rise and is a risk factor for Type II diabetes.

olfactory: Having to do with the sense of smell; the chemoreception of molecules suspended in air.

omnivore: An animal that eats both meat and vegetation.

oncogene: A cancer-causing gene.

organ: An organized assembly of various tissues performing some major body function; for example, the heart, brain, liver.

organic molecule: A molecule containing carbon and generally produced by living organisms.

orgasm: In humans, the climax of sexual excitement, usually accompanied in men by ejaculation and in women by rhythmic contractions of the cervix.

origin: 1. Evolutionary ancestry. 2. The fixed skeletal attachment of a muscle or tendon.

oscillator: The internal mechanism that is the clock in a biological rhythm.

ovary: 1. In animals, the organ in which oogenesis occurs and in which eggs mature. 2. In flowering plants, the enlarged, rounded base of a pistil, consisting of a carpel or several united carpels, in which ovules mature and megasporogenesis occurs.

ovulation: The release of one or more eggs from an ovary.

oxidation: 1. The loss of electrons from an element or compound. 2. The loss of hydrogens from a compound.

oxidative respiration: The breakdown of biochemicals to produce cellular energy, utilizing oxygen as the final electron acceptor.

pancreas: A gland located in the abdomen that produces both digestive enzymes (exocrine pancreas) and hormones (endocrine pancreas). Key hormones produced by the pancreas are insulin and glucagon, which play roles in regulating blood glucose levels.

parasite: An organism living in or on another living organism from which it obtains its organic sustenance to the detriment of its host.

patches: Regions of localized concentrations of resources.

pathogen: An organism that is capable of causing disease in another organism; generally refers to viruses and parasitic bacteria and fungi.

peptide: A chain of two or more amino acids linked by peptide bonds, too short to be coagulated by heat or precipitated by saturated ammonium sulfate; most often seen as a partial digestion product or a protein or polypeptide.

peptide hormone: Any hormone consisting of one or more amino acids.

perception: The analysis and interpretation of sensory information.

perennial: 1. Continuing or lasting for several years. 2. A plant that lives for an indefinite number of years, as compared with annual or biennial.

period: The duration of one cycle of a biological rhythm.

phase: A specified, recognizable portion of an activity cycle.

phenotype: The observable characteristics of an organism that result from the influence of both the organism's genotype and environmental factors.

pheromone: A species-specific odor cue released by animals that influences the behavior and/or physiology of conspecifics.

photon: A quantum of electromagnetic radiant energy.

photoperiodism: The response of an organism to photoperiods, involving sensitivity to the onset of light or darkness and a capacity to measure time.

photopigment: A molecule in visual receptor cells that responds to light energy.

photoreceptors: Sensory cells that contain photopigments and respond specifically to light energy.

photosynthesis: The organized capture of light energy and its transformation into usable chemical energy in the synthesis of organic compounds.

phototaxis: Orientation with respect to light.

phylogeny: The evolutionary history of a group of organisms.

physiology: 1. A branch of biology dealing with the processes, activities, and phenomena of individual living organisms, organs, tissues, and cells. 2. The normal functioning of an organism.

pigment: Any chemical substance that absorbs light, whether or not its normal function involves light absorption: for example, chlorophyll, cytochrome *c,* hemoglobin, and melanin.

pineal gland: An endocrine gland located near the midline of the brain that produces melatonin, a hormone involved in biological rhythms, particularly in annual cycles.

pituitary gland: The master gland of the endocrine system of vertebrate animals. Located directly below the hypothalamus of the brain, the pituitary produces or releases a variety of hormones that target other endocrine glands of the body.

placebo: A substance having no pharmacological effect but administered as a control in experimentally or clinically testing the efficacy of a biologically active preparation.

placenta: 1. In mammals other than monotremes and marsupials, the organ formed by the union of the uterine mucosa with the extraembryonic membranes of the fetus, which provides for the nourishment of the fetus, the elimination of waste products, and the exchange of dissolved gases. 2. In flowering plants, the part of the ovary to which the ovule and seeds attach.

plasmid: In bacteria, a small ring of DNA that appears in addition to the main bacterial chromosome.

platelets: Minute blood cells associated with clotting.

pleistocene: The geologic epoch that lasted from about 1.6 million to 10,000 years ago.

pleiotropic: A description of a gene or set of genes that influences the phenotype of more than one characteristic.

pleiotropy: The situation in which one gene has many effects.

polarized: A description of a membrane that has a potential difference due to an unequal distribution of ions across the membrane.

polypeptide: A continuous string of amino acids in peptide linkage, longer than a peptide.

polysaccharide: A polymer of sugar subunits.

population: Usually a local or breeding group; a group in which any two individuals have the potential of mating with each other.

population genetics: The scientific study of genetic variation within populations, of the genetic correlation between related individuals in a population, and of the genetic basis of evolutionary change.

positive feedback: A process in which a positive change in one component of a system brings about changes in other components, which in turn bring about further positive changes in the first component.

potential energy: Energy stored in chemical bonds, in nonrandom organization, in elastic bodies, in elevated weight, or any other static form in which it can theoretically be transformed into another form or into work.

predation: 1. The act of catching and eating. 2. Being caught and eaten; for example, subject to predation. 3. A mode of life in which food is primarily obtained by killing and eating other animals.

predator: An animal that habitually preys on other animals; a carnivorous animal.

primary immune response: The slower, initial response against invasion of the body by organisms or foreign molecules, during which immature, inactive lymphocytes are activated into specialized B- and T-cell lymphocytes.

primates: An order of placental mammals, mostly arboreal, with two suborders: the anthropoids and the prosimians.

primitive: A character or state characteristic of the original condition of the group under consideration; ancestral; not derived; of or like the earliest state within the group considered.

prion: A little-known disease agent; a protein shell capable of penetrating and killing cells.

progesterone: A type of steroid hormone produced mainly by the ovaries and placenta that is needed to prepare for and maintain pregnancy.

prokaryote: Any organism of the kingdom Monera having no nucleus and a single circular chromosome of nearly naked DNA; a eubacterium or archaebacterium.

promoter: A DNA sequence to which RNA polymerase must bind in order for transcription to begin.

prostaglandin: Any of a group of hormone-like substances derived from long-chain fatty acids and produced in most animal tissues.

prostate gland: A gland in the lower abdomen of men that contributes to the formation of seminal fluid.

proteins: Molecules composed of chains of amino acids.

protoeukaryote: A hypothetical predatory microorganism capable of the engulfment of prey, which by the successive engulfment of protomitochondrion, a protochloroplast, and perhaps a protocilium evolved into the ancestral eukaryotic cell perhaps a billion years ago.

proton: 1. One of the two particles composing the atomic nucleus in ordinary matter having an electrostatic charge of +1 and a mass 1,837 times that of an electron, and by its numbers determining the chemical properties of the atom. 2. A hydrogen ion.

proton pump: An active transport system using energy to move hydrogen ions from one side of a membrane to the other against a concentration gradient, as in chemiosmosis.

psychobiology: The study of the mechanism and function of the central nervous system from both psychological and biological perspectives.

psychoneuroimmunology: The field that studies the interaction between the mind, body, and social systems and how this interaction influences health and healing.

psychopharmacology: The study of the brain's behavior in terms of chemical, physiological, and psychological parameters.

puberty: The age at which an organism can first reproduce.

pulmonary circuit: The passage of venous blood from the right side of the heart through the pulmonary arteries to the capillaries of the lung, where it is oxygenated and from which it returns by way of the pulmonary veins to the left atrium of the heart.

punctuated equilibrium: The theory that evolution does not occur gradually but that life continues over long periods of time with little evolutionary change and is interrupted periodically by great changes.

receptors: Molecules that sit on cell surfaces and play a role in chemical "communication." For example, insulin cannot allow glucose into our cells unless the receptors on the cells respond properly to the insulin.

recessive: Describing a trait that is expressed only when the organism is carrying two copies of the underlying hereditary material (two copies of the responsible gene).

reciprocal altruism: Behavior functions that increase the fitness of the individual insofar as they increase the likelihood that the individual will be the recipient of beneficial behavior at another time.

recombinant DNA: A general term for laboratory-manipulated DNA. DNA molecules or fragments from various sources are severed and combined enzymatically and reinserted into living organisms.

red blood cells: Also called corpuscles, these are vertebrate blood cells without nuclei and containing hemoglobin.

Red Queen hypothesis: The hypothesis that sexual reproduction has evolved because the genetic variation that results from it is adaptive in the evolutionary "arms race" between hosts and their pathogens and parasites as well as between predators and prey.

refractory state: A brief period when a neuron cannot generate a second impulse.

rejection phenomenon: When tissue is transplanted from one body to another, the immune system of the recipient xenophobically identifies the new tissue as a "stranger" and attacks it. Rejection is a threat to the success of transplantation, and researchers are now looking at better ways to reduce biological rejection and also how to make two systems more "info-energetically" friendly to one another.

releasing factors: Hormones or neurosecretions from the hypothalamus that travel either via the hypothalamic-pituitary portal system or along axons between the hypothalamus and the pituitary, where they exert their effect in terms of production and release of hormones.

releasing hormone: A chemical messenger released by the hypothalamus that stimulates hormonal release by the pituitary.

REM sleep: A normal period of sleep during which the muscles are very relaxed but the eyes move rapidly under closed lids; accompanied by high electrical activity in the brain.

repair enzyme: Any of several different complexes of enzymes that recognize improper base pairing in DNA, excise a region of one of the strands, and rebuild the DNA according to the rules of Watson-Crick pairing or that otherwise repair mutational damage, including double-strand chromosome breaks.

replication: The capacity of DNA to generate copies of itself in the nucleus of a cell.

reproductive success: The production of viable offspring that reproduce in turn; levels of reproductive success may differ between individuals.

respiration: 1. The physical and chemical process by which an organism supplies oxygen to its tissues and removes carbon dioxide. 2. The energy-requiring metabolic transformation of food or food storage molecules yielding energy.

resting state: A state of seeming activity in a neuron, but one in which the membrane activity maintains a polarized state in preparation for conduction.

restriction enzyme: In bacteria, an enzyme that recognizes and serves a specific, short DNA sequence, thus protecting the cell from all but a few highly adapted, host-specific viruses; such enzymes have proved useful for experimental DNA manipulation.

retrovirus: A single-strand RNA virus that, after undergoing reverse transcription and producing double-strand DNA from its RNA coding, inserts into the host chromosome, where it is replicated through many host cell generations. It may later escape from the chromosome to enter a period of viral reproduction and cell lysis.

RNA (ribonucleic acid): A compound found with DNA in cell nuclei and chemically close to DNA; transmits genetic code from DNA to direct the formation of proteins. May take two forms: messenger RNA (mRNA) or transfer RNA (tRNA).

savanna: A tropical or subtropical grassland with scattered trees or shrubs, usually maintained by such human activities as burning and foraging for firewood.

secondary immune response: A rapid response to a second or subsequent invasion of the body by organisms or foreign molecules, during which memory cells quickly produce large numbers of active, specialized B- and T-cell lymphocytes.

self-propagating: A description of the events occurring during an action potential, with each regional depolarization by sodium voltage-gated channels causing a similar event at an adjacent area downstream.

senescence: The biological characteristics of aging.

sensation: The process of transducing environmental stimuli or energy into action potentials.

sensory adaptation: A process that occurs at the level of the sensory receptors and that consists of a slowing down or cessation of nerve impulses transmitted to the central nervous system.

sensory deprivation: A withholding of all or a specified portion of the sensory input that an animal would normally be receiving.

sensory filter: Neural circuits that selectively transmit some features of a sensory input and ignore other features.

sensory neuron: A neuron that is modified to respond to a particular set of stimuli.

serum (plasma): A clear liquid component of blood that carries the red blood cells, white blood cells, and platelets.

sex chromosomes: Those chromosomes that carry genes that control sex (maleness or femaleness).

sex hormone binding globulin (SHBG): A protein produced in the liver that binds most sex hormones in the bloodstream and tempers their effects on cells.

sex-linked trait: An inherited trait coded on the sex chromosomes, and thus having a special distribution related to sex.

sinoatrial (SA) node: The heart's rhythmic center. It is a tiny patch of tissue in the heart's back wall near the top of its right atrium that is the center of the "cardiac conduction system." It functions as the heart's own internal pacemaker and is central to the complex "nervous system" of the heart.

smooth muscle: The muscle tissue of the glands, viscera, iris, piloerection, and other involuntary functions consisting of masses of uninucleate, unstriated, spindle-shaped cells occurring usually in thin sheets.

society: A group of individuals belonging to the same species and organized in a cooperative manner. The group's ties are usually assumed to extend beyond sexual behavior and parental care of offspring.

sociobiology: A study that involves the application of the principles of evolution to the social behavior and social systems of animals.

sodium ion gate: Either of the two gates controlling sodium ion passage through an ion channel, including an activation gate and inactivation gate.

sodium/potassium ion exchange pump: A poorly understood molecular entity in the plasma membrane capable of actively transporting sodium out of a cell and potassium into a cell, at a cost of ATP energy.

somatic: Having to do with body cells, i.e., those that do not produce gametes.

speciation: The process of two populations that share a common descent evolving in different ways so that they ultimately do not interbreed and therefore remain different species.

species: A group of populations of organisms that are enough alike in structure and behavior so that individuals can interbreed and produce fertile offspring if they have access to one another. Individuals from one species are reproductively isolated from those in other species.

spleen: An abdominal organ consisting of lymphoid, reticular, and endothelial tissues in which the blood supply and red blood cells circulate freely in intercellular spaces; its functions include the scavenging of debris and the maintenance of blood volume.

stabilizing natural selection: Natural selection that operates during periods when the environment is stable and that maintains the genetic and phenotypic status quo within a population.

stasis: A period of evolutionary equilibrium or inactivity.

stem cell: A self-renewing type of cell that also produces differentiated products.

steroid: A family of lipid molecules, including cholesterol and the sex hormones estrogen and testosterone.

steroid hormone: A class of hormones consisting of the steroid molecule with carious side group substitutions, believed to freely pass across the cell membrane and, once bound by a specific carrier protein, to interact directly with the chromatin in gene control; included are the vertebrate sex hormones.

strategy: In the special zoological sense, a complex of adaptations that brings about an effective and efficient means of reproduction or resource use. No conscious choice is implied.

stimulus: An aspect of the environment that influences the activity of a living organism or part of an organism, especially through a sense organ.

stomach: A muscular dilation of the alimentary canal in vertebrates, between the esophagus and the duodenum, that functions in temporary storage, preliminary digestion, sterilization, and physical breakdown of ingested food.

stop codon: In mRNA, one or more of the codons UAA, UAG, or UGA, signaling the end of polypeptide translation.

structural protein: Protein that is incorporated into cellular or extracellular structures.

sugar: A form of carbohydrate that provides calories and raises blood glucose levels. There are a variety of sugars, such as white, brown, confectioners', invert, and raw. Fructose, lactose, sucrose, maltose, dextrose, glucose, honey, corn syrup, molasses, and sorghum are also sugars.

sugar substitutes: Sweeteners used in place of sugar. Note that some sugar substitutes have calories and will affect blood glucose levels, such as fructose and sugar alcohols like sorbitol and mannitol. Others have very few calories and will not affect blood glucose levels, such as saccharin, acesulfame-K, and aspartame (NutraSweet).

superoxide dismutase (SOD): An enzyme that combats free radical production.

suppressor T cell: Specific subpopulation of T cells whose role is to moderate, slow, and stop specific immune responses.

suprachiasmatic nucleus (SCN): A brain nucleus involved in the visual pathway that has been associated with biological rhythms mediated by photoperiod.

symbiosis: Two species living together in intimate association.

synapse: A junction between two neurons or between a neuron and muscle fiber in which action potentials along the presynaptic membrane will influence the postsynaptic membrane.

synaptic cleft: The minute space between the synaptic knob of one neuron and the dendrite or cell body of another into which neurotransmitters are released in the transmission of nerve impulses between cells.

synergism: The interaction of two or more agents or forces so that their combined effect is greater than the sum of their individual effects, as when two hormones combine to affect target tissues.

T cell: A lymphocyte of a variety that matures in the thymus and interacts with invading cells and other cells of the immune system.

taxis: A directed reaction to a stimulus involving an orientation of a long axis of the body in line with the stimulus source.

telomere: A cap on the end of chromosomes that does not contain a genetic code for proteins but has a protective function.

temperature-compensated rhythm: The relative insensitivity of biological rhythms to the effects of temperature; this contrasts with the fact that many chemical reactions double in rate for every 10°C. increase in temperature.

terrestrial: Adapted to living on the ground.

territorial behavior: Defense of any area by animals.

territory: An area occupied exclusively by an animal or group of animals that is defended.

testosterone: The male sex hormone, which is mainly produced by testes.

thalamus: A large subdivision of the diencephalon, consisting of a mass of nuclei in each lateral wall of the centrally located third ventricle of the brain.

theory: A proposed explanation that is still conjectural, in contrast to well-established propositions that are often regarded as facts. Theory and hypothesis are often used colloquially to mean an untested idea or opinion. A theory is a more or less verified explanation accounting for a body of known facts or phenomena, whereas a hypothesis is a conjecture put forth as a possible explanation of a specific phenomenon or relationship that serves as a basis for argument or experimentation.

thermiogenesis: In endothermic animals, the production of body heat through an increase in the metabolic rate, that is, the release of energy from fuels.

thermodynamics: 1. The branch of physics that deals with the interconversions of energy as heat, potential energy, kinetic energy, radiant energy, entropy, and work. 2. The processes and phenomena of energy interconversions.

thermoreceptors: Sensory cells that are sensitive to changes in temperature.

thermoregulation: 1. An animal's control over its internal temperature. 2. The physiological mechanisms that maintain a body at a particular temperature in an environment with a fluctuating temperature.

threshold: The minimum stimulus necessary to initiate an all-or-none response.

thrombin: In blood-clotting reactions, a proteolytic enzyme that catalyzes the conversion of fibrinogen to fibrin by the removal of two short peptide segments and, in turn, is produced from prothrombin by the action of thromboplastin.

thymus: A glandular body above the lungs involved in T-cell lymphocyte development.

thyroid gland: An endocrine gland located in the throat region whose major endocrine products are protein hormones involved in regulation of cellular metabolism.

tissue: A group of associated cells identical in structure and function.

transcription: The process of RNA synthesis as an RNA nucleotide sequence is directed by specific base pairing with the nucleotide sequence of a transcribed strand of a DNA cistron.

transformation: In a bacterium, the direct incorporation of a DNA fragment from its medium into its own chromosome.

Type I diabetes: A form of diabetes that tends to develop before age 30 but may occur at any age. It's caused by an immune system attack on insulin-producing beta cells which, when they are destroyed, prevent the pancreas from producing insulin. People who have Type I diabetes must take insulin to survive.

Type II diabetes: This form of diabetes usually occurs in younger people, especially among minorities. Most people who develop Type II diabetes are insulin resistant. However, some simply cannot produce enough insulin to meet their bodies' needs, and others have a combination of these problems. Many people with Type II diabetes control the disease through diet and exercise, but some must also take oral medications or insulin.

ultradian rhythm: A cyclical rhythm of less than 24 hours.

ultraviolet light: Electromagnetic radiation having a shorter wavelength than visible light and a longer wavelength than X-rays.

urine tests: Tests that measure substances in the urine. Urine tests for blood glucose provide a general idea of a person's blood glucose level several hours before the test. Urine tests for ketones are the only tests that measure ketones and are important in preventing ketoacidosis.

uterus: 1. In female mammals, a muscular, vascularized, mucous-membrane-lined organ for containing and nourishing the developing young prior to birth and for expelling them at the time of birth. 2. An enlarged section of the oviduct of various vertebrates and invertebrates modified to serve as a place of development of the young or of eggs.

vascular system: 1. The circulatory system of an animal. 2. The xylem and phloem of a vascular plant.

vascular tissue: Plant tissues specialized for conducting water and foods.

ventricle: A cavity or a body part or organ, either one of the large muscular chambers of the four-chambered heart or one of the systems of communicating cavities of the brain, consisting of two lateral ventricles and a median third ventricle.

virus: A noncellular organism consisting of DNA and RNA enclosed in a protein coat, often together with a few enzymes; it replicates only within a host cell and utilizes host ribosomes, enzymes, and energy.

vitamin: Any organic substance that is essential to the nutrition of an organism, usually by supplying part of a coenzyme.

voltage-gated channels: Ion-specific channels that open only in response to a specific polarity across the cell membrane.

wave/particle duality: The quantum physics principle that everything in the cosmos, and the cosmos itself, is both "stuff" and "process," both "matter" and "energy." All particles are waves and vice versa; whether the particle or wave nature of something is observed is determined by what is being looked for and when.

zeitgeber: Any entraining agent that plays a role in setting or resetting an internal biological clock. Examples include sunrise or sunset.

I N D E X

acetylcholine, 133
acidophilus, 188
Ackerman, Diane, 117
addiction, 112–13
adenosine triphosphate, 63
adrenal gland, 51
aggression
  and genetic link, 106–07
  and serotonin resistance, 105–06
aging, 1, 4, 6, 54, 142, 150, 151
agricultural revolution
  and carbohydrate supply, 26–27, 34–35,
    71, 151–52
  disease consequences of, 72–74
  and reproduction, 71–72
alcohol consumption, 24, 110, 113, 114–16
Allen, Woody, 9–10
alphalipoic acid, 187
American Anthropology, 126
American Cancer Society, 18
American Heart Association, 18
American Medical Association, 190
amino acids, 175, 179
amygdala, 11–12
amylase, 167, 175
andropause, 147
angiotensin I and II, 93
antibiotics, 28, 127
antidepressants, 97, 107, 108–09
antifreeze, 84
apes
  carbohydrate consumption of, 151–52
  longevity of, 156
appetite
  for carbohydrates, 64–66, 83, 91
  and HPA axis, 51
  and neurotransmitters, 60
arteriosclerosis, 124
artificial light, 3, 5
  and carbohydrate consumption, 18,
    19–20, 22–23, 62, 83

  in cold periods, 43–45
  Edison's development of, 28–29
  and extended day, 3, 26, 66–67, 79, 101,
    123
  fire, 26, 34, 43, 44–45, 66–68
  and hibernation instinct, 81–82
  and hormonal change, 34
  levels, 164
  and mental illness, 99–100, 101
  night-shift work, 22
  price-performance curve for, 21
  and reproduction, 67, 68
  in rural *vs.* urban areas, 29
Ashkenazic Jews, and breast cancer, 140
Asimov, Isaac, 35–36, 44
aspartame, 172
Association of Sleep Disorders Center,
    "Project Sleep", 78
Atkins, Robert C., 11, 165, 169, 188, 189,
    190, 191
atrial naturetic peptide (ANP), 135

bacteria
  and heart disease, 127–28
  and immune system, 48–51, 53
Baker, Samm Sinclair, 188
barbecued meat, 176
Barton, Catherine, 134
Beattie, Gillian, 86
Bell's theorem, 136
Bernstein, Leonard, 53
bipolar disorder, 98
blood sugar, 23, 94, 162–63
body temperature, and melatonin, 55–56,
    148
brain
  –body connection, 47–48
  and depression, 119
  expansion of, 68, 70
  fat in, 179
  –heart communication, 119, 131–37

343

T. S. Wiley and Bent Formby are researchers currently working together who met while volunteering at the Breast Resource Center in Santa Barbara, California.

Wiley presented the team's own research on the role of progesterone deficit and cancer in July of 1997 in Kingston, Ontario, at the World Conference on Breast Cancer. Formby and Wiley most recently presented their original research on the role of estrogen and insulin synergy in breast cancer at the American Diabetes Association National Conference in Chicago in the summer of 1999.

They are currently proposing a cancer protocol to clinically test their progesterone theories at Cottage Hospital in Santa Barbara, California. Their coauthored experiments are presented for academic peer review to mainstream scientific journals. The November 1998 issue of the *Journal of Clinical and Laboratory Sciences* features their work on apoptosis and natural progesterone. They at present have two more papers out for publication, one on the role of the newly discovered gene survivin, and one on the role of natural progesterone and the gene P21.

T. S. Wiley is an anthropologist and medical theorist. She is a member of the New York Academy of Sciences and has been a guest investigator at Sansum Medical Research Institute. She's done research and restoration work at the Metropolitan Museum of Art and the Brooklyn Museum. In the news department of the NBC-TV affiliate in St. Louis, Missouri, Wiley was an investigative reporter. As of 1995, she turned to medical research, with a special interest in endocrinology and evolutionary biology. She lives with her husband of twenty-five years and five children in East Hampton, Santa Barbara, and Santa Fe.

Dr. Formby holds doctorates in biochemistry, biophysics, and molecular biology from the University of Copenhagen in Denmark. He has worked for the last seventeen years in California, first at the University of California at San Francisco in cancer research, and most recently as an independent researcher affiliated with the Sansum Medical Research Institute in Santa Barbara. Dr. Formby has published more than one hundred peer-reviewed papers over the course of his career, covering both cancer and diabetes research. In his off hours, he writes poetry in his native language and paints in oils. He is the proud father of two young men.

Kept in the Dark is a combined effort of creative insight and astute research crossing multiple disciplines. Only an approach covering a broad range of medical theory and encompassing clinical and anecdotal evidence across cultures could hope to solve the ongoing American health crisis. Wiley and Formby's collaboration on *Kept in the Dark* has produced the last pieces of startling evidence necessary to complete a seemingly unsolvable fifty-year old puzzle. Their next joint work for a general audience is entitled *Sex, Lies, and Menopause: The Truth about Hormone Replacement.*